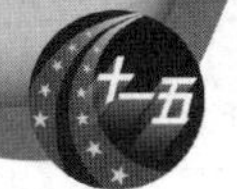

普通高等教育“十一五”国家级规划教材

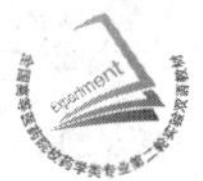

全国高等医药院校药学类专业第二轮实验双语教材

微生物学实验与指导

(第4版)

主　　编　周长林

副 主 编　陈向东　徐旭东　徐　威

编　　者　(以姓氏笔画为序)

马晓楠(沈阳药科大学)

王卓娅(广东药科大学)

王艳红(山西医科大学)

陈向东(中国药科大学)

周长林(中国药科大学)

徐　威(沈阳药科大学)

徐旭东(东南大学)

窦　洁(中国药科大学)

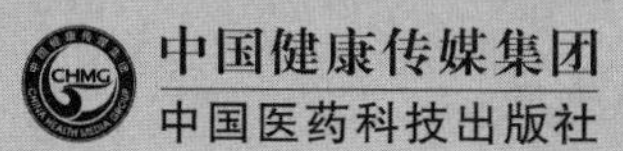

中国健康传媒集团

中国医药科技出版社

内 容 提 要

本教材为“全国高等医药院校药学类专业第二轮实验双语教材”之一。全书共包括9部分61个实验，内容主要包括显微技术和微生物形态学、基本实验操作与培养技术、细菌的生理生化反应、病毒学实验、微生物遗传学实验、免疫学实验、药学微生物学实验、综合性实验以及设计性实验等。本教材为书网融合教材，即纸质教材有机融合电子教材、教学配套资源（PPT、微课、视频、图片等）、题库系统、数字化教学服务（在线教学、在线作业、在线考试），使教学资源更加多样化、立体化。

本教材供高等医药院校药学类专业微生物学实验教学使用，也可供药物质检人员参考使用。

图书在版编目（CIP）数据

微生物学实验与指导 / 周长林主编 . —4 版 . —北京 ：中国医药科技出版社，2019. 12（2025.1重印）

全国高等医药院校药学类专业第二轮实验双语教材

ISBN 978 – 7 – 5214 – 1382 – 3

Ⅰ. ①微… Ⅱ. ①周… Ⅲ. ①微生物学—实验—双语教学—医学院校—教学参考资料 Ⅳ. ①Q93 – 33

中国版本图书馆 CIP 数据核字（2020）第 000763 号

美术编辑 陈君杞

版式设计 南博文化

出版 **中国健康传媒集团** | 中国医药科技出版社

地址 北京市海淀区文慧园北路甲 22 号

邮编 100082

电话 发行：010 – 62227427 邮购：010 – 62236938

网址 www. cmstp. com

规格 889 × 1194mm 1/16

印张 17½

字数 289 千字

初版 2004 年 1 月第 1 版

版次 2019 年 12 月第 4 版

印次 2025 年 1 月第 4 次印刷

印刷 三河市万龙印装有限公司

经销 全国各地新华书店

书号 ISBN 978 – 7 – 5214 – 1382 – 3

定价 49.00 元

获取新书信息、投稿、为图书纠错，请扫码联系我们。

序

Preface

教学是学校人才培养的中心环节，实验教学是这一环节的重要组成部分。“全国高等医药院校药学类专业实验双语教材”是中国药科大学坚持药学实践教学改革，突出提高学生动手能力、创新思维，通过承担教育部“世行贷款21世纪初高等教育教学改革项目”等多项教改课题，逐步建设完善的一套与药学各专业学科理论课程紧密结合的高水平双语实验教材。

本轮修订，适逢“全国高等医药院校药学类专业第五轮规划教材”及《中国药典》（2020年版）、新版《国家执业药师资格考试大纲》出版，整套教材的修订强调了与新版理论教材知识的结合，与《中国药典》（2020年版）等新颁布的法典法规结合。为更好地服务于新时期高等院校药学教育与人才培养的需要，在上一版的基础上，进一步体现了各门实验课程自身独立性、系统性和科学性，又充分考虑到各门实验课程之间的联系与衔接，主要突出了以下特点。

1. 适应医药行业对人才的要求，体现行业特色，契合新时期药学人才需求的变化，使修订后的教材符合《中国药典》（2020年版）等国家标准及新版《国家执业药师资格考试大纲》等行业最新要求。

2. 更新完善内容，打造教材精品。在上版教材基础上进一步优化、精炼和充实内容。紧密结合“全国高等医药院校药学类专业第五轮规划教材”，强调与实际需求相结合，进一步提高教材质量。

3. 为适应信息化教学的需要，本轮教材全部打造成为书网融合教材，即纸质教材与数字教材、配套教学资源、题库系统、数字化教学服务有机融合，为读者提供全免费增值服务。

4. 坚持双语体系，强调素质培养教材以实践教学为突破口，采用双语体系编写有利于加快药学教育国际接轨，提高学生的科技英语水平，进一步提升学生整体素质。

“全国高等医药院校药学类专业第二轮实验双语教材”历经15年4次建设，在各个时期广大编者的努力下，在广大使用教材师生的支持下日臻完善。本轮教材的出版，必将对推动新时期我国高等药学教育的发展产生积极而深远的影响。希望广大师生在教学实践中对本套教材提出宝贵意见，以便今后进一步修订完善，共同打造精品教材。

吴晓明

全国高等医药院校药学类专业第五轮规划教材常务编委会主任委员

2019年10月

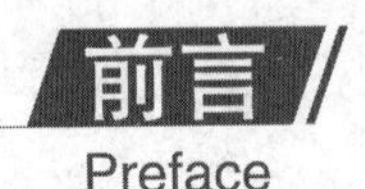

前言
Preface

本教材为“全国高等医药院校药学类专业第二轮实验双语教材”之一。全书共分9部分61个实验，内容主要包括显微技术和微生物形态学、基本实验操作与培养技术、细菌的生理生化反应、病毒学实验、微生物遗传学实验、免疫学实验、药学微生物学实验、综合性实验以及设计性实验等。本版教材为第3版修订，具体编写分工如下：第一部分的实验一、实验二和第二部分由马晓楠编写；第一部分的实验三至实验十三和第九部分的实验五十六由周长林编写；第三部分、第八部分的实验四十九和第九部分的实验五十四由徐旭东编写；第四部分的实验二十四和二十六由王卓娅编写；第五部分、第八部分的实验五十一和第九部分的实验五十三、实验五十五、实验五十七由陈向东编写；第六部分和第九部分的实验五十九、实验六十、实验六十一由窦洁和王艳红编写；第四部分的实验二十五，第七部分，第八部分的实验四十八、实验五十和第九部分的实验五十二、实验五十八由徐威和马晓楠编写；附录由徐旭东编写。本书英文部分由中国药科大学外语系陈菁老师校稿。

本教材的实验编排包括实验目的、实验原理、实验材料、实验方法、结果与讨论五个部分，力求使学生在实验中有明确的实验思路。结果与讨论部分旨在培养学生分析问题和全面总结实验结果的能力，培养独立思考的习惯，以期进一步消化和巩固所学的理论知识。实验所需的染料、培养基配方、试剂及缓冲液配制和微生物学实验的英文词汇等均列于附录中。

本教材为书网融合教材，即纸质教材有机融合电子教材、教学配套资源（PPT、微课、视频、图片等)、题库系统、数字化教学服务（在线教学、在线作业、在线考试)，使教学资源更加多样化、立体化。

本教材是微生物学教学同仁多年教学实践的结晶，具有药学微生物学实验教学的显著特色，实验内容可根据教学需要适当选做，期望在药学生的素质教育方面能尽微薄之力。由于编者水平有限，在实验内容编排和中英文表述方面定有欠妥之处，恳请批评指正。

编　者

2019年10月

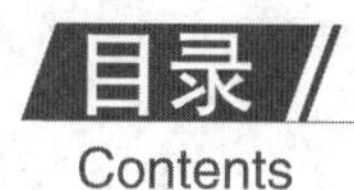

Contents

第一部分　显微技术和微生物形态学

微生物学的研究对象是肉眼无法直接分辨的微小生物，正是由于微生物的这个特性，使得显微镜成为这个学科中最为重要的工具之一。因此，显微镜的使用方法和如何制备标本也是必须掌握的实验技能。本单元共包括两部分：显微技术——从最常用的明视野光学显微镜入手，讲述了光学显微镜的构造和原理，及其使用方法，并对暗视野光学显微镜的使用也进行了介绍；微生物形态学——描述了如何利用显微镜对不同微生物（包括特殊结构）的形态、大小和运动性进行观察与测量的方法。本单元最后以常见微生物的菌落形态观察结尾。

实验一　明视野光学显微镜

扫码“学一学”

【实验目的】

（1）掌握明视野光学显微镜的使用方法、尤其是油镜的使用。

（2）熟悉明视野光学显微镜的结构和工作原理。

（3）了解观察微生物染色标本的方法。

【实验原理】

明视野光学显微镜（以下简称“明视野显微镜”）是最常用的光学显微镜。之所以叫它“明视野”，是因为它就像你现在所看到的本页书上的文字一样，能够在较亮的背景下形成一个比较暗的图像。

1. 明视野显微镜的结构　明视野显微镜的基本结构如图 1 – 1 所示，分光学系统和机械系统两部分。

（1）光学系统　主要包括物镜、目镜、聚光器和光源等。

① 显微镜有两种放大镜头，一种是目镜，一种是物镜。每一部分都对载物台上的标本起放大作用。显微镜的放大倍数由物镜和目镜的乘积决定。用转换器可以将物镜进行转换，因而也就改变了显微镜的放大倍数。转换器上共有四个物镜，分别是 4 倍的扫描物镜（红色）、10 倍的低倍镜（黄色）、40 倍的高倍镜（蓝色）和 100 倍的油镜（白色）。需要注意的是这些物镜之所以用颜色进行标记是为了更容易进行辨认。在必要情况下镜头只能用擦镜纸进行清洁。

② 光圈和聚光器位于载物台下方。聚光器将穿过标本的光线进行汇聚，而光圈则用于调节穿过标本的光线强弱。

③ 光源位于显微镜的基座上，由开关控制并对其亮度进行调节。显微镜不使用的情况下应将光源关掉。

（2）机械系统　主要包括镜座、镜臂、载物台、物镜转换器和调节旋钮等。

① 镜座是显微镜的底座，是支撑显微镜全部重量的部件。

② 镜臂用以支撑载物台和光学镜筒。需要注意的是在搬运显微镜时，需要一手握住镜

扫码"看一看"

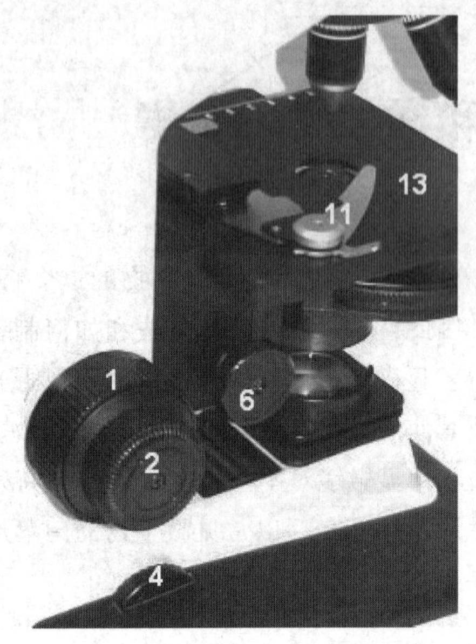

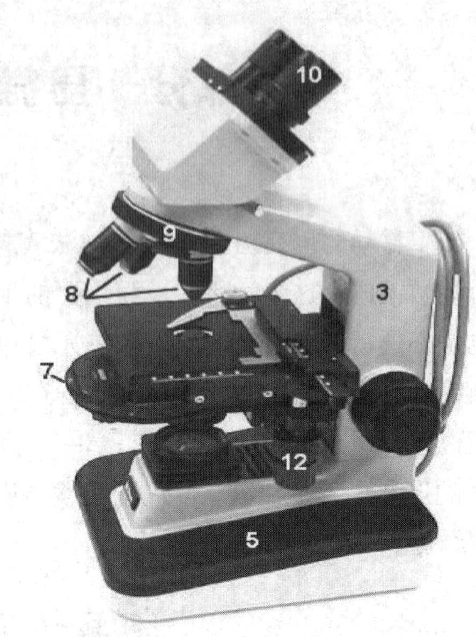

图1-1　明视野显微镜

1. 粗调节旋钮；　2. 细调节旋钮；　3. 镜臂；　4. 电源开关（亮度调节旋钮）；　5. 镜座；　6. 聚光器调节旋钮；
7. 光圈；　8. 物镜；　9. 物镜转换器；　10. 目镜；　11. 玻片夹；　12. 标本推动旋钮；　13. 载物台

臂，一手支撑底座。

③ 载物台用以放置被检标本，在载物台的中央有一小孔，可以使光线穿过。载物台上装有一对玻片夹，镜检时用来固定标本。.

④ 物镜转换器位于光学头的下半部，是一个带有物镜的可旋转圆盘。

⑤ 较大的粗调节旋钮位于镜臂两侧，用于快速升降载物台，进行粗略调焦，使用时应记住升高或降低载物台的旋钮旋转方向。较小的细调结旋钮用于载物台高度的细微调节，位于粗调节旋钮的中间。

2. 显微镜的分辨率和油镜的使用　显微镜所观察到的应是放大且清晰的图像。其清晰度由分辨率来决定。分辨率（R）是指能够将非常靠近的两点进行区分的能力。分辨率越小，其分辨能力越高。下面的方程式显示了决定分辨率的主要参数：

$$R = 0.61\frac{\lambda}{\mathrm{NA}}$$

其中，λ 是所用的光线波长，NA 叫做数值孔径。由方程可见，所用波长越小，成像越清晰，电子显微镜所具有的高分辨率就与此有关。分辨率的另一个决定因素是数值孔径。数值孔径是用来描述镜头改变光线方向的相对有效性的数学常数。数值孔径的大小如下面方程显示：

$$\mathrm{NA} = n\sin\theta$$

其中，n 代表物镜与样本间介质的折射率，θ 则定义为穿过样本进入镜头的光锥角度的 1/2，即镜口角（图1-2）。

由于数值孔径越大，分辨率效果越好。所以要提高数值孔径，可以通过提高 n 和 $\sin\theta$ 来达到。空气的折射率是1，并且由于 $\sin\theta$ 不会大于1，所以任何透镜在空气中的数值孔径都不会大于1。要使数值孔径大于1的唯一可行方法就是通过使用香柏油是一种无色液体，来提高折射率，香柏油与载玻片具有相同的折射率。当用香柏油代替空气时，入射光线就

不会发生反射和折射。因此，就能够得到较大的数值孔径和更好的分辨效果（图1－3）。

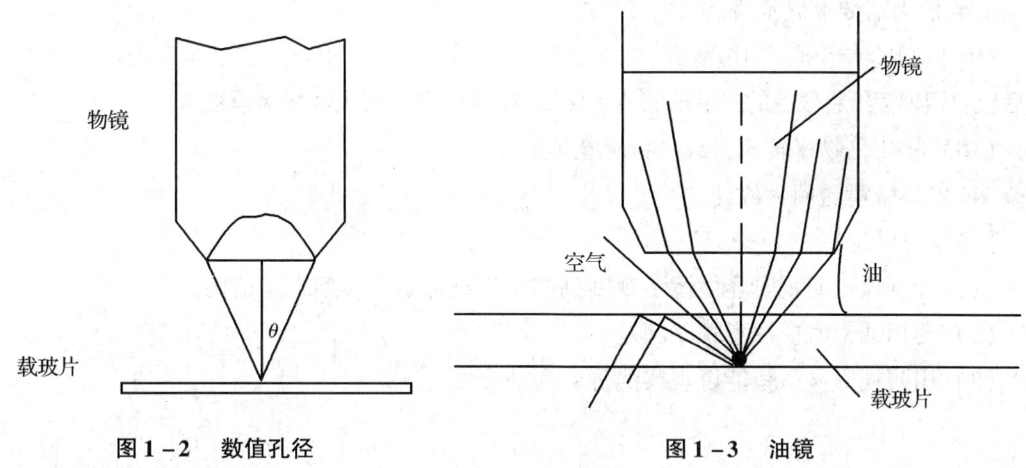

图1－2　数值孔径　　　　图1－3　油镜

【实验材料】

1. 载玻片标本

（1）细菌基本形态标本　金黄色葡萄球菌、唾液链球菌、大肠埃希菌、枯草芽孢杆菌、霍乱弧菌。

（2）细菌特殊结构标本　芽孢（枯草芽孢杆菌、破伤风梭菌）、鞭毛（伤寒沙门菌）、荚膜（肺炎链球菌）。

（3）真菌基本形态标本　酿酒酵母。

2. 仪器与试剂　明视野显微镜、二重瓶（内装香柏油和二甲苯）、擦镜纸、吸水纸。

3. 其他　擦镜纸、吸水纸。

【实验方法】

（1）一手握住镜臂，一手托住镜座，取出显微镜置于实验台上，镜座距实验台边缘约3～4cm。为减少疲劳，镜检者应姿势端正，两眼睁开。一般用左眼观察，右眼便于绘图或记录。

（2）将标本用玻片夹固定在载物台上，通过调节标本推动旋钮将涂有标本的位置置于载物台光源通过孔的正上方。

（3）适当调节光圈、聚光器和光亮度，使视野得到均匀照明。

（4）先用低倍镜（即10倍物镜）进行观察，将载物台上升至载玻片与物镜下方距离大约为5mm处，然后用粗调节旋钮缓慢下降载物台，同时从目镜中观察，直至视野中出现图像。这样做可以防止在观察过程中物镜与载玻片接触而损坏物镜。当视野中出现图像时，改用细调节螺旋将图像调至清晰。注意：细调节旋钮不可沿同一方向过度调节。

（5）转至高倍镜（即40倍物镜），此时标本仍应在视野中，只不过比原来大了4倍。用细调节旋钮将物像调至清晰。少数显微镜在从低倍镜转至高倍镜时，仍需要按步骤（4）再次进行调节。真菌标本用高倍镜即可观察清楚。

（6）用油镜观察细菌的染色标本　降低载物台，在载玻片上光源透过的位置加一滴香柏油，然后将100倍物镜（即油镜）转入光路，用粗调节旋钮升高载物台，并从侧面观察，使镜头浸入油中并几乎与载玻片接触。注意：不可用力过猛，以免压碎玻片，损坏镜头。

（7）从目镜中进行观察，同时将光亮度升至最大。用粗调节旋钮缓缓下降载物台至出现物象时，改用细调节旋钮调整至物像清晰。

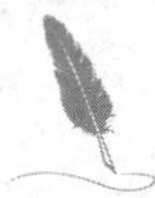

（8）当使用油镜时，一旦镜头接触香柏油，就不要再将高倍镜转入。否则高倍镜头会因为沾到油而需要彻底清洗。

（9）当观察结束时，用擦镜纸擦除油镜上残留的香柏油，也可用二甲苯来进行此步骤，但最后也要用擦镜纸将残留的二甲苯擦掉。显微镜镜头只能在必要时用擦镜纸清洁。

（10）将 4 倍物镜转入，载物台降至最低。

（11）显微镜送回存放处。

【结果与讨论】

（1）分别绘出明视野显微镜下观察到的微生物标本的典型形态结构。

（2）使用油镜时应注意哪些问题？

（3）用明视野显微镜能否观察病毒？为什么？

PART ONE Microscopic Techniques and Microbial Morphology

Microbiology is the study of organisms invisible to the naked eye. Because of this characteristic of microbes, microscope is an essential tool in this discipline. Thus, to understand how microscope works and the way to prepare the specimens are of great importance. This part begins with the most commonly used microscope – bright – field light microscope, including its structure, principle and use. Dark – field microscope is also introduced. The second section is about how to use light microscope to observe the morphology and motility of different microbes. This part closes with microbial colony observation.

EXPERIMENT 1 Bright – Field Light Microscope

Purpose

(1) To grasp how to correctly use a microscope, especially the oil immersion lens.

(2) To be familiar with the structure and principle of bright – field light microscope.

(3) To understand the way to observe several stained microorganism specimens.

Principles

Bright – field light microscope (or “bright – field microscope”) is the most commonly used type of light microscope. It is so named “bright – field” because it forms a dark image against a brighter background just like the words on a printed page.

1. The structure of bright – field microscope

As illustrated in Fig. 1 – 1, the fundamental structure of a bright – field microscope includes optical system and mechanical system.

(1) Optical system: mainly includes objective lens, ocular, condenser and light source.

①There are two magnifying lenses in the microscope. One magnifying lens is in the ocular and one is in the objective. Each contributes to the magnification of the object on the stage. The total magnification of any set of lenses is determined by multiplying the magnification of the objective by the magnification of the ocular. When rotating the nosepiece, there is change in the objective and consequently in magnification. On the nosepiece, a 4 × objective lens (red), a 10 × low power objective (yellow), a 40 × high power objective (blue), and a 100 × oil immersion lens (white) can be found. Note that these lenses are color – coded for easy identification. Only lens paper is allowed to clean the lens when necessary.

②The iris diaphragm and condenser are located under the stage. The condenser focuses the light passing through the specimen and the iris diaphragm is used to regulate the amount of light passing through the specimen.

③An electric light source is mounted on the base of the microscope, and is controlled by an on – off switch which can also adjust the brightness. Please turn off the light when the microscope is not in use.

(2) Mechanical system: mainly includes base, arm, stage, nosepiece and adjustment knobs.

①The base is the main support for the microscope.

②The arm supports the stage and the optical head. Note that the proper way to carry a microscope is to grasp the arm with one hand and support the base with the other hand.

③The stage is a flat area upon which the specimen is placed. It has a hole in the center through which light may pass. Mounted on the stage is a pair of stage clips. This is designed to immobilize the slide during observation.

④The nosepiece is a revolving plate on the lower side of the optical head which holds the objective lenses.

⑤A pair of large knobs located on both sides of the arm are coarse adjustment knobs that permit rapid raising or lowering of the stage. Please memorize the direction of rotation to lower or raise the stage. A pair of smaller knobs located "inside of" the coarse adjustment knobs are fine adjustment knobs that permit minor adjustments in the stage height.

2. Microscope resolution (resolving power) and the oil immersion objective

Microscope is used to provide a magnified and clear image. Resolution (R) is essential for this. Resolution is the capacity of an optical system to distinguish or separate two adjacent objects or points form one another. The smaller the resolution, the better the resolving ability. The following equation expresses the main determining factors in resolution:

$$R = \frac{0.61\lambda}{\mathrm{NA}}$$

In the equation, lambda (λ) is the wavelength of light used to illuminate the specimen and NA is the numerical aperture. From the equation, it indicates that a major determinant of resolution is the wavelength of the light used. The shorter the wavelength is, the clearer the image will be. This will help to understand the high resolution of the electron microscope introduced in later parts. Another determinant of resolution is NA. NA is a mathematical constant that describes the relative efficiency of a lens in bending light rays. It could be expressed as:

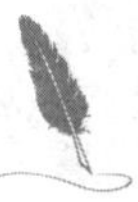

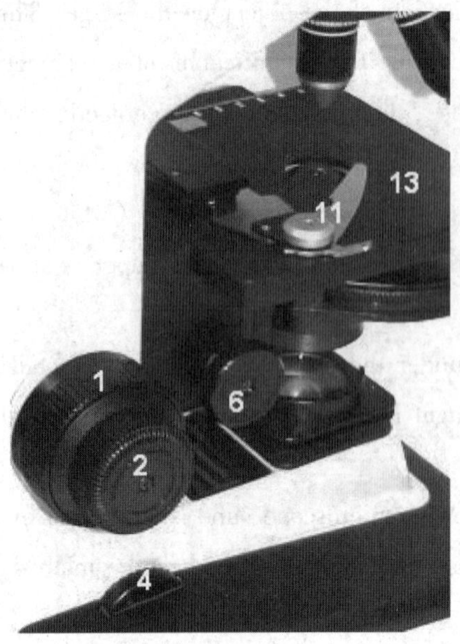

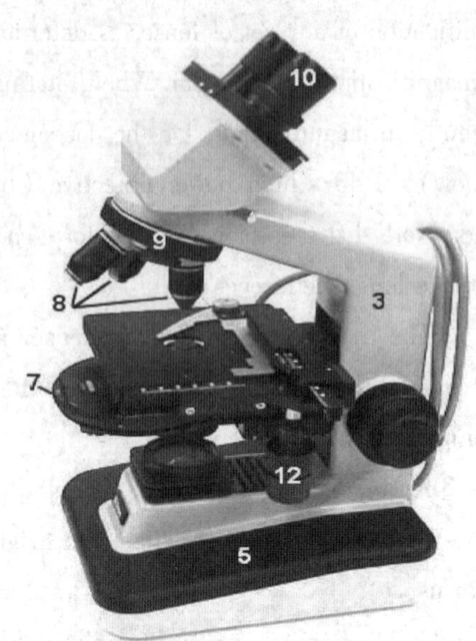

Fig. 1 - 1 Bright - field microscope

1. Coarse adjustment knob; 2. Fine adjustment knob; 3. Arm; 4. Power switch/ brightness control 5. Base; 6. Condenser knob; 7. Iris diaphragm; 8. Objective lens; 9. Revolving nosepiece; 10. Ocular eyepiece lens; 11. Stage clips; 12. Stage motion knobs; 13. Stage

$$NA = n \sin\theta$$

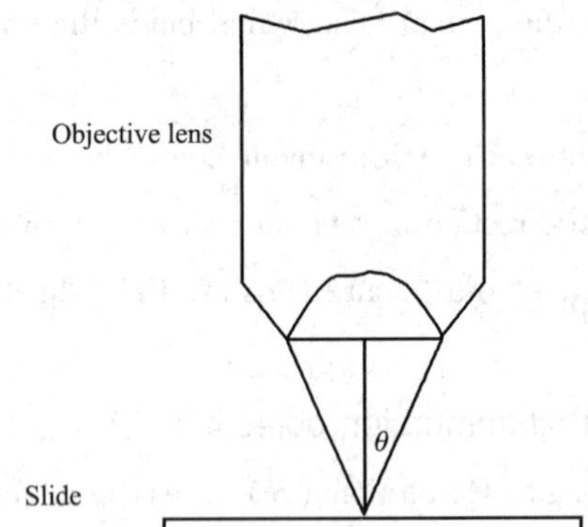

Fig. 1 - 2 Numerical aperture

In the equation, n represents the refractive index of the medium between the objective and the specimen. θ is defined as 1/2 the angle of the cone of light that enters a lens from a specimen (Fig. 1 - 2).

Remember that a higher NA can provide a better resolution. An increase in either n or $\sin\theta$ or both can result in a higher NA. The refractive index for air is 1.00. Since $\sin\theta$ cannot be greater than 1.00, no lens working in air can have a NA higher than 1.00. The only practical way to make NA above 1.00 is to increase the refractive index with immersion oil, a colorless liquid with the same refractive index as the slide. When air is replaced with immersion oil, reflection and refraction of the light from the condenser to the objective will be avoided effectively. Thus, an increase in numerical aperture and resolution is achieved (Fig. 1 - 3).

Materials and Apparatus

1. Specimens on glass slides

(1) The basic morphology of bacteria—*Staphylococcus aureus*, *Streptococcus salivarius*, *Escherichia coli*, *Bacillus subtilis* and *Vibrio cholerae*.

(2) The special structures of bacteria—endospore (*Bacillus subtilis*, *Clostridium tetani*), flagella (*Salmonella typhosa*) and capsule (*Streptococcus pneumoniae*).

(3) The basic morphology of fungi—*Saccharomyces cerevisiae*

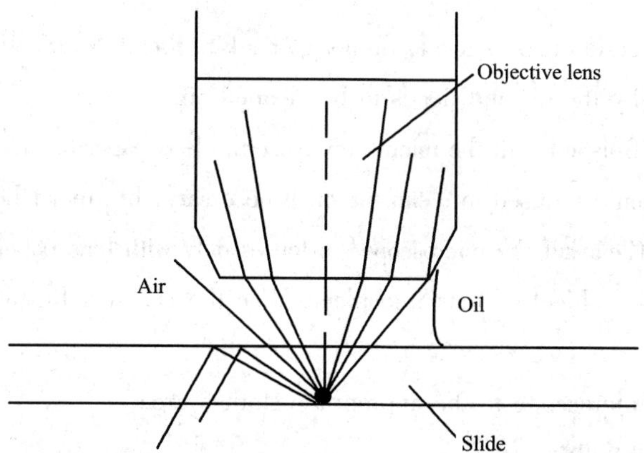

Fig. 1 – 3　The oil immersion objective lens

2. Apparatus and reagents　bright – field microscope, dual – bottle (with immersion oil and xylene) .

3. Others　lens paper, water – adsorption paper.

Procedures

(1) Always carry the arm of the microscope with one hand and support the base with the other hand. Place it on the desk 3 to 4 cm away from the desk edge. In order to reduce fatigue, observers should posture properly and open both eyes. Usually use the left eye to observe and use the right eye to take records.

(2) Place a slide on the stage, and secure it firmly using the stage clips. Try to guesstimate the location of the specimen on the slide, and place it above the hole through which the light passes.

(3) Adjust the iris diaphragm, condenser, and brightness of light carefully to get suitable illumination.

(4) With the low – power objective (10 × objective) in position, raise the stage until the tip of the objective is at a distance of 5mm from the slide. Then lower the stage slowly using the coarse adjustment knobs while looking at the microscope until the object comes into view. This can avoid striking the objective to the slide. Once the object is in view, switch over to the fine adjustment knob to focus the desired image. Note: Do not overuse the fine adjustment knob in one direction.

(5) Rotate the high – power objective (40 × objective) in position. Your specimen should still be in the field of vision, but 4 times larger now. Use your fine adjustment knobs to clarify the image. For some microscopes, when switch over to the high – power objective, same manipulation as step 4 is still necessary. Fungi specimen can be observed clearly with the high – power objective.

(6) Use the oil immersion lens to examine the stained bacteria samples provided. Lower the stage and place a single drop of immersion oil on the slide right over where the light is coming through the stage. Then rotate the 100 × objective (oil immersion lens) into position. Raise the stage with the coarse adjustment knob while looking at the objective from the side until the lens immerses in oil and just touches the slide. Note: Do this gently to avoid breaking the slide and the objective.

(7) Now look through the oculars and adjust the light for maximum illumination. Lower the stage slowly with the coarse adjustment knob. Once the object is in view, use the fine adjustment

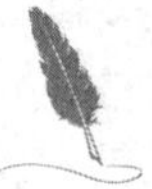

knob to focus clearly.

(8) Once oil immersion lens is used, do not go back to the 40 × objective. Otherwise, the objective will be polluted by the oil and needs to be cleaned off.

(9) After you are finished with the microscope, use the lens paper to wipe the oil from the 100 × objective lens. Xylene could be used to clean the oil if necessary, but remember to remove xylene with the lens paper as well. Clean all the microscope' s lenses only with lens paper if necessary.

(10) Rotate the 4 × objective lens into place. Use the coarse adjustment knobs to lower the stage to the bottom.

(11) Return the microscope to the appropriate storage area.

Results and Discussion

(1) Draw the typical morphologies of microorganisms you observed by using the bright – field microscopes.

(2) What should be paid attention to when you use the oil – immersion lens?

(3) Can you observe virus with a bright – field microscope? Why?

实验二　暗视野光学显微镜

扫码“学一学”

【实验目的】

(1) 了解暗视野光学显微镜的基本原理。

(2) 熟悉暗视野光学显微镜的使用方法。

【实验原理】

暗视野光学显微镜（以下简称“暗视野显微镜”）与明视野显微镜相比，除聚光器外其他结构都相同。如果将明视野显微镜的聚光器镜头下方安装一个暗视野光阑，就可以将其改造成一个暗视野显微镜（图2-1）。

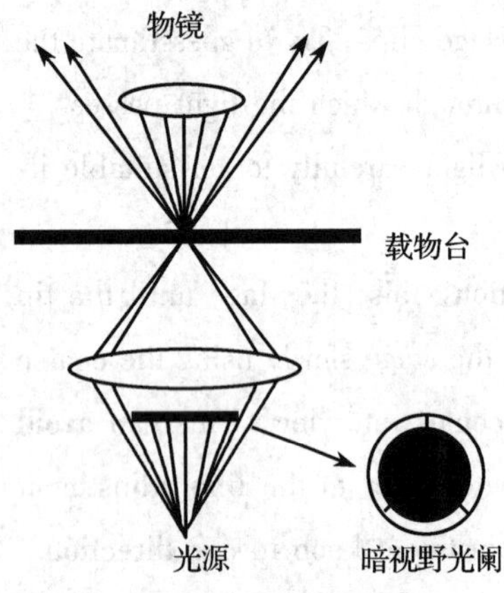

图2-1　暗视野显微镜光路

暗视野光阑使得只有由标本反射或折射的光线才能进入到物镜中。当光线经过暗视野聚光器时，形成了一个中空的光锥照射在标本上并成像。此时标本周围的视野呈黑色，而标本本身被照亮。由于在黑色背景下观察亮的物体总是比在相反条件下所看到的图像更清晰，因此暗视野显微镜更适于观察未染色或难于染色的微生物标本，同时也适用于观察微生物的外部轮廓以及判断细胞的运动性。暗视野显微镜的分辨能力也比明视野显微镜要高得多。

【实验材料】

1. **菌种**　酿酒酵母液体培养物，枯草芽孢杆菌液体培养物。
2. **仪器与试剂**　暗视野显微镜，无菌水，二重瓶。
3. **其他**　载玻片，盖玻片，擦镜纸，吸水纸。

【实验方法】

(1) 直接在暗视野聚光器上滴加一滴香柏油。

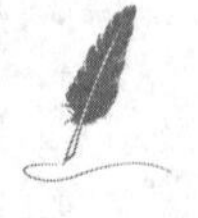

（2）制备酵母细胞水浸片。然后将标本片放于载物台上，使标本处于光源上方。

（3）小心上升聚光器，直至油滴接触到载玻片。

（4）先用低倍镜进行观察，然后转至高倍镜，用粗调节旋钮和细调节旋钮将图像调至清晰。

（5）按照相同步骤观察枯草芽孢杆菌标本，最后用油镜进行观察。

【结果与讨论】

（1）分别记录酿酒酵母与枯草芽孢杆菌观察结果。

（2）与明视野显微镜相比，暗视野显微镜更适于观察活细胞微生物。为什么？

EXPERIMENT 2 Dark – Field Light Microscope

Purposes

(1) To understand the principles of dark – field light microscope.

(2) To be familiar with how to use dark – field light microscope correctly.

Principles

Dark – field light microscope (abbreviated as "dark – field microscope") has the same structure as bright – field microscope except the condenser. A bright – field microscope can be converted to a dark – field microscope by placing a dark – field stop underneath the condenser lens (Fig. 2 – 1).

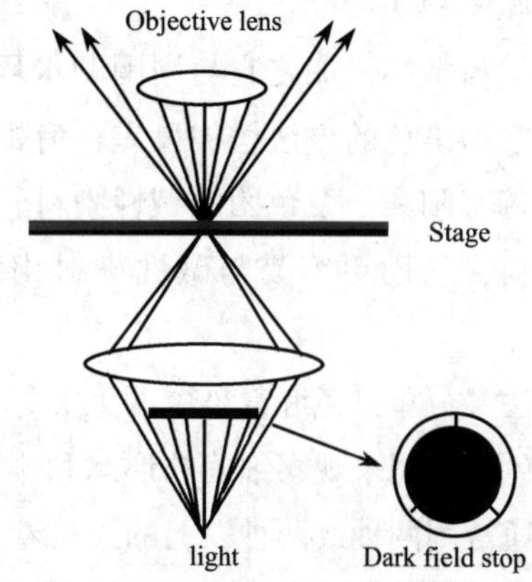

Fig. 2 – 1 Light pathway of a dark – field microscope

The stop blocks all light from entering the objective lens except the light that has been reflected or refracted by the specimen. A hollow cone of light is focused on the specimen and forms an image. The field surrounding the specimen appears black, while the object itself is brightly illuminated. Since light objects against a dark background are seen more clearly by the eye than the reverse, dark – field microscopy is useful in observing both unstained living microbes and microbes that are difficult to stain. It can outline the organism's shape and identify cellular motility. The resolving ability of dark – field microscopy is much higher than that of bright – field microscopy.

Materials and Apparatus

1. Cultures broth cultures of *Saccharomyces cerevisiae* and *Bacillus subtilis*.

2. Apparatus and reagents dark – field microscope, sterile water, dual – bottle.

3. Others slide, cover slip, lens paper, water – adsorption paper.

Procedures

(1) Place a drop of immersion oil directly on the dark – field condenser lens.

(2) Prepare a wet mount of yeast cells. Then put it on the stage and make sure that the specimen is justabove the light source.

(3) Raise the condenser carefully until the oil just touches the slide.

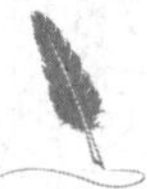

(4) Observe with the low - power objective first and then switch to the high power objective. Focus with the coarse and fine adjustment knobs.

(5) Do the same with *B. subtilis* specimen. And then use the oil immersion lens to observe.

Results and Discussion

(1) Record the observation results of the two specimens respectively.

(2) Compared with bright - field microscope, the dark - field microscope is more suitable for observing living microorganisms. Why?

实验三 单染色法

扫码"学一学"

【实验目的】

(1) 熟悉细菌单染色标本的制备过程。

(2) 掌握油镜观察细菌的形态结构。

【实验原理】

由于细菌微小，加之它与周围的水环境光学性质相近，从而用一般光学显微镜不易看到它。通常用染色的方法增加反差，有助于细菌标本的观察。染料有带阴离子发色团的酸性染料和带有阳离子发色团的碱性染料。由于在一般生理条件下（pH7.4 左右）细菌菌体都带负电荷，从而更容易与碱性染料相结合。常用的碱性染料有结晶紫、亚甲蓝和碱性复红。

染色法又分单染色和复染色两大类。单染色法即仅用一种染料着色，所有的细菌均被染成一种颜色，可用来观察细菌的形态和排列方式，但无鉴别细菌的作用。复染色法又称鉴别染色法，通常用两种或两种以上的染料着色，由于不同种类的细菌或同种细菌的不同组成结构对染料有不同的反应性而被染成不同的颜色，从而有鉴别细菌的作用。

【实验材料】

1. **细菌** 金黄色葡萄球菌斜面培养物 1 支，大肠埃希菌斜面培养物 1 支。

2. **试剂** 吕氏亚甲蓝染色液，复红染色液，香柏油，生理盐水，二甲苯。

3. **其他** 载玻片，吸水纸，接种环，酒精灯，擦镜纸，显微镜。

【实验方法】

1. **涂片**

(1) 取载玻片一张，拭净。

(2) 接种环火焰灭菌，取生理盐水一滴，放在载玻片中央（如被检材料是液体，可不加生理盐水）。

(3) 左手斜持菌种管，右手持接种环，经火焰灭菌后，用右手小指拔开菌种管棉塞，管口通过火焰，将接种环插入管中取菌少许（切不可多，更不可将培养基刮下）。

(4) 管口再通过火焰，塞好棉塞。

(5) 将接种环上的细菌加入载玻片上之水滴内，磨匀，涂成直径约 1cm 大小的薄菌膜。

(6) 接种环经火焰灭菌。

2. **干燥** 涂片置于空气中，使其自然干燥。

3. **固定** 干燥后将涂片在火焰上缓缓通过 3 次，此为"固定"。目的是使细菌粘于载

玻片上，染色和水冲时不易脱落；且细菌为蛋白质，被热凝固可保持完整形态。

4. 染色

（1）在固定后的标本上加吕氏亚甲蓝染液（或复红染液）以覆满标本为度，染 1 ~2 分钟。

（2）用细流水自载玻片一端徐徐冲洗。

（3）待其自然干燥或用吸水纸轻轻吸干。

5. 油镜观察　吕氏亚甲蓝染色者，菌体呈蓝色；复红染色者，菌体呈红色。

细菌单染色法见图 3 –1。

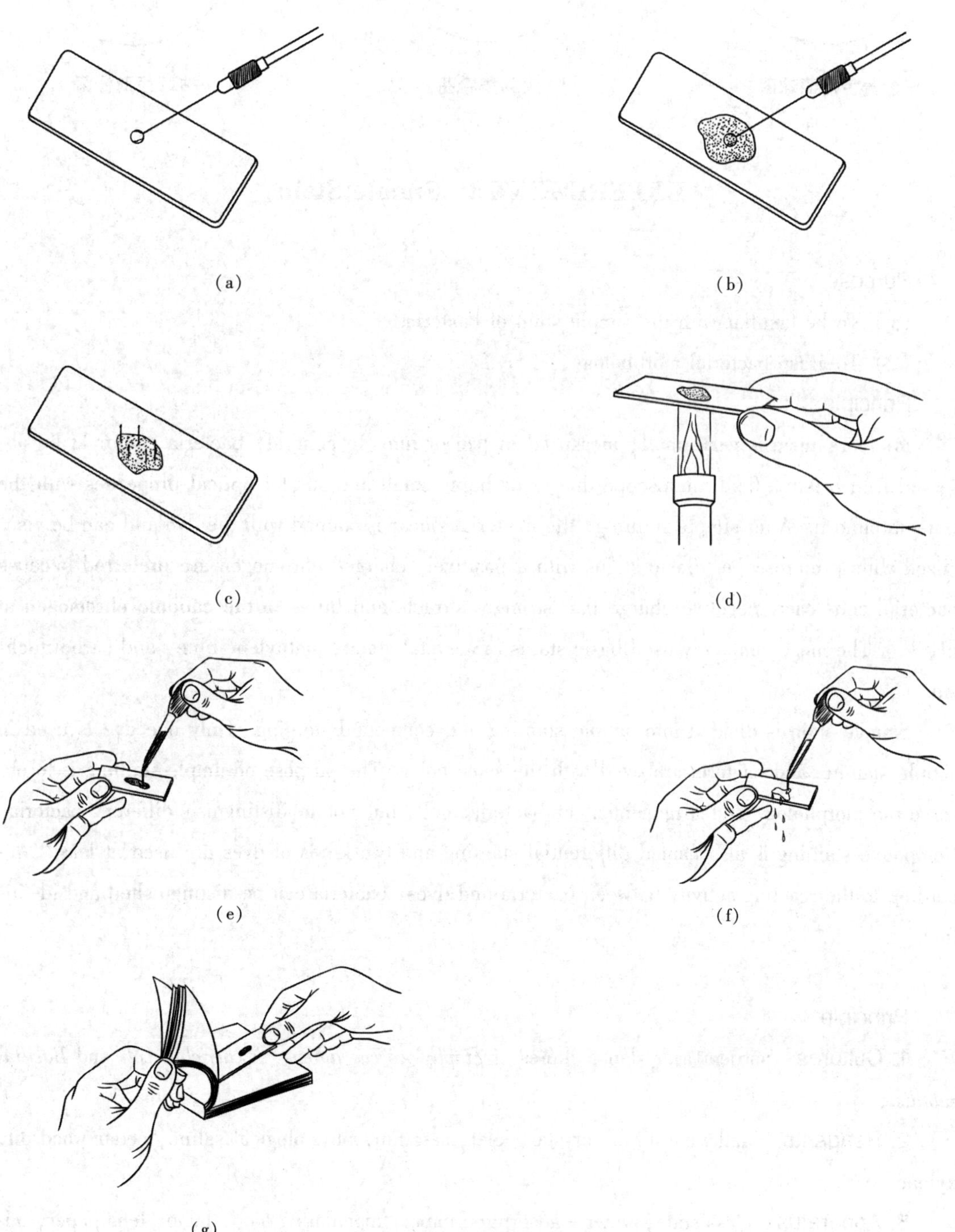

图 3 –1　细菌单染色法

（a）取菌；（b）涂片；（c）干燥；（d）固体；（e）染色；（f）冲洗；（g）吸干

【结果与讨论】

(1) 说明细菌单染色法的原理。

(2) 分别绘出下列细菌细胞的形态。

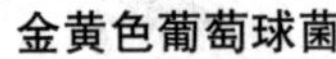

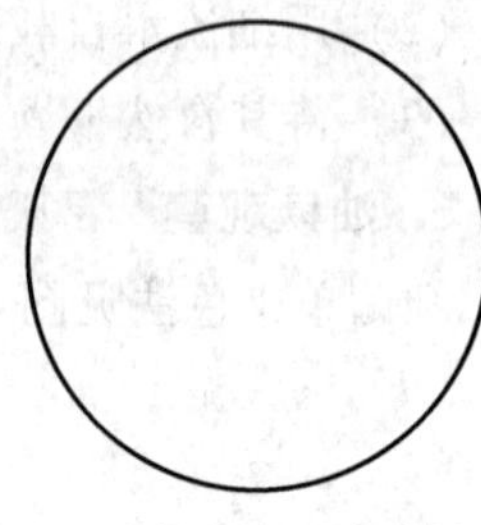

金黄色葡萄球菌　　大肠埃希菌　　枯草芽孢杆菌

EXPERIMENT 3　Simple Stain

Purpose

(1) To be familiar with the simple stain of bacteria.

(2) To grasp bacterial morphology.

Principle

Microorganism is very small, measured in μm or nm. In general, bacteria couldn't be observed with bright-field microscope due to its being small and similar optical properties with the water around it. After simple staining, the bacterial smear is stained with the dye and can be visualized with a microscope. Basic stains with a positively charged chromogen are preferred because bacterial cells carry negative charge that strongly attracts and binds to the cationic chromogen at pH 7.4. The most commonly used basic stains are crystal violet, methylene blue, and carbol fuchsin.

Sample stain is divided into simple staining and compound staining. Only one dye is used in simple staining and bacteria are dyed with the same color. The purpose of simple staining is to observe the morphology and arrangement of bacterial cells but not to distinguish different bacteria. Compound staining is also named differential staining and two kinds of dyes are used at least. According to the reacting activity between bacteria and dyes, bacteria can be distinguished and identified.

Principle

1. Cultures　nutrient agar slant cultures of *Staphylococcus aureus*, *Escherichia coli* and *Bacillus subtilis*.

2. Reagents　Methylene blue, crystal violet, safranin, physiological saline, cedar wood oil, xylene.

3. Apparatus　glass slide, water-adsorption paper, inoculating loop, lamp, lens paper, microscope.

Procedures

1. Preparation of bacterial smears disposable

(1) Clean a glass slide and place it on the staining tray. Drop a blob of physiological water on the center of glass slide unless the sample is liquid media.

(2) Flame the inoculating loop until the wire becomes red – hot. Sterilize the metal handle.

(3) Remove the cap from tube and keep the cap between the palm and the small fingers. Flame the neck of the culture tube. Allow the loop to cool. Take some bacteria from slant with the sterilized loop.

(4) Flame the neck of the tube and recap.

(5) Place the bacteria on the loop into physiological water, stir and smear it to form a bacterial membrane of approximate 1 cm diameter.

(6) Sterilize the inoculating loop again.

2. Air dry Let the smear to air dry.

3. Fixation While holding the glass slide at one end, slowly pass the smear over the flame of the lamp three times. Fixation of bacteria on the surface of the glass slide is necessary for preventing dissociation during sample dying and washing and for keeping the intact form of bacteria while cell protein is being heat – denatured.

4. Staining

(1) Stain the smear with methylene blue or crystal violet or safranin for 1 to 2 minutes.

(2) Wash the smear with tap water from one side of the glass slide to remove excess stain.

(3) Air dry or adsorb water with paper but do not wipe the slide.

5. Examine all stained slides under oil immersion.

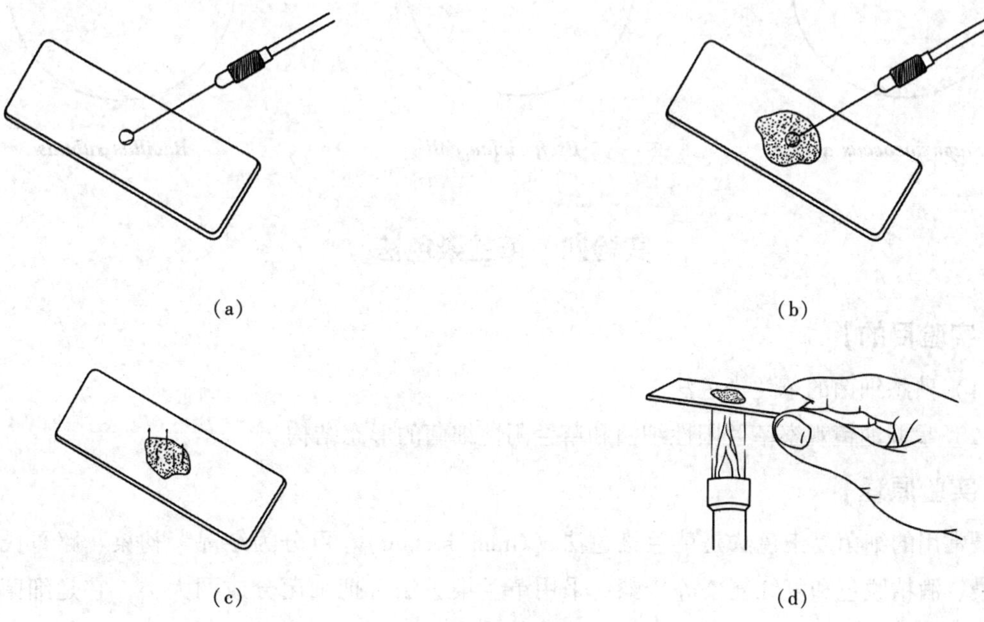

Fig. 3 – 1

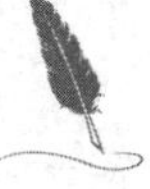

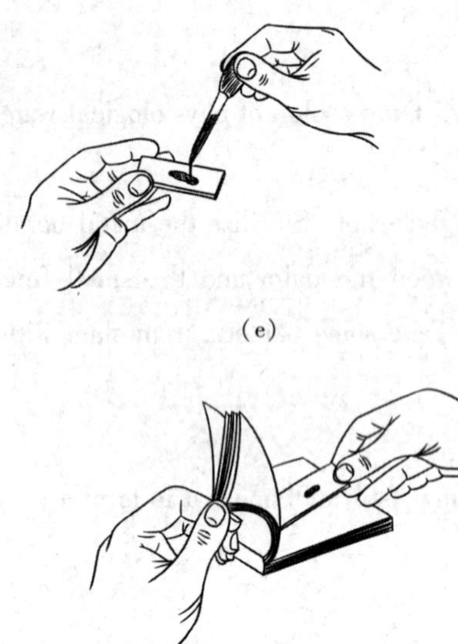

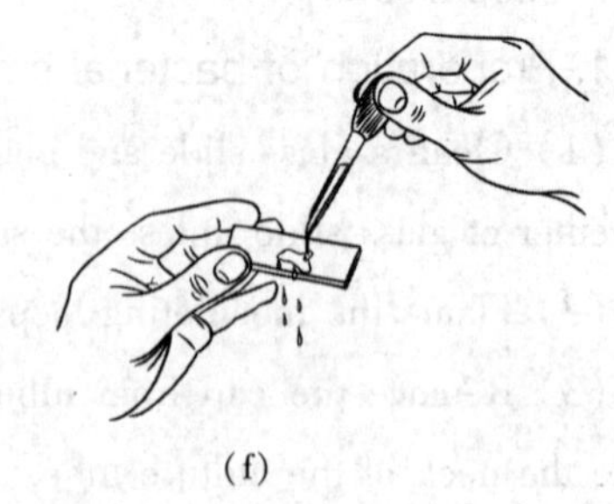

(e)　　(f)

(g)

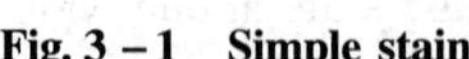

Fig. 3 – 1　Simple stain

(a) Take some bacteria; (b) Preparation of bacteria smears; (c) Air dry; (d) Fixation; (e) Staining; (f) Wash the smear; (g) Absorb the water

Results and Discussion

(1) What's the principle of simple staining?

(2) Draw a representative morphology for each organism.

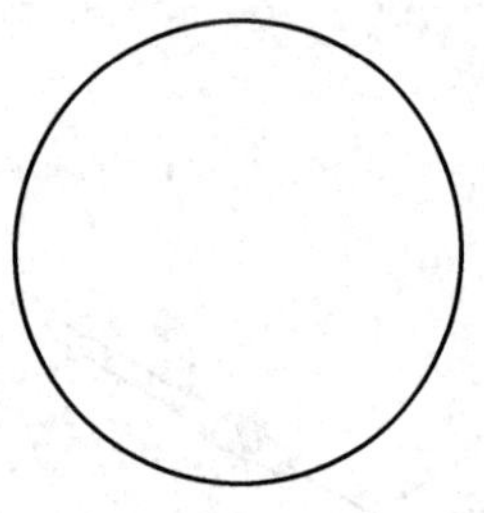

Staphylococcus aureus

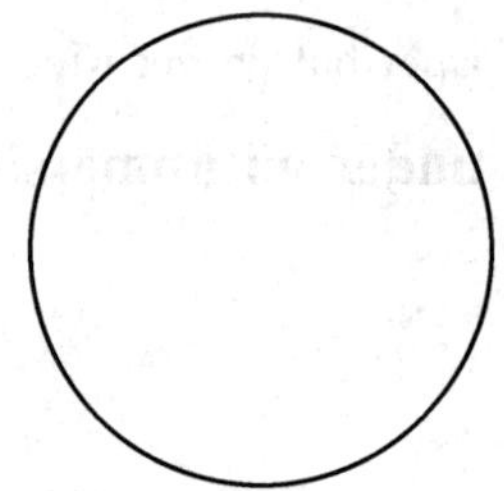

Escherichia coli

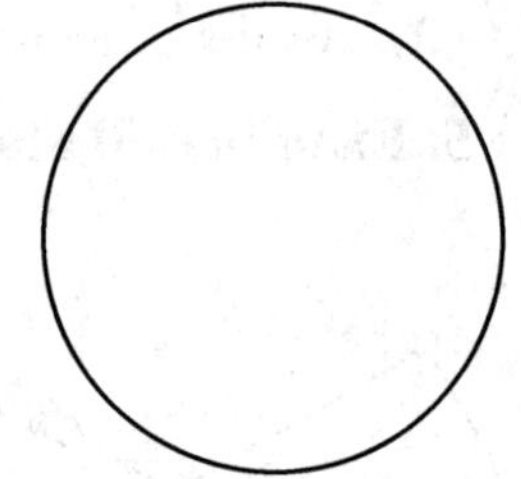

Bacillus subtilis

实验四　革兰染色法

扫码“学一学”

【实验目的】

(1) 熟悉细菌的革兰染色法。

(2) 掌握油镜观察革兰阳性细菌和革兰阴性细菌的形态结构。

【实验原理】

最常用的细菌复染色法是革兰染色法（Gram's stain）。可分为结晶紫初染、路哥氏碘液媒染、酒精脱色和复红复染等步骤。采用革兰染色法可把细菌分成两大类，它是细菌分类和鉴定的基础。凡能使第一种染料结晶紫保留蓝紫色的细菌叫做革兰阳性（G^+）细菌，凡被酒精脱色后染上对比颜料沙黄或稀释复红而呈红色的细菌叫做革兰阴性（G^-）细菌。

一般认为，革兰染色法与下列诸因素有关：① 革兰阳性细菌等电点低（pI = 2 ~ 3），

而革兰阴性细菌等电点高（pI = 4 ~ 5），因此在一般生理条件下（pH7.4 左右），革兰阳性细菌所带的负电荷要比阴性菌多得多，从而与碱性染料结晶紫结合牢固。② 革兰阴性细菌细胞壁有外膜结构，含有较多的脂质成分，对酒精作用敏感。脂质被酒精溶解，造成细胞壁破损，结晶紫－碘复合物容易被抽提出来而脱色。③ 革兰阳性细菌细胞壁脂质含量低，对酒精作用不敏感。且革兰阳性细菌细胞壁含有多层致密（交联度大）的肽聚糖层以及带有大量负电荷的磷壁酸，乙醇脱色处理时，因失水反而使网孔缩小，把结晶紫－碘复合物牢牢留在细胞内，使其仍呈紫色。

扫码“看一看”

【实验材料】

1. **细菌**　金黄色葡萄球菌斜面培养物 1 支，大肠埃希菌斜面培养物 1 支。
2. **试剂**　结晶紫、95% 乙醇溶液、路哥碘液、稀释复红各 1 瓶，香柏油，二甲苯，生理盐水。
3. **其他**　载玻片，吸水纸，接种环，酒精灯，擦镜纸，显微镜。

【实验方法】

1. **涂片、干燥、固定**　同单染色法。
2. **初染**　加结晶紫染液于标本上，使其覆满标本，染 1 ~ 2 分钟，细水冲洗。
3. **媒染**　加路哥碘溶液经 1 分钟，细水冲洗。
4. **脱色**　加 95% 乙醇溶液于载玻片上，脱色约 30 秒，倾去酒精，细水冲洗。
5. **复染**　加稀释复红染液复染约 1 分钟，水洗，待其自然干燥或用吸水纸轻轻吸干。
6. **镜检**　油镜观察。

细菌革兰染色法见图 4－1。

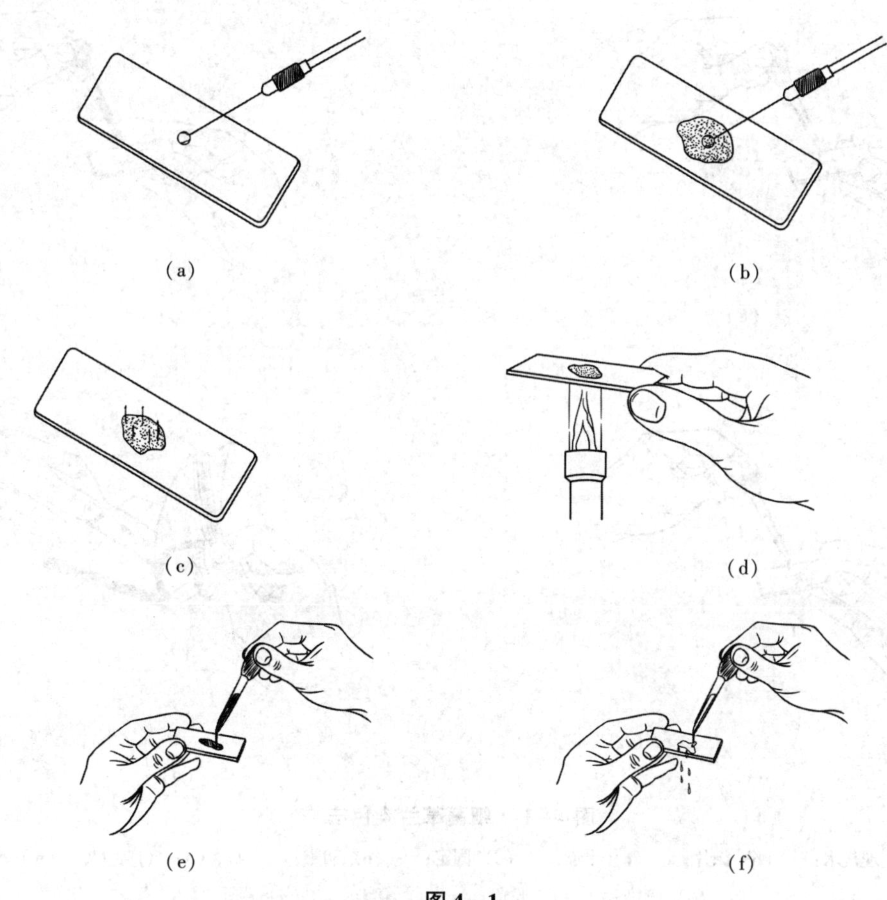

图 4－1

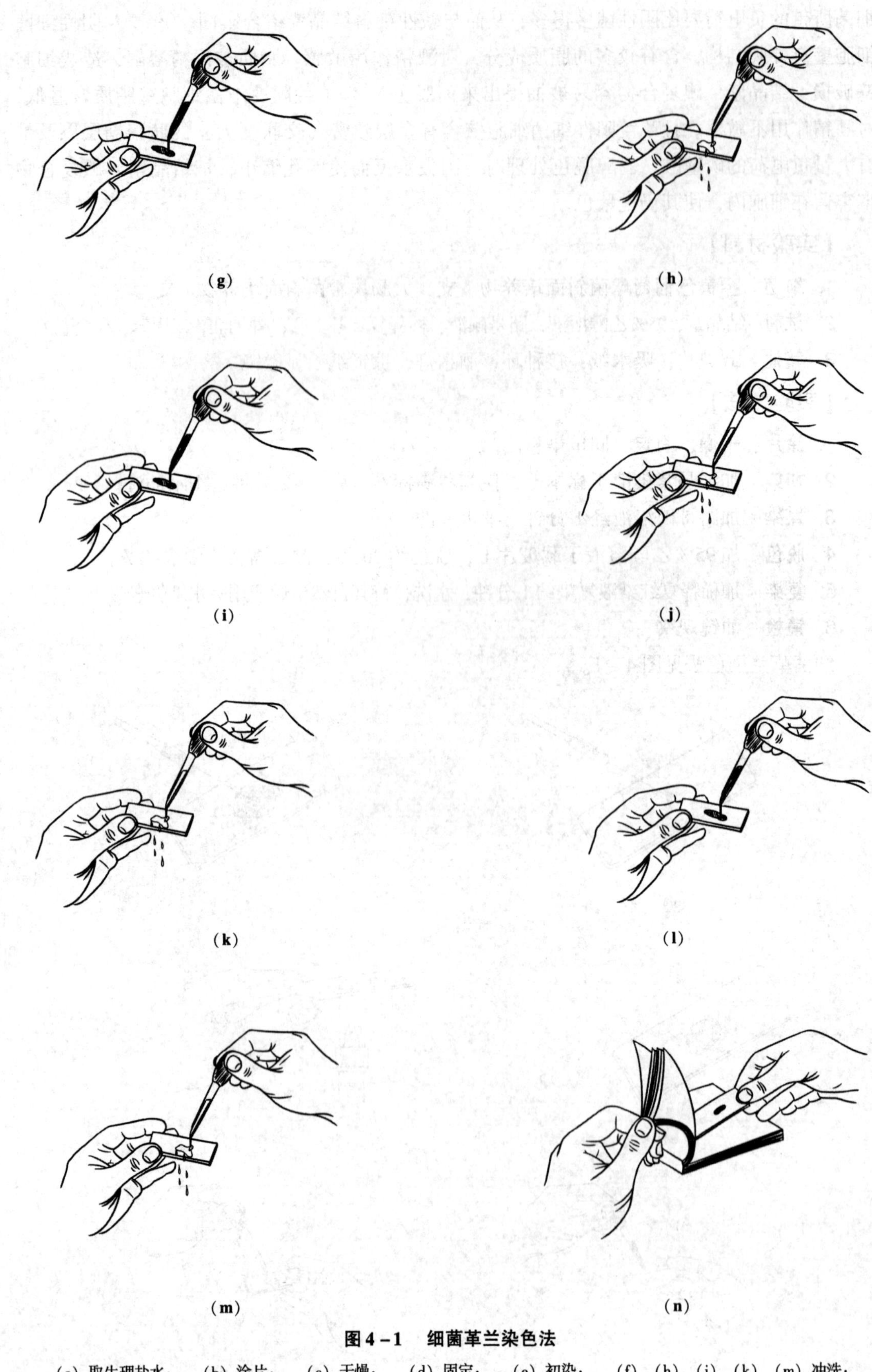

图 4－1　细菌革兰染色法

(a) 取生理盐水；　(b) 涂片；　(c) 干燥；　(d) 固定；　(e) 初染；　(f)、(h)、(j)、(k)、(m) 冲洗；
(g) 媒染；　(i) 脱色；　(l) 复染；　(n) 吸干

【结果与讨论】

（1）说明细菌革兰染色的原理。

（2）分别绘出下列革兰阳性细菌和革兰阴性细菌的形态。

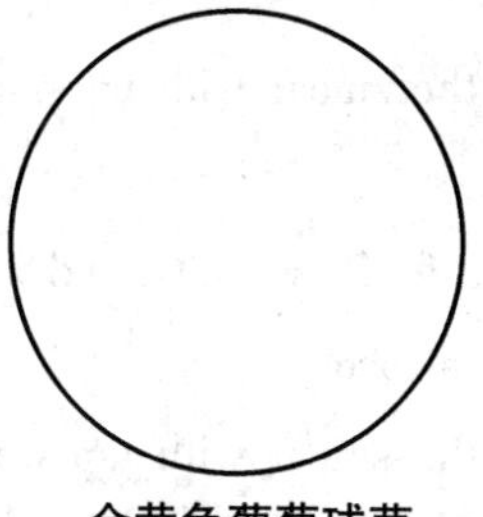

金黄色葡萄球菌

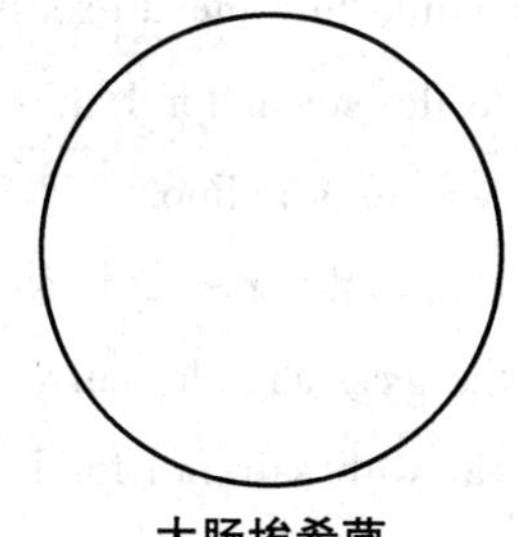

大肠埃希菌

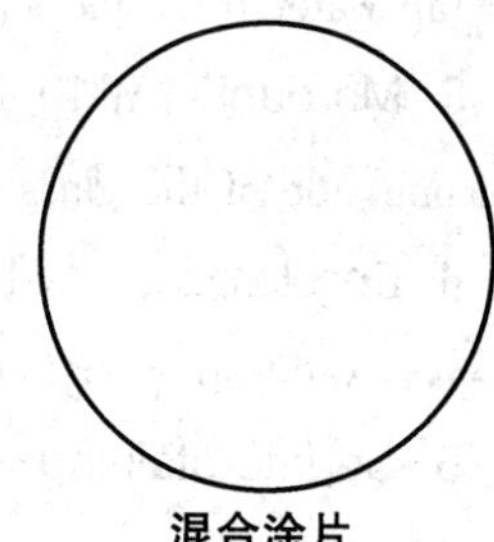

混合涂片

EXPERIMENT 4　Gram's Stain

Purpose

(1) To be familiar with Gram's stain.

(2) To grasp the morphology of gram - positive and gram - negative bacteria.

Principle

Gram's stain is a popular compound staining technique that includes primary stain with crystal violet, addition of Lugol's iodine, decolorization with 95% ethyl alcohol and counterstaining with safranin. It divides bacterial cells into two major groups named gram - positive (G^+) and gram - negative (G^-), which makes it an essential tool for classification and differentiation of microorganisms. After Gram's stain, gram - positive bacteria appear violet because they bind crystal violet and can't be decolorized by 95% ethyl alcohol, while gram - negative bacteria appear red because they bind safranin and can be decolorized by 95% ethyl alcohol.

Generally, the principle of Gram's stain involves: ① The isoelectric point of gram - positive bacteria is lower ($pI = 2 \sim 3$) than that of gram - negative bacteria ($pI = 4 \sim 5$). So it contains much more negative charges and bind to crystal violet tightly. ② The cell wall of gram - negative bacteria is composed of outer membrane containing much lipid composition, which is sensitive to ethyl alcohol. When decolorizing with 95% ethyl alcohol, the complex of crystal violet and iodine is extracted from cell wall. ③ The cell wall of gram - positive bacteria contains less lipid composition that is insensitive to decolorization with ethyl alcohol. In addition, it contains peptidoglycan multilayer and teichoic acid with large amount of negative charges. The complex of crystal violet and iodine binds to cell tightly and can't be extracted by 95% ethyl alcohol. So it appears purple after staining.

Materials and Apparatus

1. Cultures　24h nutrient agar slant cultures of *Staphylococcus aureus* and *Escherichia coli*.

2. Reagents　Crystal violet, 95% ethyl alcohol, Lugol's iodine, safranin, physiological saline, cedar wood oil, xylene.

3. Apparatus　glass slide, water - adsorption paper, inoculating loop, lamp, lens paper, microscope.

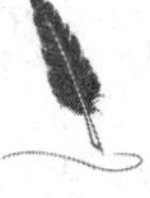

Procedures

1. Preparation of bacterial smears, air dry and fixation the same as simple staining techniques.

2. Primary stain Stain the smear with crystal violet for 1 to 2 minutes, and wash the smear with tap water from one side of the glass slide to remove excess stain.

3. Mordant Add Lugol's iodine to the smear for 1 min, and wash the smear with tap water from one side of the glass slide to remove excess iodine.

4. Decolorizing Add 95% ethyl alcohol to the smear, decolorize the smear for 30 seconds, and wash the smear with tap water from one side of the glass slide to remove excess ethyl alcohol.

5. Counterstaining Stain the smear with safranin for 1 min, wash the smear with tap water from one side of the glass slide to remove excess safranin. Air dry or adsorb water with paper but do not wipe the slide.

6. Examine all stained slides under oil immersion.

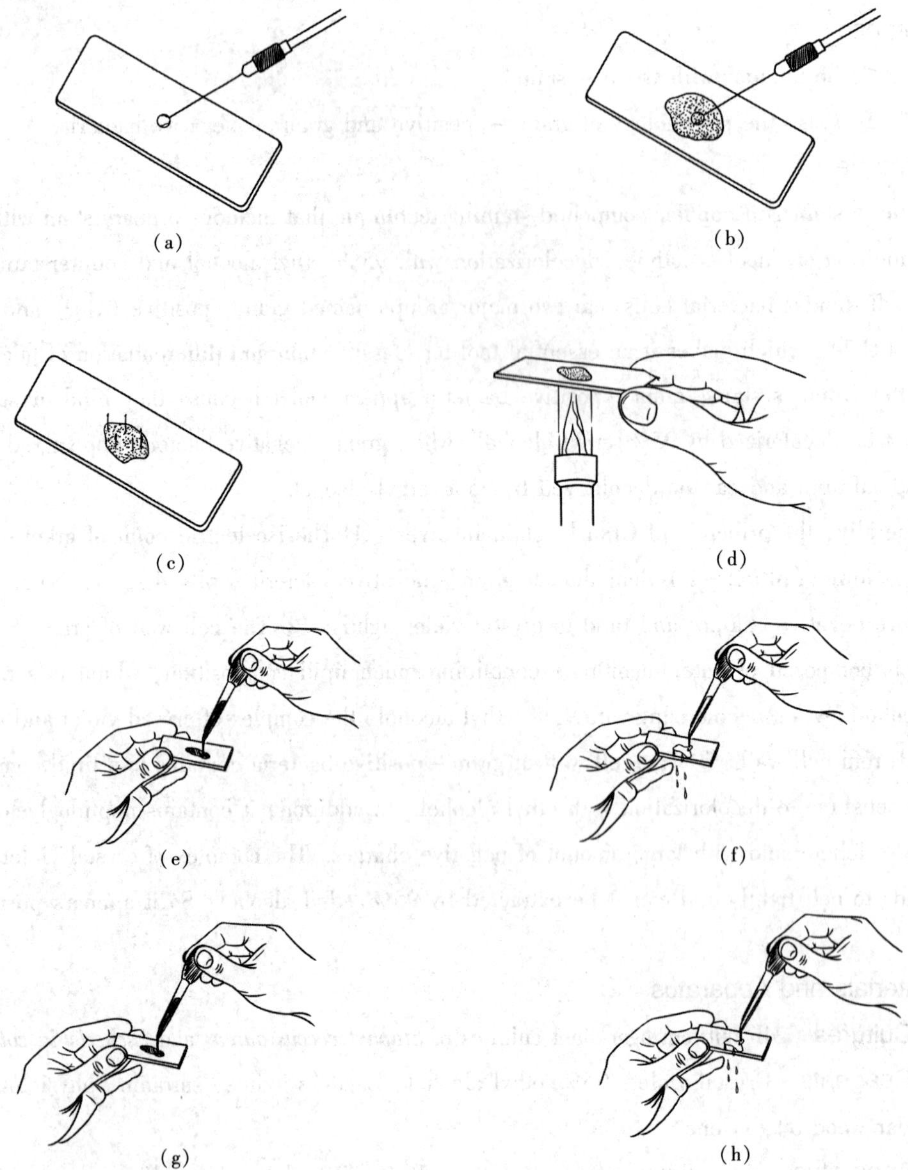

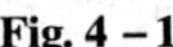

Fig. 4 – 1

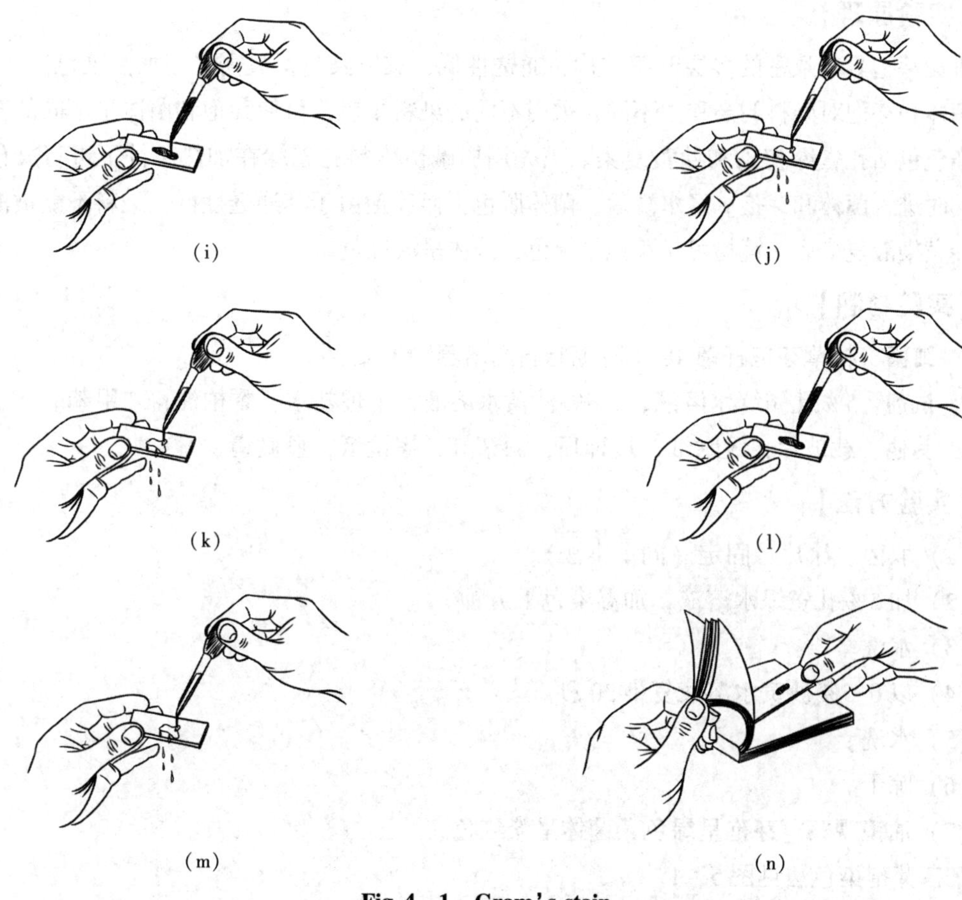

Fig. 4 - 1　Gram's stain

(a) Get some physiological saline; (b) Preparation of bacteria smears; (c) Air dry; (d) Fixation; (e) Primary stain; (f)、(h)、(j)、(k)、(m) Wash the smear; (g) Mordant; (i) Decolorizing; (l) counterstain; (n) Absorb the water

Results and Discussion

(1) What's the principle of Gram's stain?

(2) Draw a representative field for gram - positive and gram - negative bacteria.

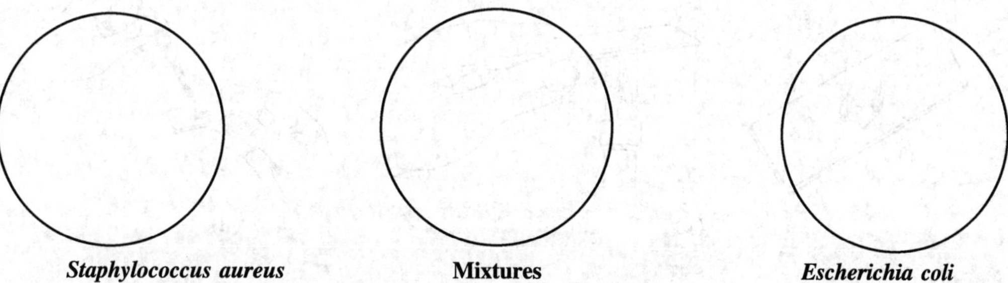

扫码“学一学”

实验五　芽孢染色法

【实验目的】

(1) 熟悉细菌芽孢的染色方法。

(2) 掌握用油镜观察细菌芽孢的形态结构。

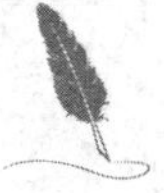

【实验原理】

细菌芽孢具有致密的多层壁膜结构，通透性低，难以染色，故需采用加温染色法。由于细菌菌体和芽孢对染料的亲和力不同，采用不同的染料染色，可使芽孢和菌体呈不同的颜色。芽孢染色包括孔雀绿初染和沙黄复染。当先用弱碱性染料孔雀绿在加热条件下进行染色时，染料同时进入菌体和芽孢。经水洗后，菌体脱色，而芽孢由于其通透性低，染料不能被洗出。当用沙黄染液复染后，镜检可见芽孢呈绿色，菌体呈淡红色。

【实验材料】

1. **细菌** 枯草芽孢杆菌48小时琼脂斜面培养物1支。
2. **试剂** 5%孔雀绿水溶液，0.5%沙黄水溶液，生理盐水，香柏油，二甲苯。
3. **其他** 载玻片，吸水纸，接种环，酒精灯，擦镜纸，显微镜。

【实验方法】

（1）取菌、涂片、固定（同单染法）。

（2）加5%孔雀绿水溶液，加温染色1分钟。

（3）水洗。

（4）以0.5%沙黄水溶液复染30秒。

（5）水洗。

（6）晾干。

（7）油镜观察，芽孢呈绿色，菌体呈淡红色。

细菌芽孢染色法见图5－1。

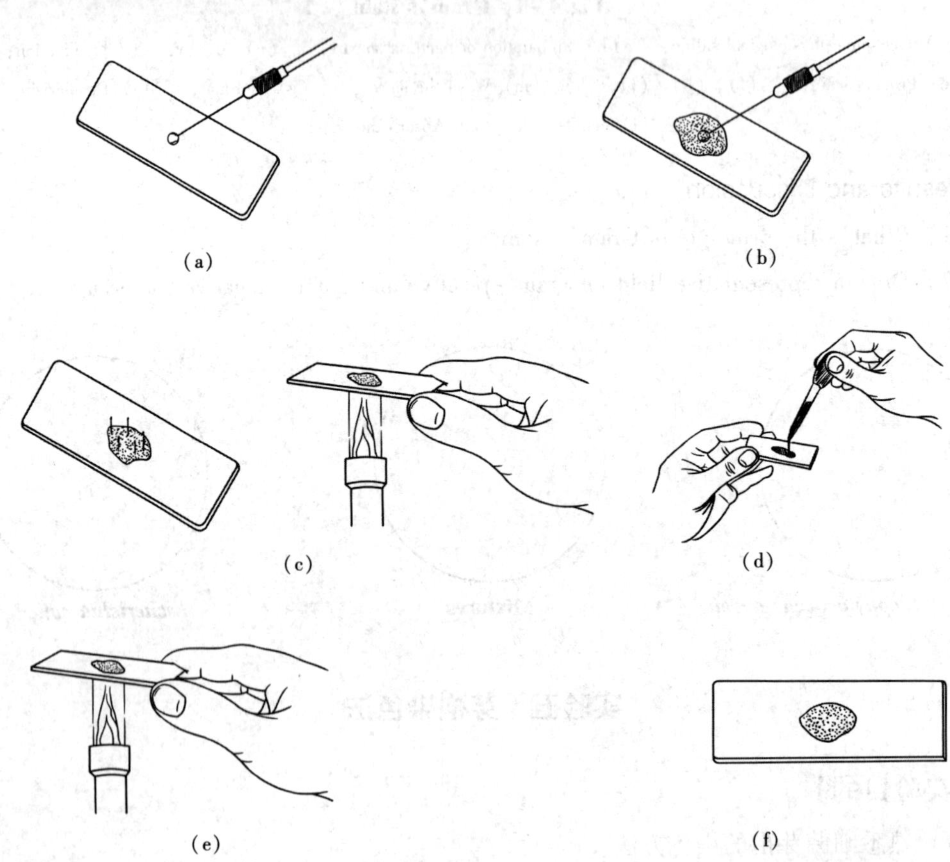

图5－1

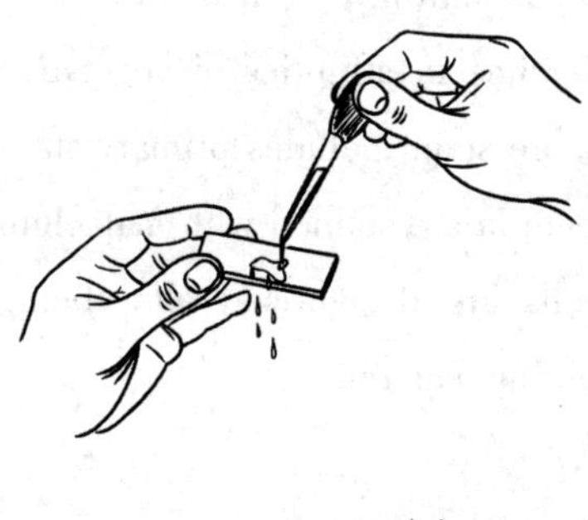

(g)

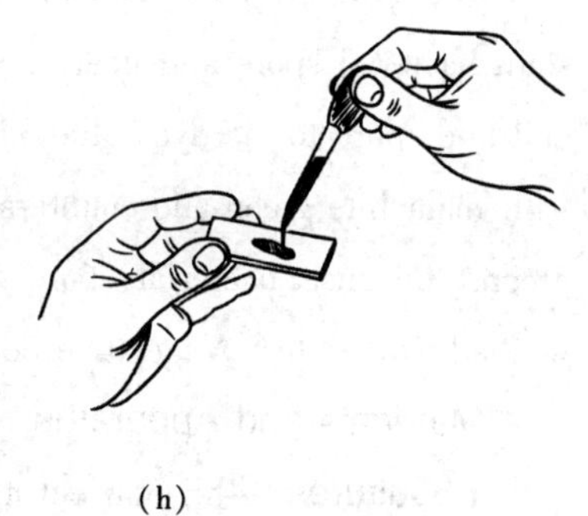

(h)

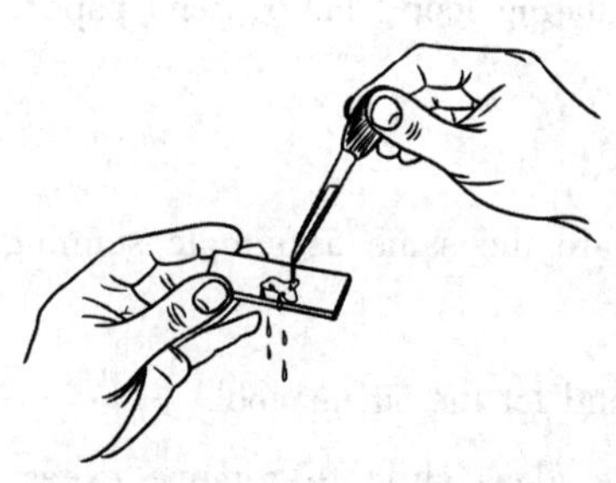

(i)

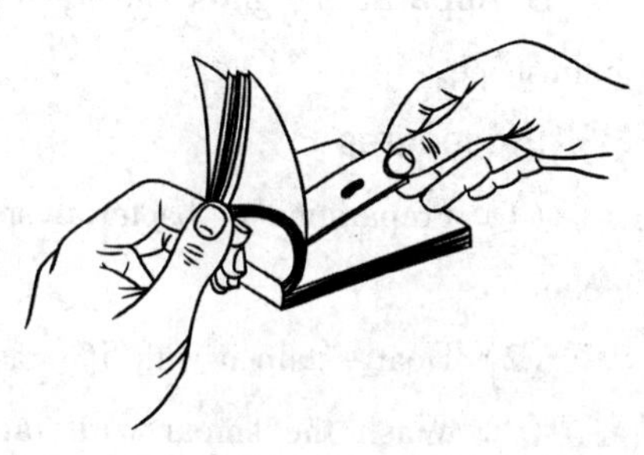

(j)

图 5-1　芽孢染色法

(a) 取生理盐水；　(b) 涂片；　(c) 干燥、固定；　(d)、(h) 染色；　(e) 加温染色；　(f) 冷却；
(g)、(i) 冲洗；　(j) 吸干

【结果与讨论】

(1) 为什么细菌芽孢需采用加温染色法？

(2) 分别绘出细菌及其芽孢的形态，并说明其所染的颜色。

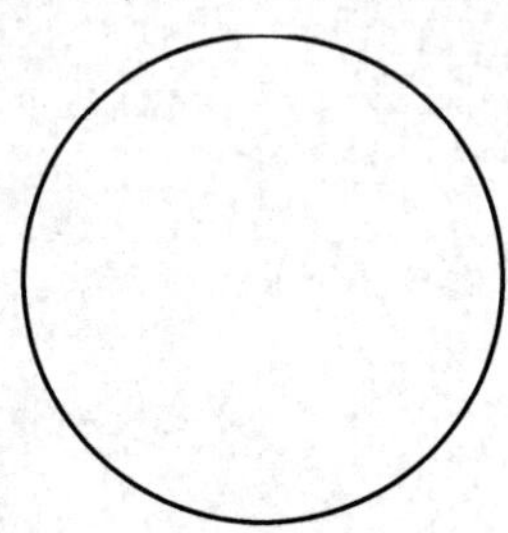

枯草芽孢杆菌

EXPERIMENT 5　Spore Stain

Purpose

(1) To be familiar with the procedures of spore stain.

(2) To grasp the morphology of bacterial spore.

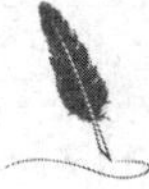

Principle

The structure bacterial spore is complex. Because of its impervious multilayers, it is difficult to stain bacterial spore and heat staining is required. Due to the difference in affinities of vegetative cell and spore to the dyes, they are stained with different colors. Spore stain includes primary stain with malachite green and counterstain with safranin. At first, the bacteria are stained with malachite green. Because bacterial spore is impervious, only vegetative cells are decolorized after being washed with water. Vegetative cells will be colorized by safranin and appear red.

Materials and Apparatus

1. Cultures 48h nutrient agar slant culture of *Bacillus subtilis.*

2. Reagents 5% malachite green, 0.5% safranin, physiological saline, cedar wood oil, xylene.

3. Apparatus glass slides, water – adsorption paper, inoculating loop, lamp, lens paper, microscope.

Procedures

(1) Preparation of bacterial smears, air dry, and fixation are the same as simple staining techniques.

(2) Heat – stain it with 5% malachite green forone minute and let the smear cool.

(3) Wash the smear with tap water from one side of the glass slide to remove excess stain.

(4) Stain the smear with 0.5% safranin for 30s.

(5) Wash the smear with tap water from one side of the glass slide to remove excess stain.

(6) Air dry or adsorb water with paper but do not wipe the slide.

(7) Examine the stained slide under oil immersion.

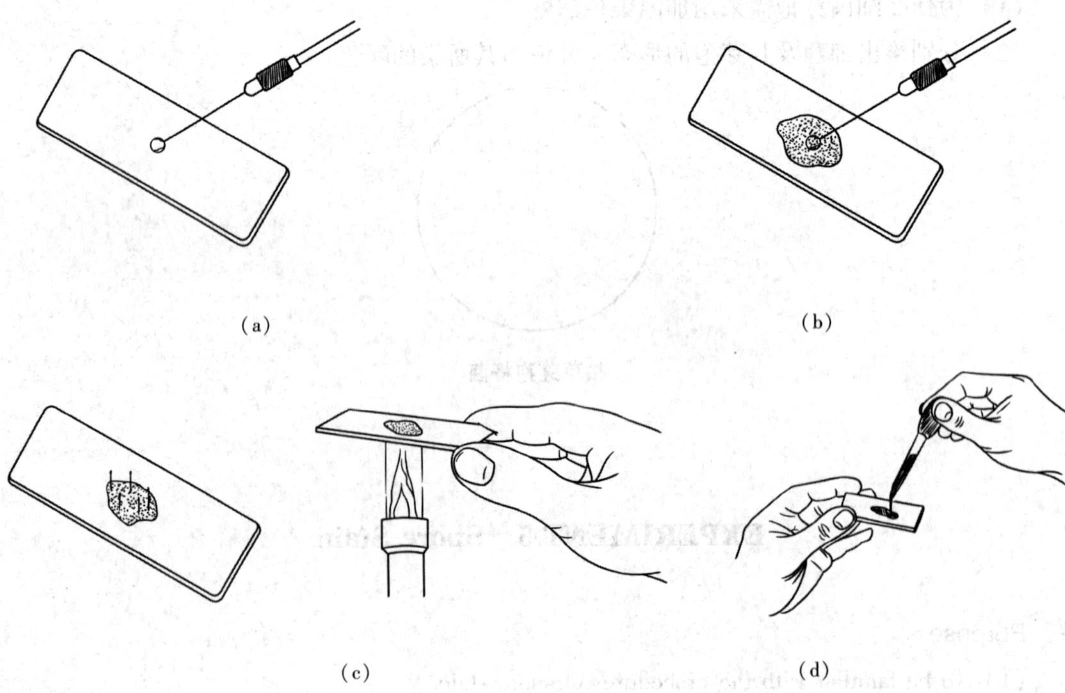

Fig. 5 – 1

(e)

(f)

(g)

(h)

(i)

(j)

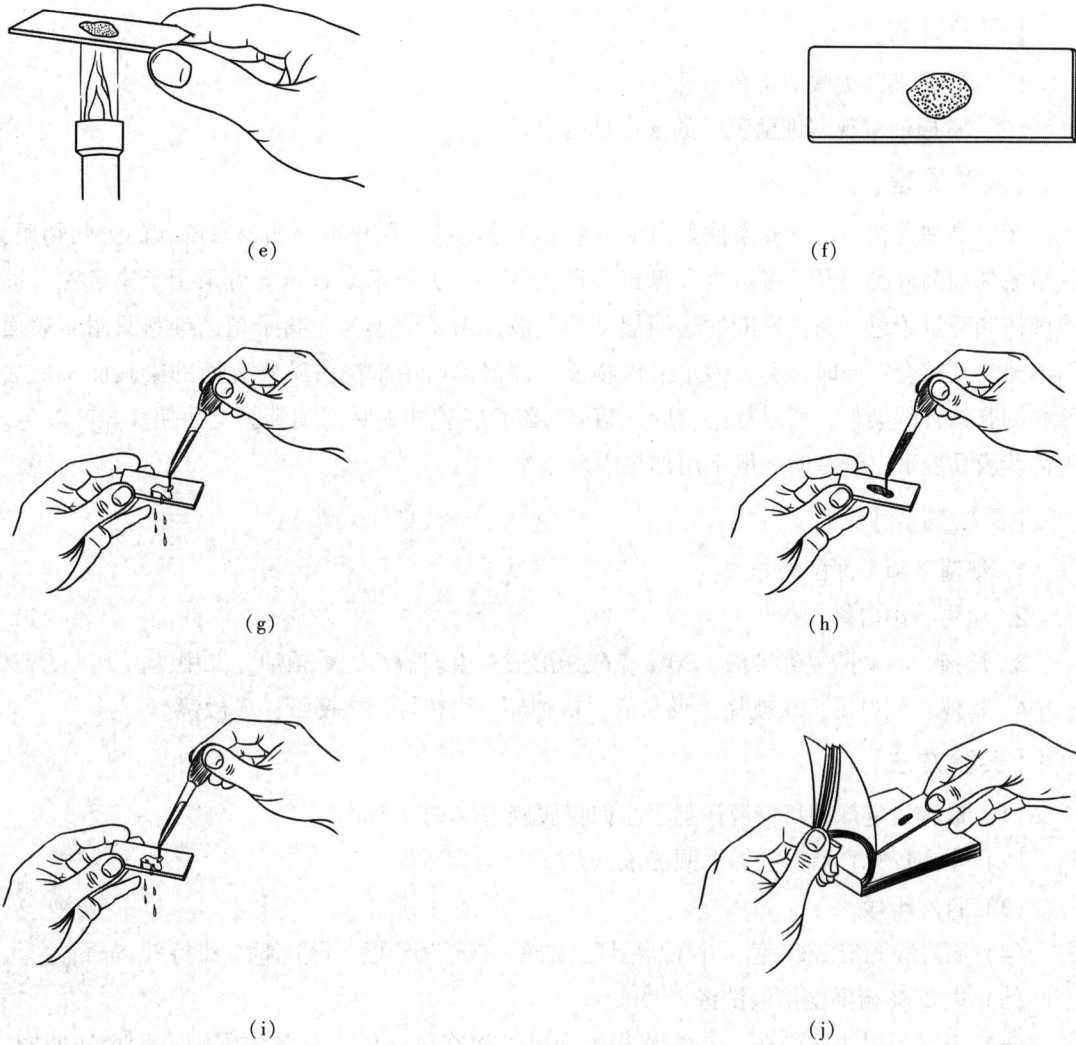

Fig. 5 – 1　Spore stain

(a) Get some physiological saline;　(b) Preparation of bacteria smears;　(c) Air dry; fixafion　(d), (h) Stain;　(e) Heat – stain;　(f) Cool down;　(g), (i) Wash the smear;　(j) Absorb the water

Results and Discussion

(1) Why is heat necessary in spore staining?

(2) Draw a representative field for the vegetative cell and bacterial spore and indicate the color of vegetative cell and the spore.

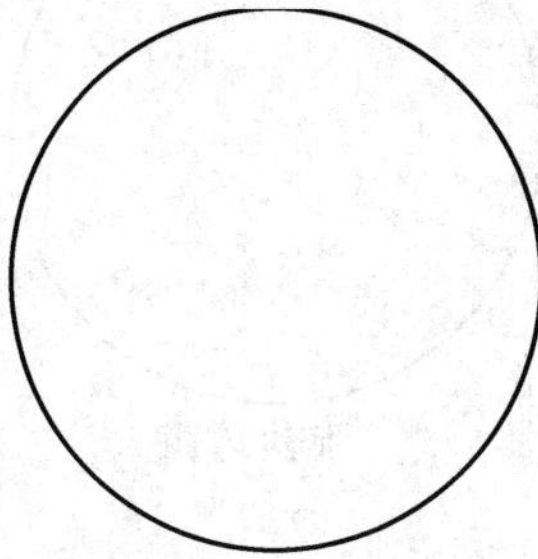

Bacillus subtilis

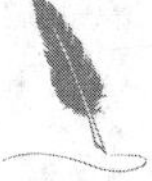

扫码“学一学”

实验六　荚膜染色法

【实验目的】

（1）熟悉细菌荚膜的染色方法。

（2）掌握油镜观察细菌荚膜的形态结构。

【实验原理】

荚膜是细菌在一定营养条件下向细胞壁表面分泌的一层松散透明、黏度大的胶状物质，其组成随细菌种类而异，多数为多糖或多肽类物质。荚膜不易着色，可采用负染色法，即将菌体和背景着色，菌体周围的透明层即为荚膜。由于荚膜为非离子型，染料只附着表面而不能与其结合；同时，荚膜为水溶性物质，硫酸铜可用来洗去荚膜表面的染料而不能去除与细胞结合的染料，所以复染色后，菌体显红色，硫酸铜吸附到荚膜上而使其显亮蓝色。细菌荚膜易变形，制片时一般不用加热固定。

【实验材料】

1. **细菌**　肺炎球菌培养液。
2. **动物**　小白鼠。
3. **试剂**　石炭酸复红染液，20%硫酸铜溶液，生理盐水，香柏油，二甲苯。
4. **其他**　注射器，载玻片，吸水纸，接种环，酒精灯，擦镜纸，显微镜。

【实验方法】

（1）取肺炎链球菌培养液注射于小白鼠腹腔中（约0.5ml）。

（2）小白鼠死亡后，立即取腹腔液涂片。

（3）自然干燥。

（4）石炭酸复红染液染色，并在酒精灯上加热至有蒸汽产生，开始计时，维持3～5min。

（5）以20%硫酸铜溶液洗涤。

（6）干燥后用油镜检查，在红色背景中可见深红色菌体，在菌体周围有无色透明圈，此为荚膜。

【结果与讨论】

（1）说明细菌荚膜染色的原理。

（2）为什么荚膜染色制片时不用加热？

（3）绘出含荚膜的肺炎链球菌的形态结构。

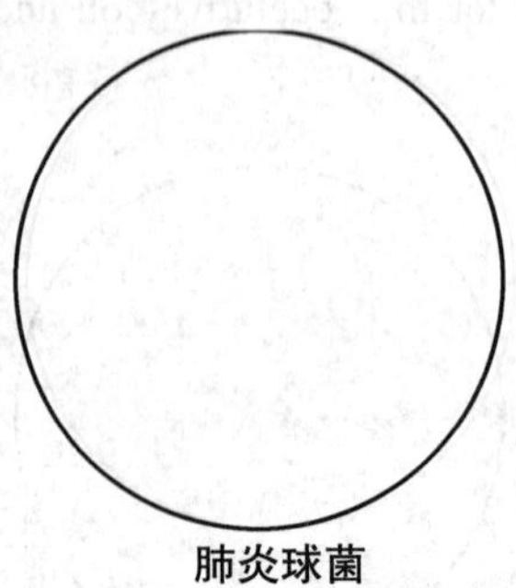

肺炎球菌

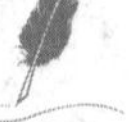

EXPERIMENT 6　Capsule Stain

Purpose

(1) To be familiar with capsule stain.

(2) To grasp the morphology of bacterial capsule.

Principle

A capsule is a gelatinous outer layer secreted by the cell that surrounds and adheres to the cells. The composition of capsule changes across bacterial species and most of bacterial capsules are composed of polysaccharides and polypeptides. Capsule is difficult to be stained and negative stain is usually required. Because the capsule is nonionic, stain only adheres to the capsule without binding to it. In addition, the capsule is water soluble, copper sulfate is used to wash the primary stain out of the capsular material without removing the stain that is bound to the cell wall. At the same time, it acts as a counterstain as it is absorbed into the decolorized capsular material. The capsule will now appear light blue in contrast to the deep purple color of the cell. Bacterial capsule is easy to be out of shape and heat fixation is not needed in smear preparation.

Materials and Apparatus

1. Cultures　culture media of *Streptococcus pneumoniae*.

2. Animal　mouse.

3. Reagents　safranin, 20% copper sulfate, physiological saline, cedar wood oil, xylene.

4. Apparatus　glass slide, water - adsorption paper, inoculating loop, lamp, lens paper, microscope.

Procedures

(1) Inject mouse (ip) with 0.5 ml of *Streptococcus pneumoniae* culture.

(2) After the mouse is dead, take a drop of abdomen and smear it.

(3) Let the smear to air dry.

(4) Stain it with safranin and heat it until steam appears, maintain 3 ~ 5 minutes.

(5) Wash the smear with 20% copper sulfate.

(6) Air dry or adsorb water with paper but do not wipe the slide. Examine the stained slide under oil immersion.

Results and Discussion

(1) What's the principle of capsule staining technique?

(2) Why should omit heat fixation during the preparation of smear for capsule staining?

(3) Draw a representative field for *Streptococcus pneumoniae* and indicate the color of cell, bacterial capsule and the slide background.

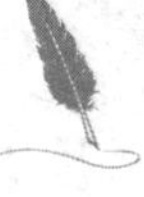

Pneumococcus pneumoniae

实验七　鞭毛染色法

扫码“学一学”

【实验目的】

（1）熟悉细菌鞭毛的染色方法。

（2）掌握油镜观察细菌鞭毛的形态结构。

【实验原理】

鞭毛是细菌菌体表面生长的纤细、弯曲、能收缩的丝状物，其主要化学组成为蛋白质。鞭毛的长度约为2～5μm，最长可达50μm，直径很细，一般为10～20nm。鞭毛可采用电子显微镜来观察，也可用特殊的鞭毛染色法在油镜下观察。

【实验材料】

1. 细菌　伤寒杆菌8小时培养液。

2. 试剂　鞭毛染色液甲（明矾饱和液20ml，20%鞣酸10ml，95%乙醇液15ml，蒸馏水10ml，复红酒精饱和溶液3ml，混合而成），鞭毛染色液乙（硼砂1g，亚甲蓝1g溶于200ml蒸馏水中），生理盐水，香柏油，二甲苯。

3. 其他　载玻片，吸水纸，接种环，酒精灯，擦镜纸，离心机，离心试管，无菌吸管。

【实验方法】

（1）取菌液2ml，加蒸馏水2ml，离心沉淀（1000r/min，10分钟），吸出上清液，再加入蒸馏水，摇匀后离心沉淀。如此操作3～4次，吸出上清液，沉淀后加入蒸馏水2ml，摇匀后待用。

（2）用接种环在玻片上滴上述制备菌液，使流成长条。

（3）干燥（在空气中自然干燥）。

（4）加鞭毛染色液甲染色5分钟，水洗。

（5）加鞭毛染色液乙染色1～2分钟，水洗。

（6）待干燥后用油镜镜检，菌体呈蓝色，鞭毛呈红色。

【结果与讨论】

（1）说明细菌鞭毛染色的原理。

（2）绘出含鞭毛的伤寒杆菌的形态结构。

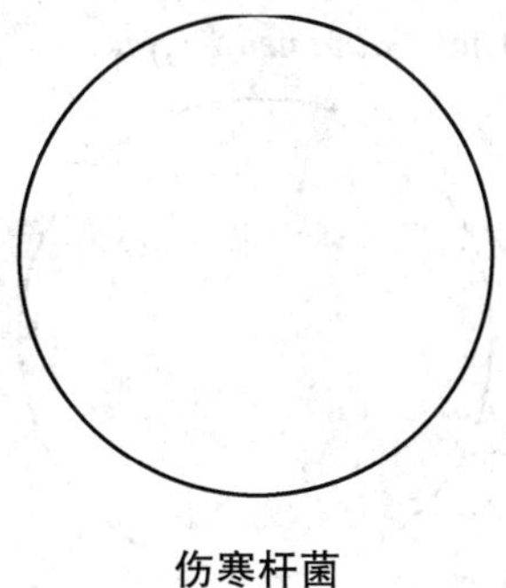

伤寒杆菌

EXPERIMENT 7　Flagella Stain

Purpose

(1) To be familiar with flagella stain.

(2) To grasp the morphology of bacterial flagella.

Principle

Flagella, the fine, threadlike organelles of locomotion, are mainly composed of protein. They are slender (about 10 to 20nm in diameter and 2 to 5μm in length). Bacterial flagella can be observed with electron microscope or light microscope after flagella staining.

Materials and Apparatus

1. Cultures 8 hours culture of *Salmonella typhi*.

2. Reagents Solution A (mixture of 20ml saturated alum solution, 10ml 20% tannic acid, 15ml 95% ethanol, 3ml safranin in ethanol), Solution B (1g methylene blue and 1g sodium borate dissolved in 200 ml distilled water), physiological saline, cedar wood oil, xylene.

3. Apparatus centrifugal machine, centrifugal tube, glass slide, water - adsorption paper, inoculating loop, lamp, lens paper, microscope.

Procedures

(1) Take 2ml culture media of *Salmonella typhi* in 2ml distilled water, centrifuge at 1000 r/min for 10 minutes, and discard the upper phase. Suspend the precipitate in 2ml distilled water.

(2) Drop a blob of *Salmonella typhi* suspension solution on a glass slide and form a line of bacterial suspension.

(3) Let the smear to air dry.

(4) Stain it with solution A for 5 minutes, wash the smear with tap water from one side of the glass slide to remove excess stain.

(5) Stain it with solution B for 1 to 2 minutes, wash the smear with tap water from one side of the glass slide to remove excess stain.

(6) Air dry or adsorb water with paper but do not wipe the slide. Examine the stained slide under oil immersion.

Results and Discussion

(1) What's the principle of flagella staining technique?

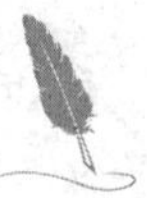

（2）Draw a representative field for *Salmonella typhi*.

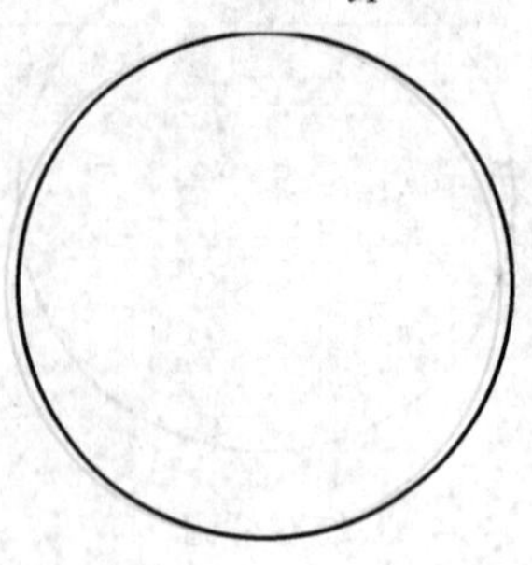

Salmonella typhi

实验八　螺旋体的染色和形态观察

扫码“学一学”

【实验目的】

（1）掌握螺旋体的染色方法。

（2）熟悉油镜观察螺旋体的形态结构。

【实验原理】

螺旋体（spirochete）是一类细长、柔软、弯曲呈螺旋状、运动活泼的原核细胞型微生物。其基本结构与细菌类似，有细胞壁和原始核，行二分裂法繁殖，对抗生素敏感。螺旋体无鞭毛，其运动有赖于轴丝。螺旋体广泛存在于自然界和动物体内，种类繁多。

螺旋体对革兰染色法不易着色，通常采用特殊染色法（如镀银法），油镜观察。

【实验材料】

1. 染料与其他试剂　方他那染液（甲、乙、丙液），生理盐水，香柏油，二甲苯。

2. 其他　干净载玻片，牙签，酒精灯，擦镜纸，显微镜。

【实验方法】

（1）以牙签挖取齿垢置于玻片上，涂成薄膜，标本自行干燥。

（2）加方他那甲液固定 1 分钟，水洗。

（3）加方他那乙液，加热至蒸汽发生，染色 30 秒，稍冷，水冲洗。

（4）加方他那丙液，加热至蒸汽发生，染色 30 秒，稍冷。

（5）自然干燥或吸干，油镜检查，染色后，背景为黄色，螺旋体及细菌呈棕色。

【结果与讨论】

（1）说明螺旋体染色的原理。

（2）绘制疏螺旋体的形态结构。

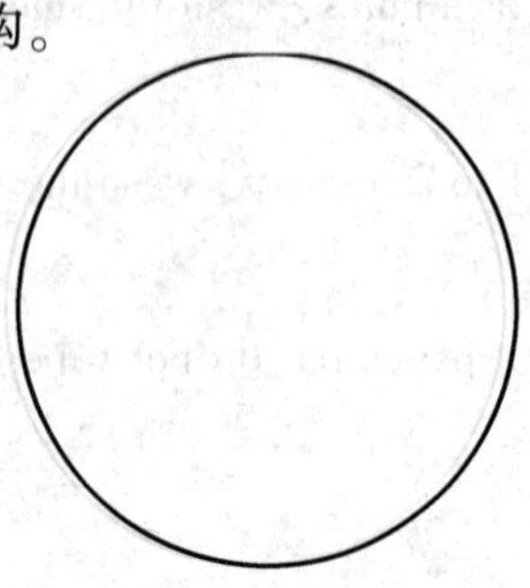

口腔奋森氏疏螺旋体

EXPERIMENT 8　Spirochetes Morphology

Purpose

(1) To be familiar with spirochetes stain.

(2) To befamilar with the morphology of spirochetes.

Principle

Spirochetes are slender, soft, curved, movable, and helical prokaryotic cells which are about 5 to 10 nm in length and 0. 2 μm in diameter. In addition to binary fission, the primary structure of spirochetes is similar to bacteria with cell wall and nucleoid. Spirochetes are sensitive to antibiotics. Their movement depends on a special axial filament rather than flagellar rotation.

Materials and Apparatus

1. Reagents　Fontana solution A, solution B, solution C, physiological saline, cedar wood oil, xylene.

2. Apparatus　glass slides, water－adsorption paper, toothpick, lamp, lens paper, microscope.

Procedures

(1) Drop a blob of physiological water on the center of a glass slide, take some tartar with toothpick into the physiological water on the glass slide and smear it, let the smear to air dry.

(2) Fix it with solution A for one minute, wash the smear with tap water from one side of the glass slide to remove excess stain.

(3) Heat－stain it with solution B for 30 seconds, cool and wash the smear with tap water from one side of the glass slide to remove excess stain.

(4) Heat－stain it with solution C for 30 seconds, cool and wash the smear with tap water from one side of the glass slide to remove excess stain.

(5) Air dry or adsorb water with paper but do not wipe the slide. Examine the stained slide under oil immersion.

Results and Discussion

(1) What's the principle of spirochetes staining technique?

(2) Draw a representative field for spirochetes.

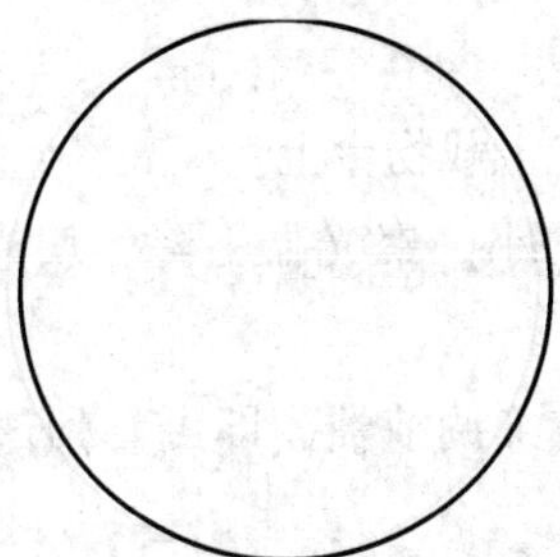

***Spirochetes* (*Borrelia vincentii*)**

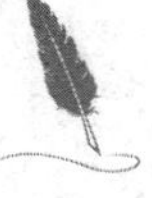

扫码“学一学”

实验九　悬滴法观察细菌的动力

【实验目的】

（1）了解不染色标本检查法。

（2）掌握悬滴法观察活细菌及其动力。

【实验原理】

细菌的鞭毛是细菌的运动器官，细菌是否具有鞭毛是细菌分类鉴定的依据之一。有鞭毛的细菌在液体中能发生位置上的变化而做真正的运动；而无鞭毛的细菌由于水分子的撞击，在原位颤动，称之为布朗运动。可采用悬滴法直接在普通光学显微镜下观察细菌是否具有运动能力，以此来判定细菌是否具有鞭毛。

悬滴法是将细菌培养液滴加在洁净的盖玻片中央，在其周围涂上凡士林，将盖玻片置于凹玻片中央，使盖玻片上的液滴悬于凹槽上方（图9－1），在光学显微镜下观察细菌的运动情况。

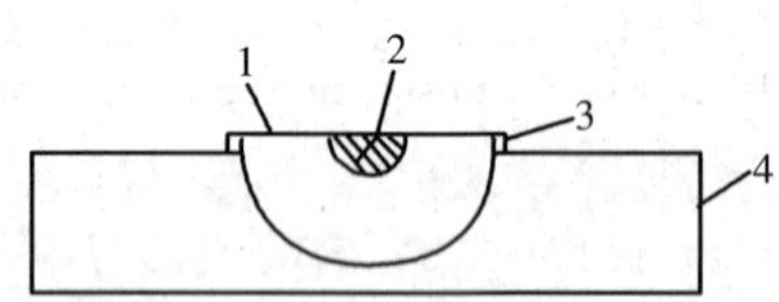

图9－1　悬滴法示意图

1. 盖玻片；　2. 菌液；　3. 凡士林；　4. 凹玻片

扫码“看一看”

【实验材料】

1. **细菌**　枯草芽孢杆菌和金黄色葡萄球菌的8小时液体培养物。

2. **其他**　凹玻片，盖玻片，牙签，接种环，酒精灯，凡士林，显微镜。

【实验方法】

1. 悬滴标本的制备

（1）用灭菌的接种环挑取细菌液体培养物一环，加于平放桌上之洁净盖玻片中央。

（2）在洁净凹玻片的凹面周围用牙签涂上少许凡士林（或浆糊）。

（3）将凹玻片凹面向下，覆盖在已滴加有菌液的盖玻片上，轻压，使盖玻片粘在凹玻片上。

（4）迅速反转凹玻片，使盖玻片上之菌液悬于凹玻片之凹面中。

2. 显微镜检查

（1）将制备好的悬滴标本固定于载物台上。

（2）先用低倍镜对光（光圈缩小，聚光器下降，使光线较暗），找到菌液之边缘，并调至视野中央。

（3）转换高倍镜，再轻轻调节细调节器，即可看到透明的菌体。观察两种细菌的不同运动特征。

【结果与讨论】

（1）分别描述金黄色葡萄球菌和枯草芽孢杆菌的运动特征。

（2）检测细菌是否具有动力的方法有哪些？

EXPERIMENT 9 Observation of Bacterial Motion with Hanging Drop

Purpose

(1) To be familiar with the preparation of unstained specimen.

(2) To grasp how to observe the motion of living bacteria.

Principle

Flagella are Motion "organelles" of bacteria. Bacteria with flagella can move from one place to another in culture solution. Bacteria without flagella will vibrate due to water collision. That is called Brown's motion. Hanging drop method is used to observe the motion of living bacteria with bright - field microscope. As shown in Fig. 9 - 1, a drop of bacteria liquid culture is suspended on the center of a cover slip.

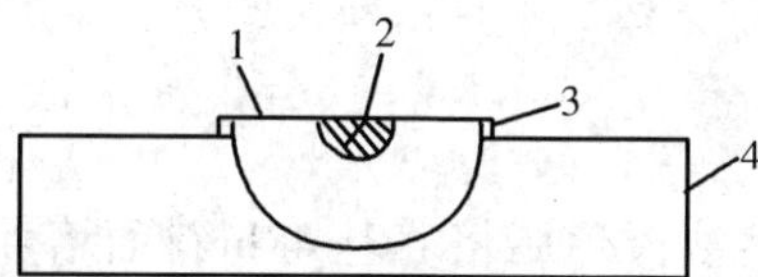

Fig. 9 - 1 Hanging drop method

1. Cover slip; 2. Bacteria liquid culture; 3. Vaselin; 4. Concavity Slide

Materials and Apparatus

1. Cultures 8 hours liquid culture of *Staphylococcus aureus* and *Bacillus subtilis*.

2. Apparatus concavity slide, cover slip, toothpick, inoculating loop, lamp, lens paper, microscope.

Procedures

1. Preparation of specimen

(1) Place a drop of liquid culture of *Staphylococcus aureus* and *Bacillus subtilis* respectively on a glass slide and mix it with inoculating loop.

(2) Smear some vaselin around the edges of the cover slip with toothpick.

(3) Place a concavity slide on the cover slide and press it softly for sticking.

(4) Reverse the specimen rapidly.

2. Observation with microscope

(1) Place the specimen on the stage.

(2) Observe it with low power lens (10 ×) and locate the edge of the drop.

(3) Observe it with high power lens (40 ×).

Results and Discussion

(1) Describe the motion characteristics of *Staphylococcus aureus* and *Bacillus subtilis*.

(2) How to decide whether bacteria can move?

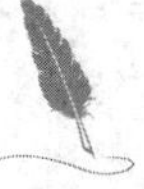

扫码“学一学”

实验十　酵母菌的形态结构观察

【实验目的】

（1）熟悉酵母菌的单染色法；酵母菌子囊孢子的观察方法。

（2）掌握观察酵母菌的形态结构。

【实验原理】

酵母菌是单细胞真菌，有圆形、卵圆形等形态，无性繁殖主要以芽殖或裂殖的方式进行，有性繁殖时形成子囊孢子。亚甲蓝是一种无毒性染料，其氧化型呈蓝色，还原型为无色。由于酵母菌的活细胞新陈代谢的作用，细胞内具有较强的还原能力，经染色的酵母菌活细胞能使亚甲蓝从蓝色的氧化型变为无色的还原型而呈无色；由于死细胞或代谢缓慢的细胞则因无还原能力或还原能力弱，从而被染成蓝色或淡蓝色。

酵母菌在其适宜的生长条件下可形成子囊孢子，葡萄糖－醋酸盐培养基特别适用于酿酒酵母子囊孢子的形成。

【实验材料】

1. 菌种　酿酒酵母改良沙氏琼脂培养基 48h 斜面培养物，葡萄糖－醋酸盐培养基的 24h 斜面培养物。

2. 试剂　0.05%和0.1%碱性亚甲蓝，石炭酸复红，3%酸性酒精，孔雀绿芽孢染液，生理盐水，香柏油，二甲苯。

3. 其他　显微镜，载玻片，盖玻片，擦镜纸，酒精灯，显微镜。

【实验方法】

1. 酵母菌细胞亚甲蓝染色法

（1）在载玻片中央滴加一滴 0.1% 碱性亚甲蓝染液，按照无菌操作法用接种环挑取在改良沙氏琼脂培养基斜面上培养 48 小时的酿酒酵母少许，于亚甲蓝染液中混匀。

（2）用镊子夹一块盖玻片，先将盖玻片的一边与液滴接触，然后将整个盖玻片慢慢放下，同时避免气泡产生。标本片静置 3 分钟。

（3）先用低倍镜观察，再用高倍镜观察酿酒酵母的形态和芽殖情况，根据细胞是否染色来区别活细胞和死细胞。

2. 酵母菌子囊孢子染色法

（1）用接种环挑取葡萄糖－醋酸盐培斜面养基上的酿酒酵母于载玻片上，涂片、干燥和固定。

（2）加石炭酸复红染液，在火焰上加温染色 5～10 分钟（避免沸腾）。

（3）3%酸性酒精洗 30～60 秒，水洗。

（4）吕氏碱性亚甲蓝数滴复染数秒后，水洗。

（5）油镜观察，酵母菌子囊孢子为红色，菌体为青色。如用孔雀绿芽孢染液单染（不加热），油镜观察可见绿色的子囊孢子。

【结果与讨论】

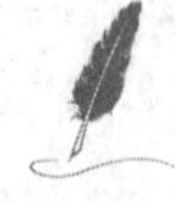

（1）为什么可用染色法区别酵母菌活细胞和死细胞？

（2）绘制酵母菌菌体和子囊孢子的形态结构。

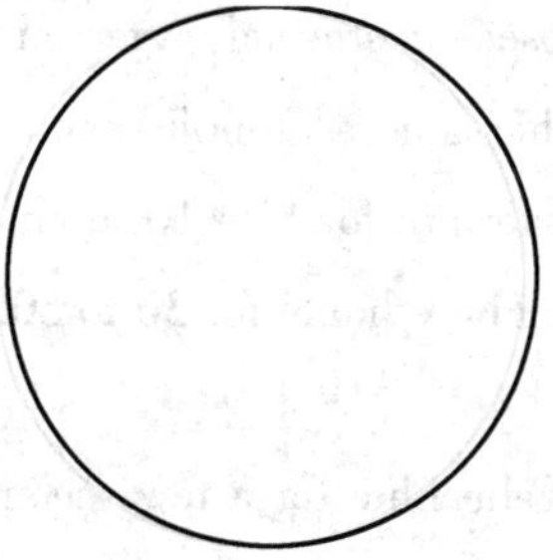

酵母菌菌体和子囊孢子

EXPERIMENT 10　Yeast Morphology

Purpose

(1) To be familiar with simple staining of yeast; ascospores staining of yeast.

(2) To grasp the morphology of yeast cells.

Principle

Yeasts are unicellular organisms. Morphologically, they may be ellipsoidal, spherical, and in some cases, cylindrical. Most yeasts reproduce asexually by a process called budding, and some yeasts may also undergo sexual reproduction by forming ascospores.

Methylene blue is a nontoxic dye which appears blue in oxidation type and colorless in reduction type. Viable yeast cells have certain reducing power due to metabolism. After stained by methylene blue, viable yeast cells reduce it to reduction type and appear uncolored. However, dead cells with little or no reducing power are stained blue or pale blue.

Yeast cells can form ascospores under appropriate conditions and glucose – acetic acid media is often used as the culture for *Saccharomyces* to form ascospores.

Materials and Apparatus

1. Cultures　48 hours Sabouraud agar culture of *Saccharomyces cerevisiae*, 24 hours glucose – acetic acid agar culture of *Saccharomyces cerevisiae*.

2. Reagents　0.05% and 0.1% methylene blue, safranin, 3% acidic ethanol, 0.5% malachite green, physiological saline, cedar wood oil, xylene.

3. Apparatus　glass slide, cover slip, tissue, inoculating loop, lamp, lens paper, microscope.

Procedures

1. Yeast stain with methylene blue

(1) Drop a blob of methylene blue on the center of a glass slide.

(2) Take some yeast cells from Sabouraud agar culture with an inoculating loop and suspend a loopful of yeasts culture into a few drops of methylene blue solution.

(3) Cover the suspension slowly with a cover slip and allow to stand for 3 minutes.

(4) Examine the slide with microscope under low and high power.

2. Ascospores stain

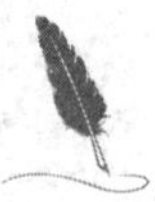

(1) Smearing of 24 hours glucose – acetic acid agar culture of *Saccharomyces cerevisiae* on a glass slide, air dry and fixation are the same as simple staining.

(2) Heat stain the smear with safranin for 5 to 10 minutes.

(3) Wash the smear with 3% acidic ethanol for 30 to 60 seconds, then wash with tap water to remove excess ethanol.

(4) Stain the smear with methylene blue for a few seconds and wash with tap water.

(5) Examine the stained slide under oil immersion.

Results and Discussion

(1) What's the principle of yeast and ascospores staining?

(2) Draw a representative field for yeast under low – power and high – power magnifications.

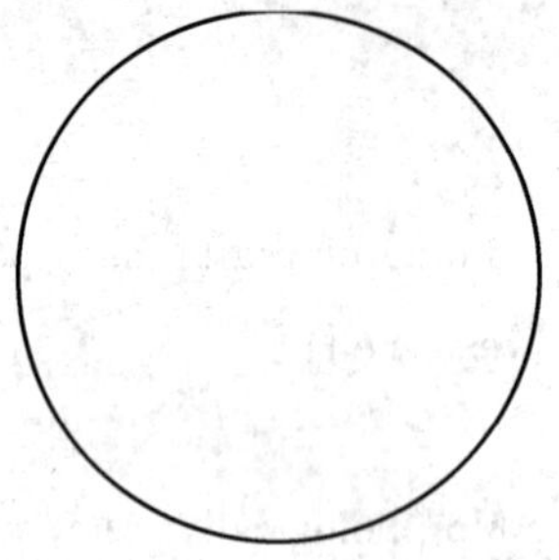

Saccharomyces cerevisiae

实验十一　微生物细胞大小测定

扫码“学一学”

【实验目的】

(1) 了解目镜测微尺和镜台测微尺的构造和使用原理。

(2) 掌握微生物细胞大小的测定方法。

【实验原理】

微生物细胞的大小是微生物重要的形态特征之一，由于菌体很小，只能在显微镜下测量。用于测量微生物细胞大小的工具有目镜测微尺和镜台测微尺。

目镜测微尺是一块圆形玻片，在玻片中央把5mm 长度刻成50 等分，或把10 mm 长度刻成100 等分。测量时，将其放在接目镜中的隔板上（此处正好与物镜放大的中间像重叠）来测量经显微镜放大后的细胞物像。由于不同目镜、物镜组合的放大倍数不相同，目镜测微尺每格实际表示的长度也不一样，因此目镜测微尺测量微生物大小时须先用置于镜台上的镜台测微尺校正，以求出一定放大倍数下，目镜测微尺每小格所代表的相对长度。

镜台测微尺是中央部分刻有精确等分线的载玻片，一般将1 mm 等分为100 格，每格长10μm（即0.01 mm），专门用来校正目镜测微尺。校正时，将镜台测微尺放在载物台上，由于镜台测微尺与细胞标本处于同一位置，要经过物镜和目镜的两次放大成像才能进入视野，即镜台测微尺随着显微镜总放大倍数的放大而放大，因此从镜台测微尺上得到的读数就是细胞的真实大小，用镜台测微尺的已知长度在一定放大倍数下校正目镜测微尺，即可求出目镜测微尺每格所代表的长度，然后移去镜台测微尺，换上待测标本片，用校正好的目镜测微尺在同样放大倍数下测量微生物大小（图11－1）。

【实验材料】

1. **细菌**　酿酒酵母（*Saccharomyces cerevisiae*）斜面菌种，枯草芽孢杆菌（*Bacillus subtilis*）染色标本片。

2. **器材**　显微镜，目镜测微尺，镜台测微尺，盖玻片，载玻片，滴管，二重瓶，擦镜纸。

【实验方法】

1. **目镜测微尺的校正**　把目镜的上透镜旋下，将目镜测微尺的刻度朝下轻轻地装入目镜的隔板上，把镜台测微尺置于载物台上，刻度朝上。先用低倍镜观察，对准焦距，视野中看清镜台测微尺的刻度后，转动目镜，使目镜测微尺与镜台测微尺的刻度平行，移动推动器，使两尺重叠，再使两尺的“0”刻度完全重合，定位后，仔细寻找两尺第二个完全重合的刻度，计数两重合刻度之间目镜测微尺的格数和镜台测微尺的格数。镜台测微尺的刻度每格长 10μm，由下列公式算出目镜测微尺每格所代表的长度。

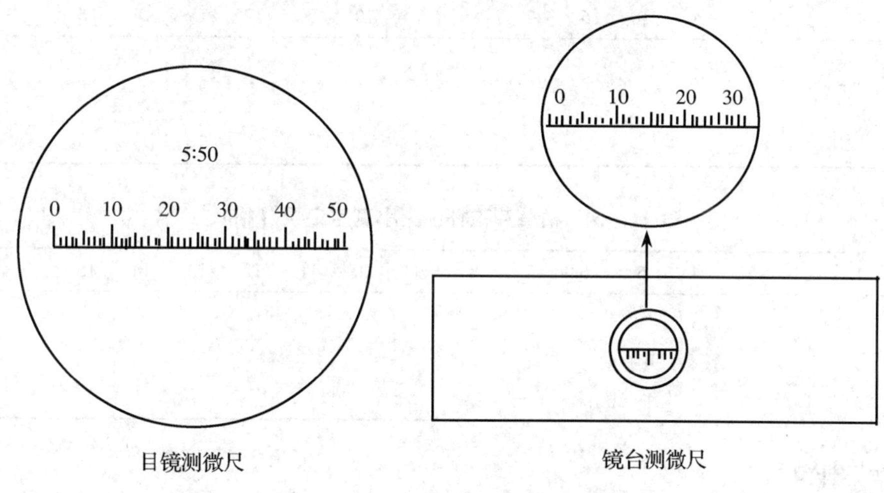

图 11－1　目镜测微尺和镜台测微尺

$$目镜测微尺每格长度（\mu m）=10\ n/m$$

其中，n 为两重合线间镜台测微尺格数；m 为两重合线间接目测微尺格数。

例如目镜测微尺 5 小格正好与镜台测微尺 5 小格重叠，已知镜台测微尺每小格为 10μm，则目镜测微尺上每小格长度为 $=5\times10\mu m/5=10\mu m$。用同法分别校正高倍镜下和油镜下目镜测微尺每小格所代表的长度。

由于不同显微镜及附件的放大倍数不同，因此校正目镜测微尺必须针对特定的显微镜和附件（特定的物镜、目镜、镜筒长度）进行，而且只能在特定的情况下重复使用，当更换不同放大倍数的目镜或物镜时，必须重新校正目镜测微尺每一格所代表的长度。

2. **细胞大小的测定**

（1）将酵母菌斜面制成一定浓度的菌悬液。

（2）取 1 滴酵母菌菌悬液制成水浸片。

（3）移去镜台测微尺，换上酵母菌水浸片，先在低倍镜下找到目的物，然后在高倍镜下用目镜测微尺测量酵母菌菌体的长，宽各占几格（不足一格的部分估计到小数点后一位数）。测出的格数乘上目镜测微尺每格的校正值，即等于该菌的长和宽。一般测量菌体的大

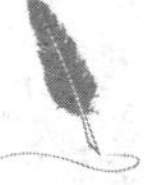

小要在同一个标本片上测定 10~20 个菌体，求出平均值，才能代表该菌的大小。而且一般是用对数生长期的菌体进行测定。

（4）同法用油镜测定枯草芽孢杆菌染色标本的长和宽。

【结果与讨论】

1. 将实验结果填入下列表格（表 11-1~表 11-3）。

表 11-1　目镜测微目尺校正结果

物镜	目尺格数	台尺格数	目尺校正值（μm）
10×			
40×			
100×			

表 11-2　酵母菌大小测定记录（格）

	1	2	3	4	5	6	7	8	9	10	11	12	13	14	15	平均值
细胞数																
长																
宽																

表 11-3　枯草芽孢杆菌大小测定记录（格）

	1	2	3	4	5	6	7	8	9	10	11	12	13	14	15	平均值
细胞数																
长																
宽																

2. 结果计算

（1）长（μm）=平均格数×校正值

（2）宽（μm）=平均格数×校正值

（3）大小表示：宽（μm）×长（μm）

EXPERIMENT 11　Determination of the Size of Microorganisms

Purpose

(1) To be familiar with the structure and principle of ocular micrometer and stage micrometer.

(2) To understand how to determine the size of microorganisms.

Principle

The size of a microorganism is one of the important morphological characteristics. As the cell is very small, it can only be measured under a microscope. Usually, we use ocular micrometer and stage micrometer.

Ocular micrometer is a circular slide, in the center of which there is a length of 5 mm carved into 50 equations. When measured, we placed it on the partition of the eyepiece to determine the

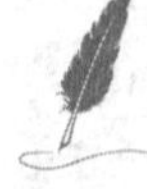

cell images amplified by the microscope. As magnifications of different combinations of Dcular eyepiecelens and Objective lens are different, each equation of the eyepiece micrometer ruler represents different actual length. As a result, before we determine the size of the microorganism, we must correct the ocular micrometer to determine the relative length each equation represents under a certain magnification.

Stage micrometer is a glass slide, in the center of which there are accurate bisectors that usually divide 1 mm into 100 parts. Each part is 10 μm, which is used to calibrate the ocular micrometer. During calibration, put the stage micrometer on the object stage.

As the stage micrometer and cell samples are in the same location, their images are magnified twice through the objective lens and eyepiece to enter the field of vision. The stage micrometer is magnified with the total magnification fold of the microscope. Thus, the reading on the stage micrometer is the real size of the cells. As a result, we use the known length of the stage micrometer to correct the ocular micrometer under certain magnification folds to determine the length each part represent. Then remove the stage micrometer, put on the sample, and determine the size of microorganism under the same magnification times.

Materials and Apparatus

1. Cultures　24h YPT agar slant culture of *Saccharomyces cerevisiae* and stained specimen of *Bacillus subtilis*.

2. Apparatus　Microscope, ocular micrometer, stage micrometer, cover slip, glass slide, dropping tube, dual bottle, lens paper.

Procedures

1. Correct the ocular micrometer

(1) Load ocular micrometer and put the stage micrometer on the object stage.

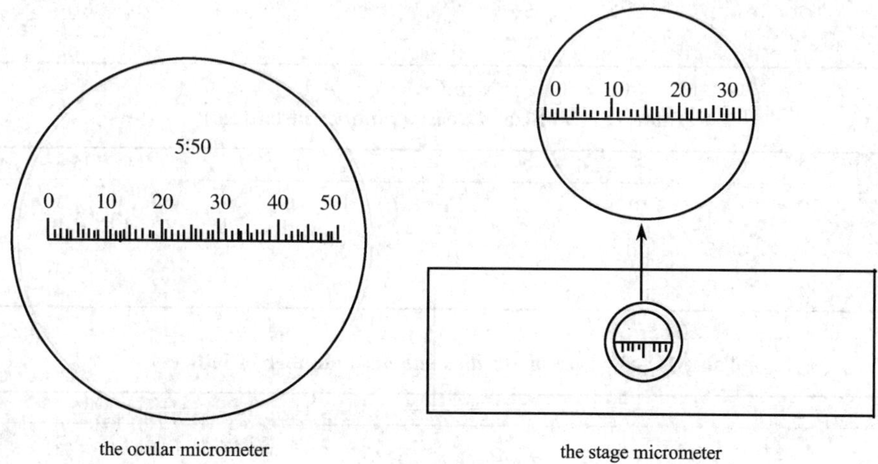

Fig. 11 －1　The ocular micrometer and stage micrometer

(2) Observe with low－power objective lens.

(3) When the ocular micrometer's graduation is clear, roll the ocular eyepiece lens, force the ocular micrometer paralleled with stage micrometer.

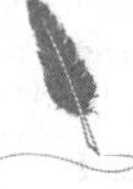

(4) Overlap the "0" of two micrometers, and then find the second scale overlapping. Count the number of the lattices between the two overlapping scale.

(5) Calculate

The length of each lattice in ocular micrometer (μm) $= 10\ n/m$

In the equation, n the number of lattices between the two overlapping scale in stage micrometer; m the number of lattices between the two overlapping scale in ocular micrometer

When observe with high - power or oil objective lens, the correct methods are the same.

2. Determination of the size of the cells

(1) Prepare cell suspension of the yeast.

(2) Prepare the slide with a drop of cells suspension.

(3) Remove the ocular micrometer, replace it with the slide. Find the object with low - power objective lens, then determine the size (length and width) under the high - power objective lens.

(4) The size of the microorganism = The number of the lattices of length / width × the correction value of the ocular micrometer.

(5) Determine 10 ~ 20 cells and calculate the average.

(6) The microorganisms are often in exponential phase.

(7) Determine the length and the width of *Bacillus subtilis* under the oil objective lens with the same method.

Results and Discussion

1. Fill the experimental results into the following tables (Table11 - 1 ~ Table11 - 3)

Table 11 - 1 Correction of Ocular Micrometer

Objective lens	Lattices of ocular Lattices of stage	Correction value micrometer	micrometer (μm)
10 ×			
40 ×			
100 ×			

Table 11 - 2 Size of yeast (number of lattices)

	1	2	3	4	5	6	7	8	9	10	11	12	13	14	15	Average
Cells number																
Length																
Width																

Table 11 - 3 Size of *Bacillus subtilis* (number of lattices)

	1	2	3	4	5	6	7	8	9	10	11	12	13	14	15	Average
Cells number																
Length																
Width																

2. Calculation of the result

(1) Length (μm) = average × correction value

(2) Width (μm) = average × correction value

（3）Size ：length（μm） × width（μm）

扫码“学一学”

实验十二 放线菌、霉菌的菌丝和孢子形态观察

【实验目的】

（1）熟悉印片法和小培养法观察菌丝和孢子的形态。

（2）熟悉观察放线菌、霉菌的菌丝和孢子形态。

【实验原理】

放线菌是一类原核单细胞型微生物，细胞的基本结构类似于细菌。放线菌具有丝状分枝，形成基内菌丝、气生菌丝和顶端部分分化而成的孢子丝，孢子丝断裂形成孢子。孢子丝可呈螺旋状、波浪状或分枝状等，有的还能分泌水溶性色素到培养基内。孢子呈圆形、杆形和椭圆形等，且具有各种颜色。气生菌丝及孢子的形态和颜色常作为放线菌分类和鉴定的重要依据。

霉菌为真核细胞型微生物，大多数为多细胞，具有分枝状菌丝体，菌丝较粗，孢子有各种不同的形状，可分为有性孢子和无性孢子。

放线菌、霉菌菌丝和孢子形态可采用印片法和小培养法来观察，其中小培养法可分为凹玻片法和插片法。

【实验材料】

1. **细菌** 放线菌和霉菌培养物。
2. **染料** 亚甲蓝染色液。
3. **器材** 盖玻片，载玻片，凹玻片，显微镜。

【实验方法】

1. 印片法观察放线菌和霉菌的菌丝和孢子形态

（1）用盖玻片在放线菌（抗生素产生菌 2809）和霉菌（青霉）菌落表面轻轻一按，即印取孢子。

（2）将印有孢子的一面朝下，放在滴有一滴亚甲蓝染液的载玻片上，静置 3 分钟，使放线菌和霉菌孢子可着色。

（3）用油镜观察放线菌和霉菌孢子、孢子丝的形态结构。

2. 凹玻片法观察放线菌和霉菌的菌丝和孢子形态

（1）取一灭菌的凹玻片，于凹窝内滴加少量熔化的固体培养基，待凝。

（2）接种少许菌种，覆盖一灭菌的盖玻片，盖玻片与凹窝间稍留一点空隙以便通气。

（3）将凹玻片置无菌平皿内，皿内垫一块潮湿的脱脂棉以维持湿度，25℃ ~28℃恒温培养 3 天。观察生长状况。

3. 插片法观察放线菌和霉菌的菌丝和孢子形态

（1）将菌种均匀的涂布在固体平板培养基上。

（2）用镊子夹一张无菌盖玻片斜插入平板内的培养基中，插入深度为盖玻片高度的 1/2 或 1/3。

（3）25℃ ~28℃恒温箱中培养 5 ~7 天。

（4）用镊子取出盖玻片放在载玻片上，用低倍镜或高倍镜观察菌丝及孢子的情况。

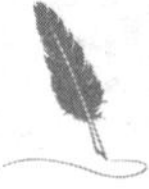

【结果与讨论】

1. 分别绘出放线菌、霉菌的孢子、孢子丝和菌丝的形态特征。

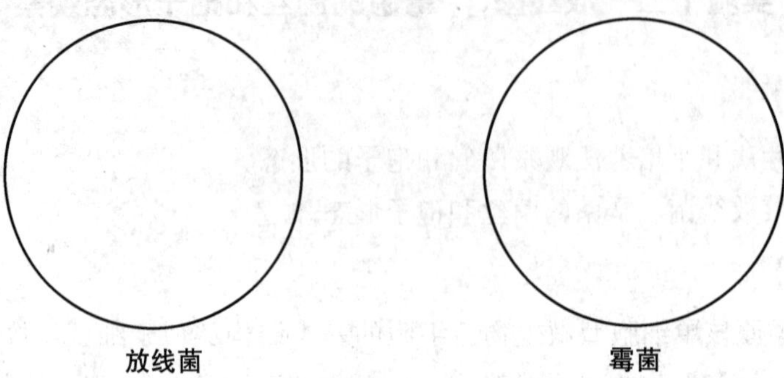

2. 放线菌、霉菌的菌丝和孢子有何区别?

EXPERIMENT 12 Morphology of Mycelia and Spore for Actinomycetes and Molds

Purpose

(1) To be familiar with the observation method of mycelia and spore.

(2) To observe the morphology of mycelia and spore of actinomycetes and molds.

Principle

Actinomycetes are prokaryotic and single cellular microorganisms. The primary cell structure of actinomycetes is similar to bacteria. Actinomycetes have filaments which contain substrate filament, aerial filament and sporebearing filament. Sporebearing filament differentiates to spore. The shape of sporebearing filament is sphere, elliptical and rod. The morphology and color of aerial filament and spore are important for the classification and characterization of actinomycetes.

Molds are eukaryotic cells and most of them are multicellular and filamented. The filament of molds is often wider than that of actinomycetes. Spores have different shapes and are divided into asexual or sexual ones.

The morphology of mycelia and spore of actinomycetes and molds can be observed by microscope and cultivated on concavity slide or cover slip.

Materials and Apparatus

1. Microorganisms Cultures of actinomycetes and molds.

2. Reagent Methylene blue.

3. Apparatus glass slide, concavity slide, cover slip, inoculating loop, lamp, lens paper, microscope.

Procedures

1. Observation of mycelia and spore of actinomycetes and molds by microscope

(1) Press a cover slip on the colony surface of actinomycetes softly to stick some spore.

(2) Place a drop of methylene blue on a glass slide. Reverse the cover slip and place it on the glass slide, allow it to stand for 3 minutes to stain the spore.

(3) Observe the morphology of mycelia and spore under oil immersion.

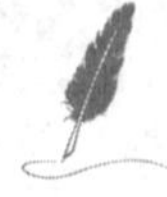

2. Observation of mycelia and spore of actinomycetes and molds by cultivation on concavity slide

(1) Place some agar media into the concavity of sterilized concavity slide and cool it off.

(2) Inoculate actinomycetes or molds with inoculating loop and place a cover slip on the concavity. Note that a little space should be kept for ventilation.

(3) Place the concavity slide and wet cotton into a sterilized plate and culture at 25℃ ~28℃ for 3 days. Record the culture state.

3. Observation of mycelia and spore of actinomycetes and molds by cultivation on cover slip

(1) Inoculate actinomycetes and molds on the culture dish.

(2) Insert 1/2 or 1/3 of a sterilized cover slip into culture media at 45℃.

(3) Culture at 25℃ ~28℃ for 5 ~7 days.

(4) Grip the cover slip with tweezers and place it on the glass slide. Observe the morphology of mycelia and spore with a microscope (low power or high power).

Results and Discussion

(1) Describe the morphological characteristics of the mycelia and spore of actinomycetes and molds.

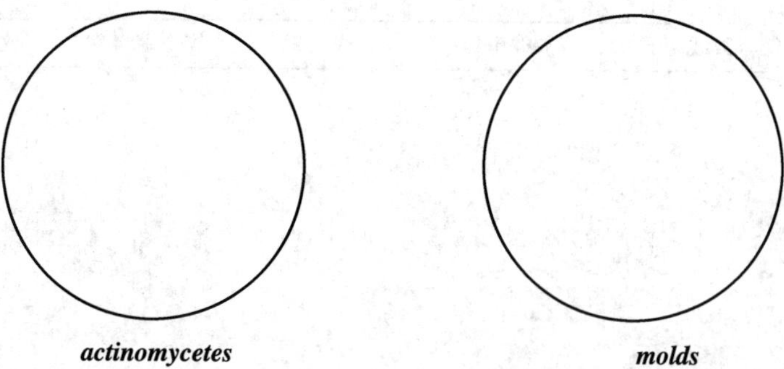

actinomycetes　　*molds*

(2) What are the differences in the mycelia and spore between actinomycetes and molds?

实验十三　细菌、放线菌、酵母菌和霉菌的菌落特征观察

扫码“学一学”

【实验目的】

熟悉通过观察培养平板，了解细菌、放线菌、酵母菌和霉菌的菌落特征。

【实验原理】

菌落是将微生物接种于固体平板培养基上，经适当温度培养后由单个细胞形成的集落。菌落特征决定于组成菌落的细胞结构和生长行为，不同的微生物具有不同的菌落特征，用以对微生物进行初步鉴定。

【实验材料】

1. 菌种　金黄色葡萄球菌、藤黄八叠球菌、大肠埃希菌、枯草芽孢杆菌、放线菌、酿酒酵母和霉菌（青霉、曲霉、毛霉、根霉）的斜面和平板培养物。

2. 培养基　普通琼脂平板，淀粉琼脂平板，改良沙氏琼脂平板。

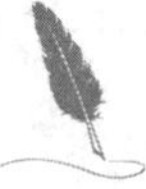

【实验方法】

（1）将金黄色葡萄球菌、藤黄八叠球菌、大肠埃希菌、枯草芽孢杆菌接种于普通琼脂平板培养基，37℃恒温培养24小时。

（2）将放线菌接种于淀粉琼脂平板培养基，28℃恒温培养5～7天。

（3）将酿酒酵母菌接种于改良沙氏琼脂平板培养基，30℃恒温培养48小时。

（4）将青霉、曲霉、毛霉、根霉接种于改良沙氏琼脂平板培养基，25℃恒温培养1～2周。

（5）菌落特征观察。

【结果与讨论】

（1）完成下列表格（表13－1～表13－3）。

表13－1　细菌的菌落特征

细菌	金黄色葡萄球菌	藤黄八叠球菌	大肠埃希菌	枯草芽孢杆菌
大小				
形态				
表面				
边缘				
颜色				
可溶性色素				

表13－2　放线菌的菌落特征

放线菌	放线菌1	放线菌2	放线菌3	放线菌4	放线菌5
大小					
形态					
表面（崎岖、皱褶或平滑）					
气生菌丝颜色及状态（粉状、绒粉状或短毛状）					
孢子丝与孢子堆的颜色					
基内菌丝的颜色					
可溶性色素					

表13－3　真菌的菌落特征

真菌	青霉	曲霉	毛霉	根霉	酵母菌
大小					
形态					
表面（崎岖、皱褶或平滑）					
气生菌丝颜色及状态（粉状、绒粉状或短毛状）					
孢子丝与孢子堆的颜色					
基内菌丝的颜色					
可溶性色素					

（2）试比较细菌、放线菌、酵母菌和霉菌菌落特征的异同。

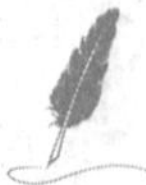

EXPERIMENT 13 Colony Characteristicsof Bacteria, Actinomycetes, Yeasts and Molds

Purpose

To be familiar with the colony morphology of bacteria, actinomycetes, yeasts and molds.

Principle

After inoculated on agar culture media and cultured at appropriate temperature for some time, microorganisms grow to form colonies from single cell that is visible to the naked eye. The characteristics of colonies depend on their cell structure and growth behavior and can be further used to identify microorganisms.

Materials and Apparatus

1. Microorganisms *Staphylococcus aureus*, *Sarcina lutea*, *Escherichia coli*, *Bacillus subtilis*, actinomycetes, *Saccharomyces cerevisiae*, molds (*Penicillium*, *Aspergillus*, *Mucor*, *Rhizopus*) .

2. Media nutrient agar slant, starch agar slant, Sabouraud agar slant.

Procedures

(1) Inoculate *Staphylococcus aureus*, *Sarcina lutea*, *Escherichia coli*, *Bacillus subtilis* on nutrient agar slant and culture at 37℃ for 24 hours.

(2) Inoculate actinomycetes on starch agar slant and culture at 28℃ for 5 to 7 days.

(3) Inoculate *Saccharomyces cerevisiae* on Sabouraud agar slant and culture at 30℃ for 48 hours.

(4) Inoculate molds on Sabouraud agar slant and culture at 25℃ for 1 to 2 weeks.

(5) Observe the colony morphology of bacteria, actinomycetes, yeasts and molds.

Results and Discussion

Table13 – 1 Describe the characteristics of bacterial colonies

Bacteria	*S. aureus*	*S. lutea*	*E. coli*	*B. subtilis*
Size				
Shape				
Surface				
Edge				
Color				
Dissolved pigment				

Table13 – 2 Describe the characteristics of actinomycetes colonies

Actinomycetes	No. 1	No. 2	No. 3	No. 4	No. 5
Size					
Shape					
Surface					
Shape and color of aerial mycelia					
Color of spore mycelia					
Color of substrate mycelia					
Dissolved pigment					

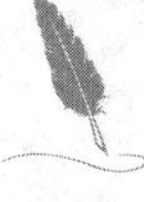

扫码“练一练”

Table13 – 3 Describe the characteristics of fungi

Fungi	*Penicillum*	*Aspergillus*	*Mucor*	*Rhizopus*	*Saccharomyces*
Size					
Shape					
Surface					
Shape and color of aerial mycelia					
Color of spore mycelia					
Color of substrate mycelia					
Dissolved pigment					

(2) Compare the colony characteristics of bacteria, actinomycetes, yeasts and molds.

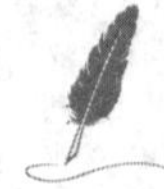

第二部分　基本实验操作与培养技术

微生物学的研究对象大部分都是用肉眼无法直接观察到的微小生物，因此要对其做研究，除了用显微镜观察其细胞形态外还涉及到对它们进行扩大培养，由于微生物在自然环境中的生活方式大多数都是杂居混生，因此对天然样本进行分离与纯化也是十分必要的。再通过对其生长过程中的多个参数进行测量达到对微生物的生长、代谢、繁殖等方面进行研究的目的。本部分介绍了微生物学研究中常用的基本实验操作与培养技术，分别是培养基的制备、灭菌；微生物的分离纯化、菌种保藏以及微生物的计数与生长曲线的测定。

实验十四　培养基的配制与灭菌

扫码“学一学”

【实验目的】

(1) 掌握培养基的配制方法。

(2) 熟悉高压蒸汽灭菌的原理与操作。

【实验原理】

微生物的生长依赖于可利用的营养物质和适宜的生长环境。实验室条件下研究微生物需要供微生物生长的培养基。培养基是用于培养、转移、储存微生物的固体、半固体或液体营养基质。培养基中必须含有微生物生长所需的全部营养物质，包括碳源、氮源、能源(有时可能与碳源相同)、无机盐、水分和生长因子。适宜的 pH 对微生物的生长也是必不可少的。

扫码“看一看”

所用培养基的物理状态有三种：液体、半固体和固体。这些培养基的主要区别是在固体和半固体培养基中加有固化剂——琼脂。琼脂是从某种海藻中得到的结构复杂的长链多糖，具有很多优良性质。当加入溶液中时，琼脂要在98℃才能融化形成有一定黏性的液体，并在42℃凝固。凝固之后要重新加热至98℃才能再次融化。琼脂具有的其他特性包括：不易被微生物降解；接近无色，因此易于观察菌落等。对于固体培养基需要加入琼脂的量约为1.5%～3%，半固体培养基需加约0.2%～0.8%。

根据培养基成分的来源不同，可将培养基分为两种：一种叫限定培养基或合成培养基，由化学成分完全了解的物质配制而成，只能满足特定微生物的基本生长需求；另一种叫天然培养基，由化学成分不清楚或不恒定的物质组成，例如肉的水解产物（蛋白胨），能够充分满足不同微生物的生长需要。天然培养基如营养肉汤培养基在实验室中通常用于培养细菌。

培养基在配制过程中会由于接触到容器、药品、称量纸或其他表面而被污染，因此必须进行灭菌，同时不能将培养基中的营养物质破坏。这就需要高压蒸汽灭菌锅（图 14－1）在121℃（即 1.05kg/cm^2 或 103.46kPa）条件下灭菌15～30分钟。在此条件下，所有微生物，包括芽孢在内，都会被杀死。当培养基中含有糖分的时候，灭菌温度也可降至113℃。

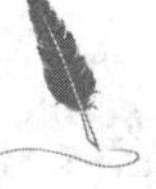

灭菌验证：培养基配制完成后，必须对灭菌效果进行验证，这将直接关系到实验结果

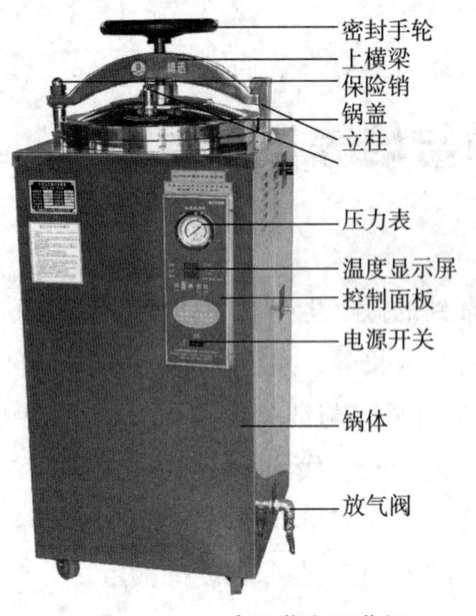

图 14－1　高压蒸汽灭菌锅

正确与否。灭菌验证方法很多，在此介绍如何利用嗜热脂肪芽孢杆菌纸片来进行灭菌验证的方法。

将嗜热脂肪芽孢杆菌纸片（以下简称菌片）用无菌镊子放入密封试管中。分别放置在高压蒸汽灭菌锅的蒸汽口处、底部排气口处及底部出水口处等不同位置，然后进行灭菌处理。灭菌后的菌片以无菌操作放入灭菌后的溴甲酚紫胨水培养基内 56℃ 培养 48h，观察颜色变化。如培养基变为黄色，说明菌片中的嗜热脂肪芽孢杆菌没有被完全杀灭，从而在培养基中生长，分解葡萄糖产酸变为黄色。如培养基颜色不变化仍为紫色，则说明芽孢菌已全部灭活。同时要用未经灭菌的菌片放入培养基内作为阳性对照，不加菌片的空白培养基作为阴性对照。

【实验材料】

1. **试剂**　牛肉浸膏，蛋白胨，氯化钠，琼脂，蒸馏水，1mol/L HCl，1mol/L NaOH。

2. **仪器**　天平，高压蒸汽灭菌锅，电炉。

3. **其他**　药匙，称量纸，量筒，烧杯，pH 试纸，三角瓶，硫酸纸。

【实验方法】

1. 营养肉汤培养基的配制

配方如下：

牛肉膏	0.5g
蛋白胨	1.0g
氯化钠	0.5g
蒸馏水	100ml
pH	7.2～7.6

（1）按照配方准确称量每一种药品。牛肉膏因为其黏性高需用硫酸纸称取。

（2）用量筒称取 100ml 蒸馏水倒入烧杯。然后将各药品加入烧杯，加热并搅拌至溶解（将称好的牛肉膏与硫酸纸一并放入烧杯中，待溶解后将硫酸纸取出）。

（3）用 1mol/L HCl 或 1mol/L NaOH 调节 pH 至 7.2～7.6。

（4）将配好的培养基分装到三角瓶（试管）中至不超过 1/2 高度处。如果配制固体或半固体培养基，将称好的琼脂直接放入三角瓶（试管）中。盖好胶塞。

（5）灭菌　用牛皮纸包装好三角瓶（试管）并写上名字。然后将三角瓶（试管）放入高压蒸汽灭菌锅中在 121℃ 灭菌 30 分钟。

（6）如果不立即使用，应将灭菌后的培养基置 4℃ 保存。

2. 灭菌——高压蒸汽灭菌

（1）向锅内加入足够的水。

（2）放入配好的培养基，注意不要装得太挤。

（3）关闭锅盖，按下开始按钮。

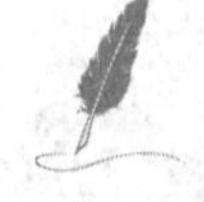

（4）打开排气阀，待冷空气完全排尽后，关上排气阀。

（5）蒸汽由夹套进入内层。于是温度开始上升，当达到121℃时，计时器开始计时15～30分钟（视所灭菌的培养基种类与体积而定）。灭菌后，锅内的液体缓慢冷却方可打开锅盖，以防止由于压力骤降引起液体喷溅。

（6）对培养基进行灭菌验证。

【结果与讨论】

（1）在配制培养细菌的培养基时为什么要将 pH 调至中性？

（2）灭菌结束后，为什么要等到灭菌锅内压力降为常压时才能打开灭菌锅盖？

PART TWO　Basic Laboratory and Culture Techniques

Most microbes are not visible to naked eyes which makes microscopy techniques necessary for microbial research. Most habitats harbor microbes in complex associations. It is often important to separate the organisms from one another so they can be identified and studied. Parameters involved in the growing process facilitate the research on microbial metabolism, production and other biological functions. This part introduces the basic laboratory techniques in microbiology, which are preparation and sterilization of culture media, purification and preservation of microbes, numeration and growth curve of microorganisms.

EXPERIMENT 14　Culture Media Preparation and Sterilization

Purposes

(1) To grasp the preparation methods of culture media.

(2) To be familiar with the principles and the operation procedures of autoclave sterilization.

Principles

The growth of microorganisms depends on available nutrients and a favorable growth environment. Laboratory studies on microorganisms require the culture media to grow the microorganisms. A culture medium is a solid, semisolid or liquid preparation used to grow, transport and store microorganisms. The medium must contain all the nutrients the microorganisms require for growth, including carbon source, nitrogen source, energy source (sometimes the same as carbon source), inorganic source, water and growth factors. A suitable pH is also needed for the microbial growth.

Culture media are classified into liquid media, semisolid media and solid media according to their physical states. The major difference among these media is that solid and semisolid media contain a solidifying agent—agar. Agar is a complex, long chain polysaccharide derived from certain marine algae and has several useful properties. When added to a solution, it melts at 98℃ and forms a slightly viscous liquid that solidifies at 42℃. After solidification, the agar will not melt unless the temperature is again raised to 98℃. Some other useful properties of agar include its resist-

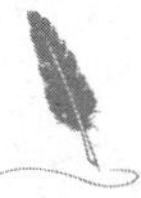

ance to microbial degradation and its translucence for easy viewing of colonies. When a solid medium is necessary, a 1.5 ~ 3% concentration of agar is typical. For semi - solid medium around 0.5 ~ 0.8% agar is employed.

According to the sources of media ingredients, two different types of media are designed. A defined or synthetic medium contains known amounts of pure chemicals which are usually the basic requirements for the growth of particular microbes. A complex medium contains undefined ingredients such as protidtemns of meat (peptones) that provide enough nutrients to sustain the growth for different microbes. Complex media such as nutrient broth is routinely used for cultivation of bacteria in the laboratory works.

Due to possible contaminations from containers, media ingredients, weighing papers, or other surfaces that come in contact with the medium, culture media should be made sterile without inactivating nutrients necessary for growth of the microorganisms. This involves the use of an autoclave (Fig. 14 - 1), in which media are sterilized by steam at 121℃ (1.05 kg/cm^2 or 103.46 kPa) for 15 ~ 30 minutes. Under these conditions, microbes, even endospores, will all be killed. The sterilization temperature could be decreased to 113℃ when sugar ingredients are involved.

Verification of sterilizing effectiveness: After sterilization, the sterilizing effect must be tested to guarantee the following experiment. Here will focus on the use of *Bacillus stearothermophilus* strip.

Put the strips into sealed test tubes and place them into the autoclave chamber where steam enters, air releases and water releases, then start to sterilize. After sterilization, aseptically transfer the strips into bromcresol purple broth and incubate at 56℃ for 48h. If the broth turns yellow, it means *B. stearothermophilus* is still alive because of acid production during bacterial growth. If the medium remains purple, sterilization is successfully done. Positive control with nonsterile strip inoculated and blank control without strip are also necessary.

Materials and Apparatus

1. Reagents beef extract, peptone, sodium chloride, agar, distilled water, 1 mol/L hydrochloric acid, 1mol/L sodium hydroxide.

2. Apparatus balance, autoclave, electric stove.

3. Others medicine spoon, weighing paper, cylinder, beaker, pH indicator paper, flask, vegetable parchment.

Procedures

1. Preparation of nutrient broth

Recipe of nutrient broth is as follows:

Beef extract	0.5g
Peptone	1.0g
Sodium chloride	0.5g
Distilled water	100ml
pH	7.2 ~ 7.6

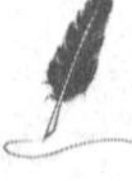

(1) Use the recipe listed above to weigh out each component required for the nutrient broth medium. For the beef extract, weigh it on a vegetable parchment because of its viscous property.

(2) Measure 100 ml water using a cylinder and then add all components into a beaker. Heat and stir until all the components are dissolved. (Add beef extract together with vegetable parchment into the beaker. After dissolving, take out the vegetable parchment).

(3) Adjust the solution pH with 1 mol/L HCl or 1 mol/L NaOH to 7.2 ~7.6.

(4) Distribute the medium to a flask (tube) to no more than 1/2 height. When solid or semi-solid medium is needed, add agar into the flask (tube) directly. Put on the plug.

(5) Wrap the flask (tube) with brown paper and write your name on it. Then put the flask (tube) into the autoclave to sterilize for 30 min at 121℃.

(6) After sterilization, preserve the sterilized media at 4℃ if they are not used right now.

2. Sterilization—autoclaving

(1) Add enough water into the autoclave.

(2) Put the media into the chamber. Note: do not pack too tightly.

(3) Lock the door of the autoclave. Press the start button to begin sterilization

(4) Open the exhaust valve until the cool air is completely exhausted then close it.

(5) Steam enters into a jacket surrounding the chamber. The temperature in the chamber will go up to 121℃. At this point, there is a counting down of 15 to 30 minutes depending on the type and volume of media. After sterilization, autoclaved liquids must be cooled slowly to avoid boiling over when the pressure is sharply released.

(6) Verification of sterilizing effectiveness.

Results and Discussion

(1) Why are media for culturing bacteria adjusted to a neutral pH?

(2) The autoclave door should not be opened after sterilization until the pressure in it lowers down to normal pressure, why?

实验十五　接种技术与微生物的分离纯化

扫码“学一学”

【实验目的】

(1) 了解纯培养物制备的原理。

(2) 掌握使用无菌操作进行接种的方法。

(3) 熟悉判断细菌在不同培养基上的生长状况的方法。

【实验原理】

通常情况下，微生物以杂居状态生长。因此要对某一种微生物进行研究，必须先将其与其他微生物进行分离。纯培养物（即由单一微生物生长得到）是进行微生物实验操作的重要材料。微生物最容易的分离方法就是进行划线分离。

当通过划线法分离单菌落时，培养物在固体培养基表面通过划线进行稀释。目的是要使细菌细胞间的间隔足够大，这样单个细胞所产生的大量后代就会形成一个菌落。由此可见，菌落就是在固体培养基表面由微生物形成的肉眼可见的细胞集团，一个菌落就代表了一个纯培养物。

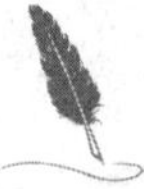

纯培养物也可以由涂布法获得。将少量微生物混合样本的稀释液加入到固体琼脂平板表面，并利用无菌涂布棒涂布均匀。如果稀释度合适，分散的细胞就会形成单菌落。

上面的分离步骤都涉及接种技术。接种所使用的器材包括接种针、接种环和移液管。接种针（环）用于将微生物从液体或斜面培养物中转移至其他培养基。接种针和接种环都由把手、金属柄、转头以及固定的镍镉或铝金属丝组成。移液管则是用来转移液体培养物，或用于微生物的梯度稀释以及配置化学药品。

分离纯培养物时，必须使用无菌操作来防止由于容器、药品、仪器和其他表面接触培养物所带来的污染。最重要的分离和接种工具就是接种针（环）。可以通过使用煤气灯火焰加热至红色来快速灭菌。

当对未知菌种进行鉴定时，首先要制备出纯培养物，然后通过微生物特征进行分析。其中最简单的是培养特征。在固体培养基上，分离出的单菌落可以通过以下参数进行观察：大小、形状、边缘、色素、质地和表面等进行观察。在液体培养基中，三种典型的生长形式包括均匀混浊生长、只在液体表面生长以及只在管底生长。半固体培养基则用于检验细菌的运动性。当在半固体培养基中央进行穿刺时，在穿刺线周围的生长状况就会显示样本的运动性（图 15－1）。如果培养基透明，只沿穿刺线生长［图 15－1（a）］，说明菌体不具有运动性；当培养基显示云雾状时［图 15－1（b）］，则说明菌体具有运动性。

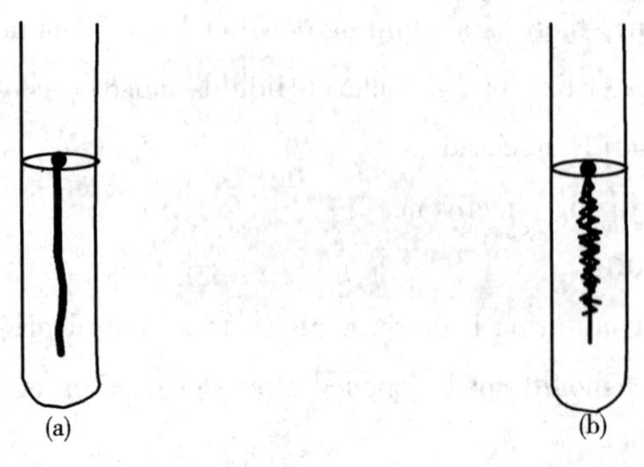

图 15－1　半固体培养基中的生长状况

【实验材料】

1. **菌种**　20 小时金黄色葡萄球菌斜面培养物，20 小时大肠埃希菌斜面培养物，20 小时藤黄八叠球菌斜面培养物，24 小时枯草芽孢杆菌斜面培养物，20 小时混合的细菌液体培养物（金黄色葡萄球菌与大肠埃希菌）。

2. **培养基**　营养肉汤琼脂斜面，营养肉汤培养基，半固体培养基，琼脂平板。

3. **仪器**　无菌平皿，接种环，接种针，无菌移液管，煤气灯。

【实验方法】

1. 接种技术

（1）将要接种的试管或平皿写好名字、日期、所用培养基和微生物名称。

（2）调整火焰至适当大小（蓝色）。如果原始培养物是液态，先要将其摇晃均匀。用左手握住原培养物试管与待接种试管。右手持接种环（针）［图 15－2（a）］。

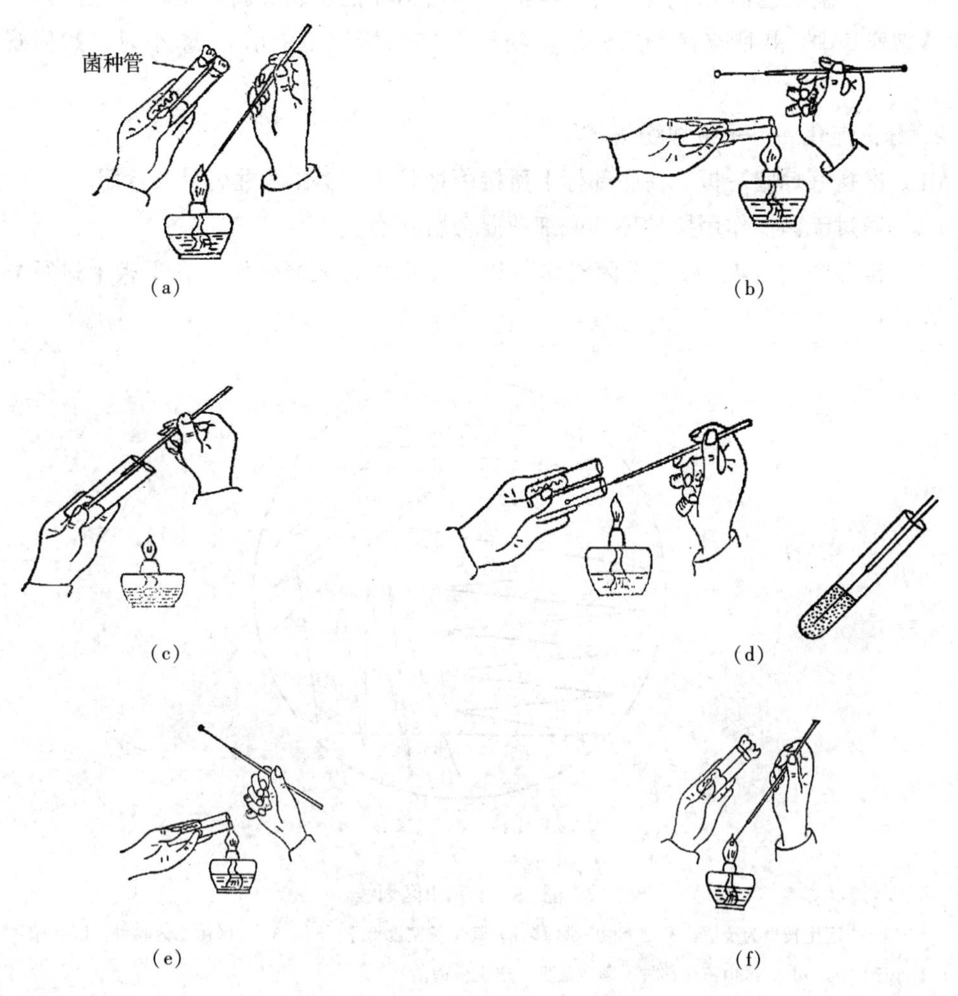

图 15 –2　无菌接种法

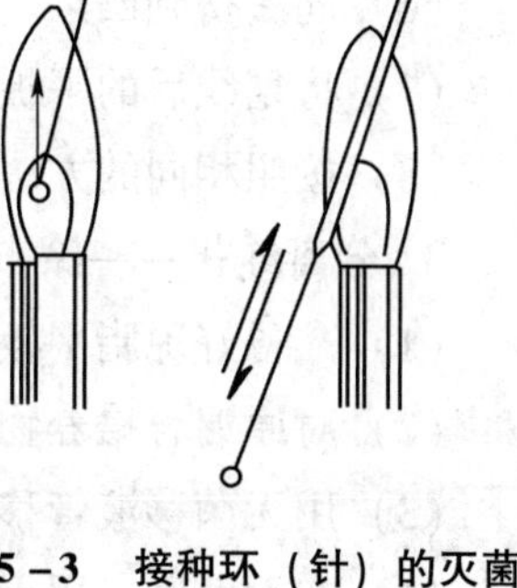

图 15 –3　接种环（针）的灭菌

(3) 用火焰加热接种环（针）至变红，然后沿金属柄向上，将能深入试管的部分依次灭菌（图 15 –3）。

(4) 待接种环（针）冷却后再取菌。否则细胞会被高温杀死。

(5) 再次确认所取微生物样本。

(6) 右手打开试管帽，于手掌与小指间夹住。在打开或盖上试管帽时都要用火焰对试管口进行灭菌［图 15 –2 (b)］。

(7) 用灭菌的接种环从原培养物试管中取一环培养物［图 15 –2（c)］加入到新的液体培养基中［图 15 –2（d)］。在这一步，也可以转移至载玻片或在斜面上划线，还可以从原始斜面培养物进行接种。

(8) 对于半固体穿刺接种，将接种针插入装有半固体培养基的试管中至 2/3 处（注意不要碰到试管壁）然后沿穿刺线拔出［图 15 –2（d)］。

(9) 重新对试管口进行灭菌［（图 15 –2（e)］。

(10) 盖上试管帽，再次灭菌接种环（针）［图 15 –2（f)］。

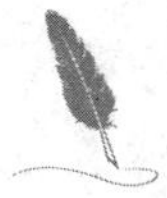

扫码“看一看”

分别接种金黄色葡萄球菌、大肠埃希菌和枯草芽孢杆菌的斜面培养物至液体培养基和半固体培养基中，将所有接种后的培养物放入37℃恒温箱中培养24小时，然后观察培养结果。

2. 分离纯化——平板划线法

（1）准备好琼脂平板，在底部标上所接菌种名称、操作者姓名以及日期。

（2）通过无菌操作用接种环移取细菌混合培养物。

（3）按照图15－4，通过无菌操作（以下操作均为无菌操作）在平板上进行划线，得到一区。

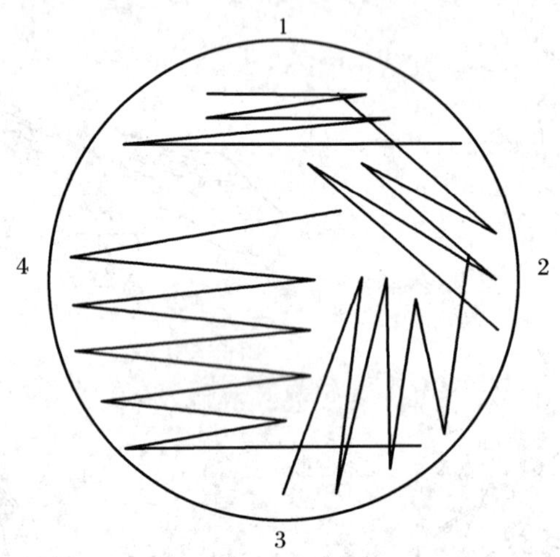

图15－4 四区划线

1. 一区生长最为茂盛；2. 二区由一区移种，其生长密度低于一区；3. 三区由二区移种，因此菌体数量小于二区；4. 四区由三区移种，菌数最少，出现单菌落

（4）将接种环移开并灭菌，杀死残留在上面的菌体。待在非接种区冷却后，从一区出发，划出二区。

（5）再次灭菌接种环，重复上一步骤，得到三区。

（6）同法得到四区。

（7）将划线后的平板倒置在37℃恒温箱中培养24小时，观察培养结果。

（8）按照相同的方法对枯草芽孢杆菌和藤黄八叠球菌的斜面培养物进行分离纯化。

3. 分离纯化——涂布法

（1）准备好琼脂平板，在底部标上所接菌种名称、操作者姓名以及日期。

（2）对原混合培养物进行10倍梯度稀释。

（3）用无菌移液管移取0.1ml细菌混合培养物至琼脂平板表面。

（4）在无菌区，用无菌涂布棒将混菌样本涂布均匀并覆盖整个平板表面。

（5）将用过的涂布棒置于指定容器内待灭菌。

（6）将平板放置在37℃恒温培养箱中倒置培养24小时，观察培养结果。

【结果与讨论】

（1）观察琼脂斜面上各细菌的生长状况。

（2）观察液体培养基中细菌生长状况，不得用力振荡培养物，将实验结果记于表15－1中。

表 15－1　液体培养基中细菌生长状况

菌　名	生长状况
金黄色葡萄球菌	
大肠埃希菌	
枯草芽孢杆菌	

（3）观察并记录细菌在半固体培养基中生长状况，将实验结果记于表 15－2 中。

表 15－2　细菌在半固体培养基中生成状况

菌　名	生长状况	运动性
金黄色葡萄球菌		
枯草芽孢杆菌		
大肠埃希菌		

（4）观察不同细菌的代表性菌落，将其菌落特点记于表 15－3 中。

表 15－3　菌落特点

菌　名	大小	形状	边缘	色素	质地	表面
金黄色葡萄球菌						
大肠埃希菌						
枯草芽孢杆菌						
藤黄八叠球菌						

（5）为从一个微生物混合材料中获得纯培养物设计两种不同的实验程序。

EXPERIMENT 15　Culture Transfer Techniques and Isolation of Pure Cultures

Purposes

(1) To understand the principles of pure culture preparation.

(2) To grasp how to correctly use aseptic techniques to transfer bacteria for sub－culturing

(3) To be familiar with how to determine the growth characteristics of bacteria on different media.

Principles

Microorganisms usually grow in complex and mixed population containing many different species. To get adequate study, single type of microbial sample has to be separated from other species. Pure culture, the growth of a single species of microorganism, is of great importance for laboratory practice involving microorganism. The best way to do this is to streak for isolation.

When streaking for single colonies, the inoculum is diluted by streaking it across the agar plate surface. The purpose is to get the inoculum diluted to the degree that there is only one bacterial cell deposited every few millimeters on the surface of the agar plate. When these individual bacterial cells divide and give rise to thousands of offspring, an isolated colony is formed. Therefore, a colony is a macroscopically visible growth or cluster of microorganisms on a solid medium and each colony represents a pure culture.

Pure culture can also be obtained by spread plate method. A small volume of dilute microbial mixture is transferred to the surface of an agar plate and spread with a sterile glass spreader. If the

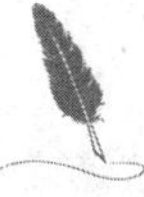

dilution is proper, the dispersed cells develop into isolated colonies.

All the above isolation procedures involve culture transfer techniques. Culture transfer instruments include inoculating needles, inoculating loops and pipette. Inoculating needles and loops are used to aseptically transfer microorganisms from broth or slant cultures to other media. Both consist of handles, a shaft, and a turret, which holds a nickel – chromium or platinum wire. A pipette is often used to transfer aliquots of culture, to prepare serial dilutions of microorganisms, and to dispense chemical reagents.

To isolate pure culture, aseptic techniques must be used to avoid contamination by containers, media ingredients, instruments and other surfaces that come in contact with the culture. The most important tool for isolating and transferring cultures is the inoculating needle or loop. It can be quickly sterilized by heating it to red hot in a Bunsen burner flame.

If an unknown bacterium sample needs to be identified, pure culture should be firstly prepared. Then different microbial characteristics including cultural characteristics, cellular characteristics, and biochemical characteristics could be examined. The simplest characterization is through cultural characteristics. On the agar plate (solid media), well – isolated colony can be observed for its size, shape, margin, pigment, texture and surface. Three typical growth patterns can be observed in nutrient broth (liquid media): even growth throughout the media to form a turbid broth, growth only on the surface and growth only at the bottom. Semisolid media are used to determine the motility of bacteria. When the medium is stabbed carefully in the center, the growth pattern around the stab line shows the motility of the sample (fig. 15 – 1). If the medium is clear with a persistent stab line (on the left), the organism is non – motile. If the medium gives a uniform cloudiness (on the right), the organism is motile.

Materials and Apparatus

1. Cultures nutrient agar slants of *Staphylococcus aureus*, *Escherichia coli*, *Bacillus subtilis* and *Sarcina lutea*, mixed broth culture of *S. aureus* and *E. coli*.

2. Media nutrient agar slants, nutrient broth, semisolid media, agar plates.

3. Others sterile plate, inoculation loop and needle, sterile pipette, burner.

Procedures

1. Culture transfer techniques

(1) Label the tubes and/or plates with operator's name, date, type of medium and the name of the organisms.

(2) Properly adjust the flame of the burner. The proper flame is a small blue cone rather than a large plume. If the primary culture is broth, mix the tube to get a uniform suspension. Place the stock culture tube and the tube for inoculation in the palm of the left hand.

(3) Flame your loop (or needle) until the wire becomes red – hot. Then sterilize the metal handle which will be inserted into the tube (Fig. 15 – 3).

(4) Allow your loop (or needle) to cool before you try to pick up the organism. Otherwise, the cells will be killed by heat.

(5) Ensure that you are transferring the correct organism into your labeled tube by double – checking the name of the organism on the stock culture from which you are collecting your inoculum.

(6) When removing the caps from tubes, always keep the caps between the palm and the small fingers (Fig. 15 – 2b) . And also flame the necks of a culture tube when you open it and before you replace the cap.

(7) With the sterile inoculation loop, transfer 1 loopful of culture from the stock culture tube (Fig. 15 – 2c) into the new broth tube (Fig. 15 – 2d) . At this point, one could also transfer to a glass slide or streak the surface of a slant. The original culture could be a slant culture as well.

(8) For the semisolid stab transfer technique, insert the inoculating needle into the semisolid media tube without touching the walls of the tube, and allow the needle to penetrate 2/3 depth of the medium. Then take the needle out along the stab line (Fig. 15 – 2d) .

(9) Re – sterilize the neck of the tubes (Fig. 15 – 2e) .

(10) Recap the tubes and sterilize the loop (or needle) (Fig. 15 – 2f) .

Inoculate *S. aureus*, *E. coli* and *B. subtilis* from the slant cultures into nutrient broth media and semi – solid media respectively. Incubate at 37℃ for 24 h. Then observe the results.

2. Isolation of pure culture—streaking – plate technique

(1) Prepare an agar plate and mark on the bottom of the plate with the name of the bacterium to be inoculated, operator's name and date.

(2) Aseptically remove a loopful of the bacterial mixture.

(3) Follow the instruction in fig. 15 – 4, streak the first section of your plate. This has to be done aseptically (the same for the following steps) .

(4) Remove the inoculation loop and kill any remaining bacteria by flaming them. Cool the loop at a non – inoculated section of the agar plate. Cross over the streaks in area 1 and streak out as shown in area 2.

(5) Flame your loop again, and repeat the streaking process for your third section.

(6) Repeat once more to make area 4.

(7) Incubate the plates upside down at 37℃ for 24 h. Then observe the isolation results.

(8) Do the same to purify *B. subtilis* and *S. lutea* from their slant cultures.

3. Isolation of pure culture—spread – plate technique

(1) Prepare an agar plate and mark on the bottom of the plate with the name of the bacteria to be inoculated, operator's name and date.

(2) Make a series of dilution tubes of the original mixed inoculum. Each succeeding dilution tubecontains approximately one – tenth of bacterial cells in the preceding one.

(3) For each dilution tube, aseptically pipette 0. 1 ml of the bacterial mixture onto the center of an agar plate.

(4) In the aseptic area, use the sterile glass spreader to spread the bacteria sample evenly over the agar surface, making sure that the whole surface has been covered.

(5) Put the spreader in a proper container to sterilize.

(6) Incubate the plates upside down at 37℃ for 24 h. Then observe the isolation results.

Results and Discussion

(1) Observe the growth patterns of cultures on agar slants.

(2) Observe the growth patterns of cultures in nutrient broth without shaking and record the

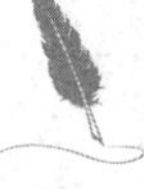

results in the following table.

Strains	Cultural characteristics
S. aureus	
E. coli	
B. subtilis	

(3) Observe the growth patterns of cultures in semisolid media and record the results in the following table.

Strain	Cultural characteristics	Motility
S. aureus		
B. subtilis		
E. coli		

(4) Observe the characteristics of the representative colonies of different bacteria and record the results in the following table.

Strains	Size	Shape	Margin	Pigment	Texture	Surface
S. aureus						
E. coli						
B. subtilis						
S. lutea						

(5) Design two different practical methods to obtain pure culture from a mixed sample.

实验十六　常用的消毒灭菌方法

扫码“学一学”

【实验目的】

(1) 熟悉巴氏消毒、紫外杀菌和干热灭菌的原理和步骤。

(2) 了解验证细菌芽孢耐热性的方法。

【实验原理】

除高压蒸汽灭菌外，对于不同物体还有其他消毒灭菌方法。本实验将介绍巴氏消毒、紫外杀菌和干热灭菌。每一种方法的使用特点与限制将通过杀菌效果展示出来。

巴氏消毒是用于对牛奶或其他液体进行加热以破坏腐败或病原微生物的消毒措施。操作温度通常在63℃～72℃，因此只能杀死营养细胞，对芽孢无效。

紫外线的波长为100～400nm。当微生物暴露在紫外光下时，DNA会吸收紫外线，并使其中相邻的胸腺嘧啶相连成二聚体。DNA复制时，无法对此二聚体进行配对，引起DNA链复制错误。换句话说，紫外照射能够引起突变并导致蛋白质合成发生错误。如果突变过多，细菌的代谢就会被阻断，从而引起微生物死亡。由此可知，紫外照射不能用于杀灭产芽孢的细菌，因为处于芽孢这一休眠时期，没有DNA复制发生。

紫外线的杀菌能力受照射时间长短的影响，照射时间越长，杀菌效果越好。同时也由所用紫外线波长决定。260nm的紫外线具有最强杀菌性，因为DNA分子的最大吸收峰在此。由于紫外照射穿透力差，只能用于表面杀菌。紫外线对眼睛和皮肤的细胞会造成伤害。

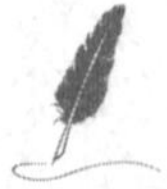

许多物品需要在干燥条件下进行灭菌，即干热灭菌。将待灭菌物品置于烘箱中160℃～

170℃灭菌1~2小时，这样能够保证彻底杀灭包括芽孢在内的一切微生物。这是因为高温能够使蛋白质氧化变性。适于干热灭菌的物品有玻璃仪器、金属仪器和粉末等水蒸气无法有效穿入并且在高温下不会被破坏的物品。

【实验材料】

1. **菌种**　24小时枯草芽孢杆菌斜面和液体培养物，20小时大肠埃希菌斜面和液体培养物。

2. **仪器**　温控水浴锅，烘箱，紫外灯，恒温培养箱。

3. **其他**　接种环，琼脂平板，营养肉汤培养基试管，无菌滴管，无菌涂布棒，镊子，星形牛皮纸等。

【实验方法】

1. 巴氏消毒

（1）分别接种枯草芽孢杆菌和大肠埃希菌到试管内的营养肉汤培养基中，再用另一管未接种的培养基作为空白对照。

（2）将3个试管共同置于63℃恒温水浴30分钟进行消毒。

（3）将试管置于37℃恒温培养24小时，观察细菌在消毒后的生长状况。

2. 紫外杀菌

（1）打开紫外灯预热10分钟。

（2）用无菌滴管分别滴加3滴两种液体培养物至两个琼脂平板表面，并涂布均匀。

（3）用灭菌后的镊子取一张无菌的星形牛皮纸。

（4）将牛皮纸放至平板中央并将边缘按压。

注：（2）~（4）步都须无菌操作。

（5）移去平板盖，在距紫外灯20cm左右距离照射30分钟。注意不要将皮肤或眼睛直接暴露在紫外灯下，以免受伤。

（6）照射后，用镊子通过无菌操作将牛皮纸取下，重新盖好，在37℃培养24小时。

（7）培养后，观察微生物的生长情况。

3. 干热灭菌

（1）将待灭菌物品［平皿、试管、吸管（无胶帽）等］放入电烘箱内，注意物品不要摆得太挤。

（2）打开烘箱开关，直至达到160℃~170℃，开始计时2小时。

（3）待电烘箱内温度降到70℃以下取出灭菌物品。

【结果与讨论】

（1）分别记录并比较63℃水浴和紫外照射对两种培养物的消毒灭菌效果。

（2）干热灭菌的注意事项有哪些？

（3）怎样才能获得枯草芽孢杆菌的芽孢悬液？

EXPERIMENT 16　Commonly Used Sterilization and Disinfection Methods

Purposes

(1) To be familiar with the principles and procedures of Pasteurization, UV radiation and dry

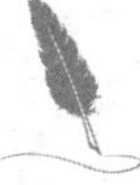

heat sterilization.

(2) To understand how to verify the heat – resistant ability of endospores.

Principles

Besides autoclaving, there are some other sterilization methods for different objects. This exercise includes Pasteurization, UV radiation and dry heat sterilization. According to the bactericidal effects, the characteristics and limitations of each method will be shown.

Pasteurization is the process of heating milk and other liquids to destroy microorganisms that can cause spoilage or disease. The manipulation temperature is usually between 63℃ to 72℃. Therefore, only vegetative cells rather than endospores can be destroyed.

The wavelength of ultraviolet ranges from 100 nm to 400 nm. When microorganisms are exposed to UV, absorption of UV by microbial DNA will cause adjacent thymine bases to covalently bond together, forming thymine – thymine dimers. When DNA replicates, the existence of thymine – thymine dimers inhibits normal base pairing, leading to mistakes in the replication of that DNA strand. In other words, UV radiation causes mutation and can lead to defect in protein synthesis. With sufficient mutation, bacterial metabolism is blocked and the organism dies. Based on this principle, UV radiation can not kill endospore – forming bacteria since there is no DNA replication in this dormancy stage.

The bactericidal activity of ultraviolet light depends on the time of exposure: the longer the exposure the higher the bactericidal activity. It also depends on the wavelength of UV used. The most lethal wavelength of UV light is 260 nm where the highest absorption of UV by DNA occurs. UV radiation can only be used for surface sterilization because of its poor penetration power. It can also damage eyes, cause burns, and cause mutations in skin cells.

Many objects are best sterilized in the absence of water by dry heat sterilization even though it is not as versatile as autoclaving. The objects are placed in an oven at 160 to 170℃ for 1 to 2 hours, which ensures thorough heating of the items and destruction of endospores. Microbial death apparently results from the oxidation and denaturation of proteins. Objects suitable for dry heat sterilization are glassware, metal instruments and powders that cannot be penetrated by steam and cannot be destroyed at high temperature.

Materials and Apparatus

1. Cultures 24h slant and broth cultures of *Bacillus subtilis* and 20 h slant and broth cultures of *Escherichia coli*.

2. Apparatus temperature – controlled water bath, oven, UV lamp, incubator.

3. Others inoculating loop, sterile agar plate, nutrient broth in tube, sterile dropper, sterile spreader, forceps, brown paper (star shape).

Procedures

1. Pasteurization

(1) Inoculate *B. subtilis* and *E. coli* to the nutrient broth tubes respectively and take another broth tube without inoculation as control.

(2) Place the three tubes together in 63℃ water bath for 30min for disinfection.

(3) Incubate the tubes at 37℃ for 24h and record the disinfection results.

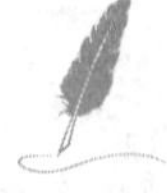

2. Ultraviolet radiation

(1) Switch on the UV lamp and allow it to warm up for 10 minutes.

(2) Use sterile droppers to add 3 drops of the two broth cultures onto the surface of two agar plates respectively and spread uniformly with sterile spreaders. All these need to be done with aseptically, which is also required for the following two steps.

(3) Sterilize the forceps and pick up a sterile brown paper in star shape.

(4) Put the brown paper on the center of the agar plate and press the edge.

(5) Remove the lid and expose the agar plate to the UV lamp at a distance of 20 cm for 30 min. Be careful not to expose your skin or eyes to the UV light directly.

(6) After exposure, take out the brown paper with sterilized forceps aseptically and recover the agar plate. Incubate upside down at 37℃ for 24 h.

(7) After incubation, observe the growth condition of the bacteria samples.

3. Dry heat sterilization

(1) Place the items (plates, tubes, straws, et al) in the oven. Note: do not pack too much.

(2) Switch on the oven and wait until the inside temperature increases to 160 ~ 170℃ and maintain for 2 h.

(3) Take out the items after sterilization when the temperature decreases to 70℃.

Results and Discussion

(1) Respectively record and compare the sterilization results of the two cultures with 63℃ water bath and UV radiation.

(2) What should be paid attention to in dry heat sterilization?

(3) How to obtain spore suspension of *B. subtilis* ?

实验十七　菌种保藏

扫码“学一学”

【实验目的】

(1) 掌握菌种保藏的目的和基本原理。

(2) 熟悉几种常用的菌种保藏方法。

【实验原理】

当某一微生物菌株得到分离纯化后，就应该以某种形式将其保存起来而不受污染。通常情况下，纯培养物应进行周期性传代以保证其连续生长。传代过程必须使用无菌操作技术。不过，由于连续传代既耗费时间又有菌种变异和污染的风险，所以必要时需要多种其他菌种保藏方法。常用的方法包括：传代保藏法、液体石蜡保藏法、沙土保藏法、低温冷冻保藏法和冷冻干燥保藏法等。

无论使用哪种方法，其基本原理都是使微生物的生命活动处于半永久性的休眠状态，也就是使微生物的新陈代谢作用限制在最低的范围内。干燥、低温和隔绝空气是使微生物代谢能力降低的重要因素，是保证获得这种状态的主要措施。现将每种方法介绍如下。

1. 传代保藏法　菌株可以通过定期从原培养物传代至新鲜培养基中的方法进行保存，这是最简单的保藏方法。培养基种类、保藏温度和传代频率因菌种而异，但需提前确认。对需氧菌可用斜面培养，对厌氧菌可进行穿刺培养，培养后于4℃冰箱内保存。此法为实验

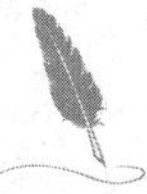

室和工厂菌种室常用的保藏法，优点是操作简单，使用方便，不需特殊设备；缺点是传代次数多，容易变异、污染杂菌。保藏时间因菌种而异，从数周至数月不等。

2. 液体石蜡保藏法 在斜面培养物或穿刺培养物上面覆盖1cm灭菌的液体石蜡后置4℃冰箱直立保存。这样可防止固体培养基中的水分蒸发而引起的菌种死亡，另一方面液体石蜡可阻止氧气进入，使好氧菌不能继续生长，从而延长了菌种保藏的时间，从数月至数年不等。此法的优点是操作简单，不需特殊设备；缺点是在保存过程中，菌种必须直立放置，所占空间较大，且菌种容易变异。

3. 沙土保藏法 去除水分可以降低微生物的代谢速度，因而这一方法对那些形成孢子的微生物比如放线菌和霉菌更加有效。因此在抗生素生产中应用最广、效果最好。操作是将微生物吸附在适当的无菌载体，如灭菌处理的土壤、沙子上，而后进行干燥处理。此法可保存约2～10年，但应用于营养细胞效果不佳。

4. 低温冷冻保藏法 也可称为液氮（－196℃）保藏法。适用于各种微生物菌种的长期保藏。处理过程中为防止低温结冰带来的对细胞的伤害，通常需要加入保护剂（甘油、二甲基亚砜等）。其优点是菌种性状不变异，保藏时间可达10～30年。但需液氮罐等特殊设备，成本较高。

5. 冷冻干燥保藏法 先使微生物在低温度（－70℃左右）下快速冷冻，然后在减压下利用升华现象除去水分（真空干燥），利用有利于菌种保藏的一切因素，使微生物始终处于低温、干燥、缺氧的条件下，因而它是迄今为止最有效的菌种保藏法之一。

用冷冻干燥保藏的菌种，其保藏期可达数年至数十年，其菌种要特别注意纯度，不能污染杂菌，这样再次使用该菌种时才不会出差错。细菌和酵母菌菌种要求培养到稳定期，一般细菌培养24～48小时，酵母菌培养3天，放线菌与霉菌一般需培养7～10天，若用对数生长期菌种进行保藏，其存活率反而会降低。此方法保存孢子比其营养体效果更好。

此法也需使用保护剂来制备细胞悬液，对于细菌的液态菌种，简便易行的方法是将液态菌种与已灭菌的80%浓度的甘油等量混合后置－20℃保存，可保存较长时间。由于本法对仪器要求较高，所以在方法中暂不介绍。

【实验材料】

1. 菌种 细菌，酵母菌，放线菌，霉菌。

2. 培养基及试剂 固体斜面培养基，灭菌脱脂牛乳，灭菌水，液体石蜡，甘油，五氧化二磷，河沙，黄土，冰块，食盐，干冰，95%酒精，10%稀盐酸，无水氯化钙。

3. 仪器 超低温冰箱（－80℃），液氮罐。

4. 其他 无菌吸管，无菌培养皿，安瓿，40目与100目筛子，油纸。

【实验方法】

1. 传代保藏法

（1）斜面低温保藏法：将对数期菌种接种于固体斜面培养基上，待菌充分生长后，移至4℃的冰箱中保藏。

（2）穿刺法：将半固体培养基注入小试管（0.8cm×10cm），使培养基距离试管口约2～3cm深。用灭过菌的接菌针无菌操作挑取培养物，在半固体培养基顶部的中央直线穿刺到半固体培养基的1/3深处，在适宜条件下培养后，熔封试管或是塞上橡皮塞，移至4℃的冰箱中保藏。

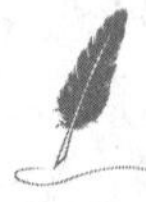

2. 液体石蜡保藏法

（1）将液体石蜡高压灭菌（1.05kg/cm^2、121.3℃）30分钟。

（2）将菌种接种至斜面培养基中培养，使其充分生长。

（3）用无菌吸管吸取液体石蜡注入斜面，其用量以高出斜面顶端1cm为准。

（4）保持试管直立，置4℃保存。

（5）从液体石蜡下面取培养物移种后，接种环在火焰烧灼时，培养物容易与残留的液体石蜡一起飞溅，应特别注意。

3. 沙土保藏法

（1）取河沙加入10%稀盐酸浸泡，去除有机杂质。

（2）倒去酸水，用自来水冲洗至中性，烘干。用40目筛子过筛，去掉粗颗粒，备用。

（3）取非耕作层的瘦黄土，磨细，100目筛子过筛。

（4）按一份土、三份沙掺合均匀，装入小试管中，每管装1cm左右，灭菌。

（5）抽样进行无菌检查，每10支沙土管抽一支，将沙土倒入肉汤培养基中，37℃培养48h，若仍有杂菌，则需重新灭菌。

（6）接种方法分干法接种和湿法接种：

干法接种（多用于保藏放线菌和部分真菌）：将斜面上已生长好的培养物，用接菌环或接菌铲刮取孢子，接种于无菌的沙土管中，搅拌均匀，注意勿接入培养基。

湿法接种：选择培养成熟的（一般指孢子层生长丰满的）优良菌种，将已生长好的菌种斜面培养物用3～5ml无菌水洗下，制成均匀的菌悬液，再用无菌吸管吸取菌悬液加到沙管中，每管约10滴约0.5ml。接种后的沙土管放于真空泵中抽干以除去沙土管中的水分，抽干时间越短越好。

（7）每10支抽取一支，用接种环取出少数沙粒，接种于斜面上，培养后观察生长情况和有无杂菌。

（8）若经检查没有问题，用火焰熔封管口，放冰箱或室内干燥处保存。每半年检查一次活力和杂菌情况。

（9）菌种复活培养时，取沙土少许移入液体培养基内培养。

4. 低温冷冻保藏法

（1）准备安瓿管：用于液氮保藏的安瓿管，需要采用硼硅酸盐玻璃制成的，能耐受温度突然变化而不致破裂。安瓿管的大小通常为7.5mm×100mm，能容1.2ml液体。将空安瓿管塞上棉塞，高压灭菌。

（2）准备保护剂与灭菌：保护剂如10%甘油或10%二甲基亚砜。含甘油溶液需经高压灭菌，含二甲基亚砜溶液则采用过滤除菌。保存细菌、酵母菌或霉菌孢子等容易分散的细胞时，则将空安瓿管塞上棉塞；若保存霉菌菌丝体用，则需在安瓿管内预先加入保护剂如10%二甲基亚砜蒸馏水溶液或10%甘油蒸馏水溶液，加入量以能浸没以后加入的菌块为限。0.1MPa高压蒸汽灭菌20分钟。

（3）接入菌种：将菌种用10%的甘油蒸馏水溶液制成菌悬液，装入无菌的安瓿管；霉菌菌丝体可用无菌打孔器，从平板内切取菌落圆块，放入装有保护剂的安瓿管内，然后用火焰熔封，浸入水中检查有无漏洞。

（4）冻结：将已封口的安瓿管以每分钟下降1℃的慢速冻结至－80℃。避免细胞急剧冷冻（在细胞内会形成冰的结晶，降低存活率）。

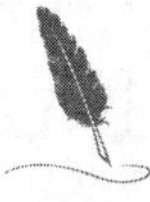

(5) 保藏：将冻结至 -80℃的安瓿管立即放入液氮冷冻保藏器的小圆筒内，再将小圆筒放入液氮保藏器内。液氮保藏器内的气相为 -150℃，液态氮内为 -196℃。

(6) 恢复培养：需要用保藏的菌种时，将安瓿管取出，立即放入38℃ ~40℃水浴急速解冻，直到全部溶化为止。再采用无菌操作技术，打开安瓿管，将内容物移入适宜的培养基上培养。

【结果与讨论】

(1) 经常使用的细菌菌种，应用哪一种方法保藏既好又简便？

(2) 细菌用什么方法保藏的时间长而又不易变异？

(3) 产孢子的微生物常用哪一种方法保藏？

EXPERIMENT 17 Preservation of Pure Cultures

Purposes

(1) To grasp the purposes and principles of pure culture preservation.

(2) To be familiar with the routine methods of pure culture preservation.

Principles

Once a microorganism has been isolated and grown in pure culture, it becomes necessary to maintain the viability and purity of the microorganism by keeping the pure cultures free from contamination. As a common practice in laboratory, the pure cultures are transferred periodically onto or into a fresh medium (sub - culturing) to allow continuous growth of microorganisms and maintain their viability. The transfer is conducted under aseptic conditions to avoid contamination. Repeated sub - culturing is time - consuming and poses the risk of genetic changes as well as contamination. As a result, some alternative methods that do not need frequent sub - culturing have been developed, including paraffin method, sand and soil method, cryopreservation, and lyophilization (freeze drying).

The basic principle of culture preservation is to keep the microorganisms in a semi - perpetual dormant state, which can minimize the metabolism activity of microorganisms. The most important factors of decreasing the metabolism are desiccation, low temperature and air isolation. This experiment will give a basic introduction to different methods for pure culture maintenance.

1. Subculture method Strains can be maintained by periodically preparing a fresh culture from the previous stock culture. This is the simplest method for preservation. The culture medium, the storage temperature, and the time intervalof the transfer all vary with the species and must be ascertained beforehand. For aerobes, they are usually cultivated on agar slants. While for anaerobes, stab culture is often performed. Store at 4℃ after incubation. The advantage of this method includes easy operation, convenience in use and no need for special equipment. However, disadvantages of genetic mutation and contamination may occur due to frequent passage.

2. Paraffin method Add 1cm depth of sterile liquid paraffin to cover the slant or stab cultures then store at 4℃. It can maintain the cultures due to the prevention of evaporation of water in solid culture medium and isolation of oxygen to stop the growth of aerobes. This method can prolong

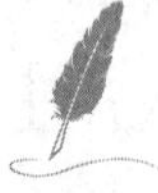

the preservation period to several months to years. This method is easy to operate and does not need special equipment, but the cultural tubes must be kept erect.

3. Sand and soil method Removal of water can reduce the rate of microbial metabolism. This method is applicable to preserve the spores of molds and actinomycetes. So it is widely used in the antibiotic industry. The procedures are to make the microorganisms adsorbed to suitable sterile carriers, such as soil or sand, then dry the specimens. They can be preserved for about 2 ~ 10 years. But the method is not suitable for vegetative cells.

4. Cryopreservation It is also called liquid nitrogen method which fit for long term preservationof all kinds of microbes. In this method, the cultured microorganisms are rapidly frozen in liquid nitrogen at -196℃ in the presence of stabilizing agents such as glycerol or Dimethyl Sulfoxide (DMSO) that prevent the cell damage by forming ice crystals and promote cell survival. The advantage is preservation for 10 ~ 30 years without causing genetic mutation. However, special and expensive equipment such as liquid nitrogen container is required..

5. Lyophilization (Freeze - Drying) Freeze - drying is a process where water and other solvents are removed from a frozen product via sublimation. Sublimation occurs when a frozen liquid goes directly to a gaseous state without entering a liquid phase. Freeze the microorganisms rapidly at low temperature (about -70℃), then remove the water under reduced pressure by sublimation (vacuum desiccation). Lyophilization is the most effective method to preserve cultures since it keeps the microorganisms under a dry, low - temperature and free - from - oxygen condition that is very favorable to culture preservation.

The cultures that are preserved by freeze - drying can be maintained for several decades, but attention must be paid to their purity to prevent contamination for later use. Bacteria and yeasts are required to be cultivated to stationary phase, generally, 24 ~ 48 hours for bacteria, 3 days for yeasts, 7 ~ 10 days for actinomycetes and molds. If cultures in logarithmic (log) phase are used, the survival rate will decrease. It is preferred for preservation of spores instead of vegetative cells.

This method involves the use ofstabilizing agents as well. For liquid cultures of bacteria, mix the culture with 80% sterilized glycerin and then preserve at -20℃. Lyophilization will not be discussed here due to the need for special instruments.

Materials and Apparatus

1. Cultures bacteria, yeasts, actinomycetes and molds.

2. Media and other materials agar slant culture, degrease milk, sterile water, liquid paraffin, glycerol, sandy and soil, ice, salt, dry - ice, 95% alcohol, 10% HCl, anhydrous $CaCl_2$.

3. Apparatus sterile pipette, sterile dish, ampoules, sieve (40 mesh and 100 mesh), oilpaper, desiccator, vacuum pump, blowtorch, lower temperature refrigerator (-30℃), ultra - cold freezer, liquid nitrogen frozen incubator.

Procedures

1. Subculturing

(1) Slant cultivation: The cultures are inoculated to the agar slant and then incubated at optimal temperature. Keep in the refrigerator at 4℃ after they are well grown.

(2) Stab cultivation: Transfer the semi - solid mediainto a small tube (0.8cm × 10cm) with a

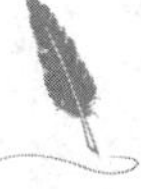

2 ~ 3cm distance away from the top of the tube. Use an aseptic inoculating needle to transfer cells from agar slants and stab into 1/3 depth of the semi – solid culture media without touching the walls. After incubating at optimal conditions, seal or plug the tube and then store it at 4℃.

2. Paraffin method

(1) Sterilize the paraffin with autoclave for 30 minutes (1.05 kg/cm^2, 121℃).

(2) Inoculate the microbial strain to an agar slant and incubate until they are well grown.

(3) Pour sterile liquid paraffin onto the agar slantto make the surface of paraffin is 1 cm higher than the top of the slant surface.

(4) Keep the tube erectly at 4℃.

Precautions should be taken when inoculating from liquid paraffin since flaming of the inoculating loop can make the cultures plash together with the liquid paraffin.

3. Sand and soil method

(1) Using 10% HCl to wash out the organic impurity in river sand.

(2) Remove the acid solution, wash the sand to neutral pH with tap water, dry and sift with 40 mesh sieve.

(3) Take non – cultivated soil and sift with 100 mesh sieve.

(4) Mix loess with sand in a ratio of 1 to 3. Put them into small test tubes with a height of 1cm and then sterilize.

(5) Carry on sterility test by randomly taking one tube out of ten. Mix the content with broth culture media and place them in a 37℃ incubator for 48h. Re – sterilize if any microbial growth appears.

(6) For inoculation, there are two methods as follows:

Dry method (for the preservation of actinomycetes and some molds): transfer a loopful of spores of well grown culture and inoculate into the soil tube with thorough mixing. Do not inoculate the culture media into the tube.

Wet method: Add 3 ~ 5ml of sterile water into the slant culture (well grown with spores) to make spore suspension. Add 10 drops (0.5ml) of the suspension to each soil tube. Put the tubes into a vacuum desiccator to remove the water as fast as possible.

(7) Take one tube out of ten and transfer some sands onto an agar slant. Incubate properly and observe the growth as well as contamination.

(8) If the result is good, seal the tubes and preserve them in a refrigerator or some dry places. Examine the viability and purity every 6 months.

(9) Inoculate the sands into liquid medium whenthe culture is rejuvenated.

4. Cryopreservation

(1) Prepare the ampoules Choose silicon borate glass ampoules that won't crack under sudden changes of temperature, The ampoules are usually 7.5mm × 100mm, with a volume of 1.2ml. Tampon the ampoules and sterilize them.

(2) Prepare the protective agents and sterilize Prepare 10% glycerol or 10% dimethylsulfoxide as protective agents. The former is sterilized by autoclaving while the latter is sterilized by filtration. As for preservation of mold mycelium, it is necessary to add the protecting agents such as 10%

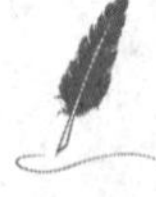

glycerol in ampoules and sterilize for 20 min at 0.1Mpa.

(3) Inoculation　Prepare spore suspension using 10% glycerol and add it into sterile ampoules. As for mold mycelium, you may cut a piece of colony block into the ampoule with protective agent. Seal the tubes and dip them into water to inspect whether they are leaking.

(4) Freezing　Freeze the ampoules slowly with 1℃ drop per minute till −30℃. (Sharp decrease in temperature should be avoided in order to prevent the formation of crystals within the cells and consequence decrease in viability).

(5) Preservation　Place the ampoules into liquid nitrogen incubator (gas nitrogen −150℃ and liquid nitrogen −196℃).

(6) Rejuvenation　During rejuvenation, take out the ampoules and put them in 38℃ ~ 40℃ water bath to ice-out rapidly until they totally thaw. Open the ampoules and transfer the culture into the proper culture media.

Results and Discussion

(1) Which method is preferred for maintenance of frequently used bacteria strain?

(2) Which method can achieve long-term preservation without causing mutation?

(3) Which method is suitable for spore-forming microbes?

实验十八　微生物计数法

扫码“学一学”

【实验目的】

(1) 熟悉对单细胞微生物进行计数的常用方法及其原理。

(2) 了解血球计数板的构造、原理，并掌握利用血球计数板测定微生物浓度的方法。

(3) 了解平板活菌计数法的基本原理和操作步骤。

【实验原理】

微生物的生长通常用群体生长量来描述而并非用单个细胞的生长作为指标。群体生长情况可以通过测定单位时间里微生物细胞数目的增加或细胞物质的增加来评价。常见的测定方法有：①显微镜直接计数法；②间接计数法——平板活菌计数法；③测量细胞生物量（如干重或湿重）；④细胞中某种成分如蛋白质、核酸等的含量测定法；⑤光电比浊法等。每种方法都有一定的适用范围，因此工作中应根据具体情况加以选择。本实验主要介绍前两种——显微镜直接计数法和平板活菌计数法，光电比浊法将在下一实验中有所涉及。

1. 显微镜直接计数法　即利用血球计数板在显微镜下直接计数，是一种常用的微生物计数方法，各种单细胞菌体的纯培养悬液、单孢子悬液以及各种微生物细胞的原生质体等均可采用血球计数板计数。将适宜浓度的孢子悬液（或菌悬液）放在血球计数板载玻片与盖玻片之间的计数室内，由于计数板上的计数室盖上盖玻片后的容积（0.1 mm^3）是一定的，所以可以根据在显微镜下观察到的细胞数目换算为单位体积内的细胞数目。

血球计数板是一块特制的厚载玻片，载玻片上有由四条槽构成的3个平台（图18-1阴影部分）。中间的平台较宽，其中间又被一短横槽分隔成上下两部分，每个半边平台上面各有一个计数室。计数室的刻度有两种：一种是计数室分为16个中方格，每个中方格又分成25个小方格（图18-2）；另一种是计数室分成25个中方格，每个中方格又分成16个小方

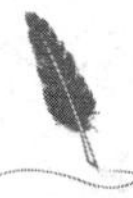

格。不管是哪一种刻度，计数室都由400个小方格组成。

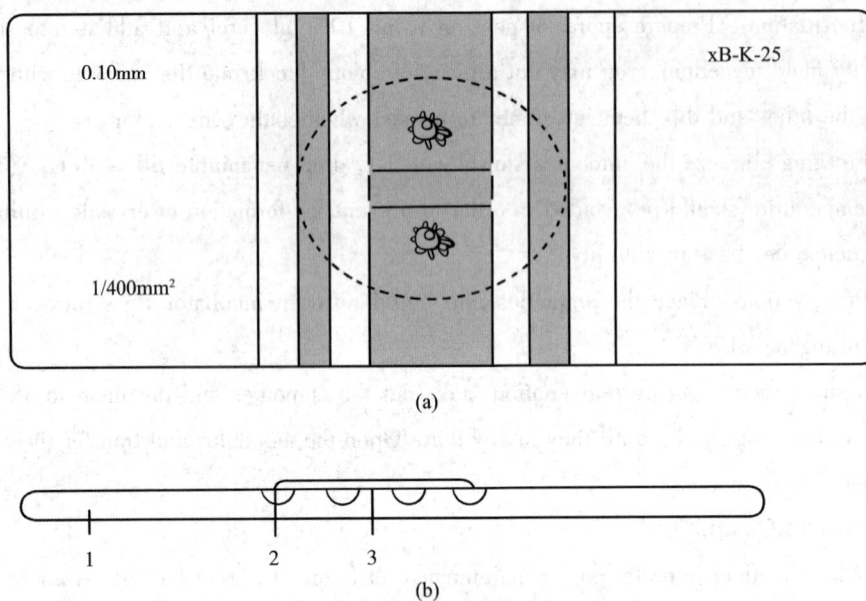

0.10mm

xB-K-25

1/400mm²

(a)

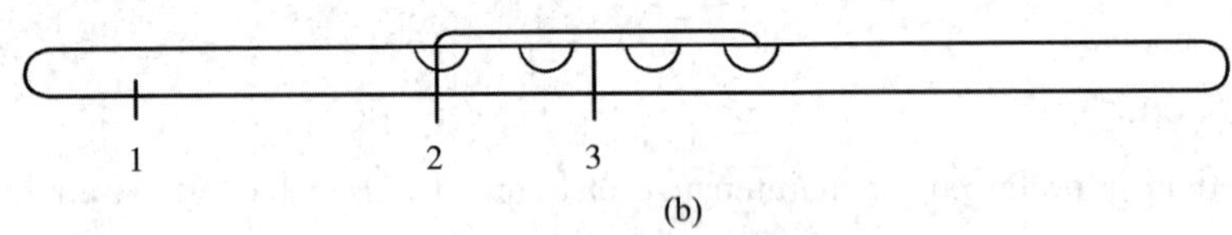

(b)

图18－1　血球计数板的构造

（a）正面图　（b）侧面图

1. 血球计数板；2. 盖玻片；3. 计数室

图18－2（a）中央为计数室，计数室的面积为$1mm^2$，盖上盖玻片后，载玻片与盖玻片之间的距离为0.1mm，所以每个计数室的体积为$0.1mm^3$。计数过程中，若计数室由16个中方格组成，一般计数左上、左下、右上、右下的4个中方格（共计100个小格）的细胞数或孢子数；如果计数室由25个中方格组成，除计数上述4个中方格外，还需计数在最中央的中方格的菌数或孢子数（共计80个小格）。在计数的过程中要不断地调节细调节旋钮，以便能看到计数室内不同深度的细胞或孢子。凡是落在中格左方和上方双线上的孢子或细胞都计算在内，而落在下方或右方双线上的孢子或细胞均不计算在内。最后可求出每小格的平均细胞数或孢子数，按照下列公式算出原细胞（孢子）悬液的细胞（孢子）浓度：

$$样品中细胞数（个/ml）=每小格的平均数\times 400\times 稀释倍数\times 10000$$

其中，10000代表1ml的容积（即$1000mm^3$）是一个计数室容积（$0.1mm^3$）的10000倍。

2. 平板活菌计数法　该法是最常用的活菌计数方法，其依据是：微生物在高度稀释条件下，在固体培养基上形成的一个菌落是由一个单细胞繁殖形成的，因此一个菌落形成单位（CFU）即代表一个细胞。在计数的时候，首先将待测样品做系列稀释，使待测样品中的微生物细胞成单个细胞状态存在，再取一定量的稀释菌液接种到固体培养基平板中（平板接种培养有涂布平板和混合平板法两种方法），使其均匀地分布于培养基表面或内部，经适宜条件培养后，单个细胞生长繁殖形成菌落，计数菌落数目，即可换算出样品中的菌浓度。

平板活菌计数法常用于生物制品的检验、土壤含菌量的测定以及食品、水源的污染程度的检验等。

【实验材料】

1. 菌种　酵母菌48小时液体培养物，大肠埃希菌18～20小时液体培养物。

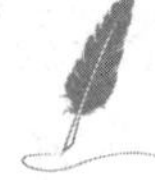

2. 培养基　营养肉汤琼脂培养基。

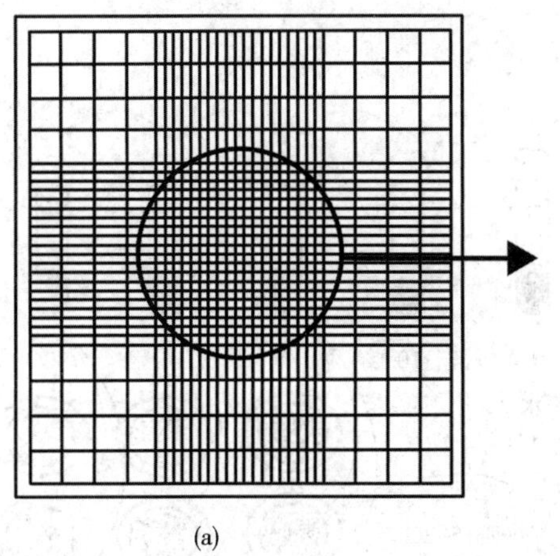
(a)

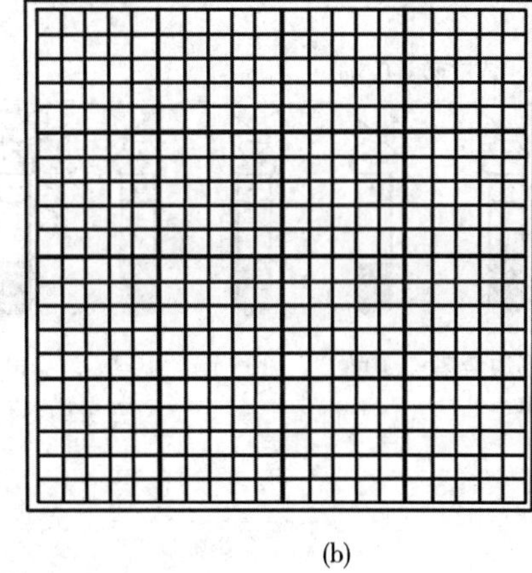
(b)

图 18－2　计数室放大图

3. 仪器　明视野显微镜，恒温培养箱。

4. 其他　血细胞计数板，滴管，擦镜纸，移液管，接种环，试管等。

【实验方法】

1. 用血细胞计数板对酵母菌悬液进行计数

（1）稀释：定量取出酵母菌液体培养物，加到无菌干燥的试管中，按照一定倍数将其稀释，稀释的程度以血细胞计数板每小格内含有 5～10 个细胞最为合适。

（2）镜检计数室：对计数室进行镜检，若有污物，则需清洗后才能进行计数。

（3）加样：将血细胞计数板盖上盖玻片，用无菌滴管从盖玻片的边缘滴 1 滴酵母菌液，则菌液会在虹吸作用下自行渗入，注意不要产生气泡。

（4）计数：静置 5 分钟，使细胞沉降不再流动，然后即可在显微镜下观察计数。先在低倍镜下找到计数室的位置，然后换成高倍镜计数。如发现菌液太浓，应重新稀释并计数。每一个样品的计数都要对两个计数室中的计算结果取平均值，以减少实验误差。

（5）清洗：计数完毕，将血细胞计数板取下，盖玻片放入指定器皿中（不回收），血细胞计数板先以 75% 乙醇清洗，再以蒸馏水淋洗，切忌用硬物洗刷，然后自然风干，镜检观察是否有细胞或其他沉积物，确认清洗干净。

2. 平板活菌计数

（1）编号：分别取 9 支盛有 4.5ml 无菌水的试管，依次标记 10^{-1}、10^{-2}、10^{-3}、10^{-4}、10^{-5}、10^{-6}、10^{-7}、10^{-8}、10^{-9}，另取无菌平皿 9 套，分别编号 10^{-7}、10^{-8}、10^{-9}各三皿。

（2）稀释液的制备：用一支 1ml 无菌移液管精确吸取 0.5ml 大肠埃希菌悬液加到 10^{-1}试管中，并用此移液管将管内悬液反复吸吹三次，使菌悬液混合均匀。另取一支 1ml 无菌移液管从 10^{-1}试管中精确吸取 0.5ml 加到 10^{-2}试管中，反复吸吹三次。其余各管依此类推。整个稀释过程见图 18－3。若待检测样品为固体时，一般准确称取待测样品 10g，放入装有 90ml 无菌水的 250ml 三角瓶中，充分振荡 20 分钟，使微生物细胞分散，静置 30 秒，即是 10^{-1}稀释液，其余稀释操作法与上述相同。

（3）制备混菌平板：用 1ml 无菌移液管精确吸取 10^{-7}的稀释液 0.5ml，对应加入已编号 10^{-7}的无菌培养皿中（共三皿）。在每皿中倒入融化并冷却至 45℃～50℃的牛肉膏蛋白胨琼脂培养基 15～20ml，迅速轻轻晃动以混匀平板，静置，待培养基凝固后倒置，于 37℃恒温培养箱中培养 48 小时后计数。10^{-8}、10^{-9}稀释度的菌液同法操作。

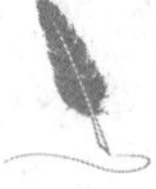

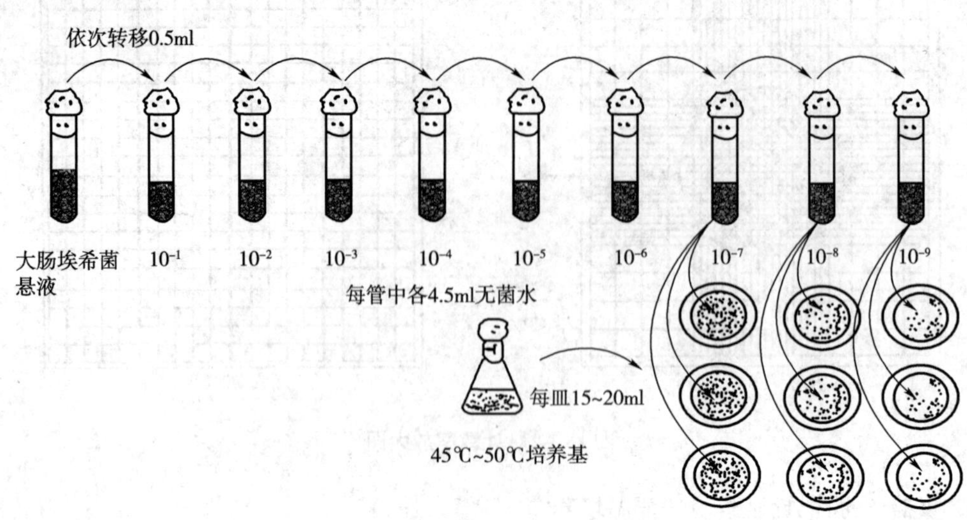

图 18－3　混合平板活菌计数法示意图

此步骤也可用平板涂布法：先将培养基融化后倒入已编号的 9 套无菌平皿中，待凝固后，用无菌移液管分别吸取 0.5ml 相应稀释度的菌液对应加到上述已制备好的无菌平板表面，然后以无菌操作技术，用无菌涂布棒将培养基表面的菌液涂均匀（每个稀释度更换一个涂布棒）；将涂布过的平板置于桌面放置 20 分钟，使菌液渗入培养基中，最后将平板倒置于 37℃培养箱中培养 48 小时。

（4）计数：待培养菌落长出后取出平板，计数同一稀释度的三个平板的菌落数，并计算其平均值，按下面公式换算每毫升样品的总活菌数。

总活菌数（个/ml）＝同一稀释度的三个平皿的菌落数的平均值×稀释倍数×2

【结果与讨论】

（1）显微镜直接计数法　将实验结果填入表 18－1，计算出每毫升酵母菌液中含有的总细胞数。

表 18－1　显微镜直接计数法实验结果

计数次数	每中格内菌数（个）						每小格内菌数	稀释倍数	样品
	1	2	3	4	5	平均值	平均值		个/ml
第一次									
第二次									
平均值									

（2）平板活菌计数法　将实验结果填入表 18－2，计算每毫升待测样品中大肠埃希菌的活菌数。

表 18－2　平板活菌计数法实验结果

稀释度	10^{-7}				10^{-8}				10^{-9}			
	1	2	3	平均	1	2	3	平均	1	2	3	平均
菌落数												
总活菌数/ml												

（3）在混合培养法中，为什么融化后的培养基要冷却至45℃～50℃才能倒平板？

（4）试比较平板活菌计数法和显微镜直接计数法的优缺点并对这两种方法进行误差分析。

EXPERIMENT 18 Counting of Microorganisms

Purposes

(1) To be familiar with the manipulations and principles of commonly used methods for microbial counting.

(2) To understand the structure and principle of blood counting chamber. Grasp the method of determining the concentration of microbes by using blood counting chamber.

(3) To understand the principle and manipulation of viable plate count.

Principles

The index of microbial growth is usuallyreflected by the growth of a cell population rather than a single cell. The growth of microorganisms can be assessed by the increase in cell numbers or in cell biomass in given time and conditions. The commonly used methods include: ① Direct microscopic count; ② Indirect count—viable plate techniques; ③Measurement of microbial biomass (dry weight or wet weight); ④ Measurement of relatively constant cellular components of cells, such as protein and nucleic acid; ⑤ Turbidimetry. Each of these methods has particular range of application, so the method selection varies in practice. This experiment focuses on the first two methods and the last method will be described in the next experiment.

1. Direct microscopic count is used to determine the total number of microbial cells under the microscope by using the blood counting chamber for various unicellular microbes including bacteria, yeasts, spores and protoplasts. Because the testing volume in the blood counting chamber covered with a cover slip is constant ($0.1mm^3$), the total microbial number can be calculated according to the cell number on the blood counting chamber.

The blood counting chamber is a special piece of thick glass slide which contains three platforms (shadow in fig. 18－1) separated by four grooves. The middle platform is divided into 2 parts with a counting chamber laid on each. There are two kinds of counting chamber: one is divided to 16 squares each of which contains 25 smaller squares; the other is divided into 25 squares with 16 smaller squares on each. Both types of blood counting chambers contain 400 small squares.

In fig. 18－2, the counting room is in the center of the left part and is magnified on the right. The volume of the counting chamber is $0.1mm^3$ because the area of each chamber is $1mm^2$, and the height between the slide and the cover slip is 0.1mm. When using a 16－square counting chamber, cells (spores) in the 4 squares located at upper left, bottom left, upper right and bottom right (in total 100 smaller squares) need to be counted. While using the 25－square counting chamber, another square in the middle also needs to be counted besides the 4 squares mentioned above (in total 80 smaller squares). When counting, the fine adjustment knob needs to be constantly adjusted in order to focus on the cells (spores) located in different depth. For the cells located on double lines of the chamber, following rules are usually applied: The cells which located on top

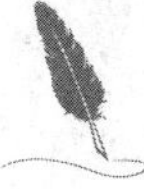

lines or left lines will be counted while the ones on bottom lines or right lines are omitted. Finally the average concentration of the original cell (spores) suspension can be calculated as follows:

Cell number/ml = average cell number in each smaller square × 400 × dilution ratio × 10000

The 10000 means that 1ml (1000mm^3) is 10000 times to the counting room volume (0.1mm^3).

2. Viable plate technique: is the most commonly used method for viable counting. Because every single colony arises from an individual cell that has undergone cell division on solid medium, one colony forming unit (CFU) represents one cell. In this method, gradient dilution of a sample is performed before inoculation on agar plates. The microbial suspension can be either spread onto the agar surfaces after solidification or mixed with the medium first and then poured into plates to solidify. After incubatingunder suitable conditions, colonies can be formed and counted. The concentration of the cells in the original sample can be calculated as well.

Viable plate counting is widely used in examining biological products, determining the number of microbes in soil and estimating the contamination degree in food and water.

Materials and Apparatus

1. **Specimens** 48h broth culture of *Saccharomyces cerevisiae*, 18 ~ 20h broth culture of *Escherichia coli.*

2. **Media** nutrient broth agar.

3. **Apparatus** Incubator, bright - field microscope.

4. **Others** blood counting chamber, dropper, lens paper, pipette, inoculation loop, tube.

Procedures

(1) Direct microscopic count with blood counting chamber:

1. **Diluting** Transfer quantitative yeast suspension to sterile dry tubes and dilute it in series until there are only 5 ~ 10 cells in each smaller square of the counting room.

2. **Examining** Observe the counting room under a microscope after to making sure the counting room is not contaminated.

3. **Loading** Cover the counting chamber with a cover slip. Siphon a drop of diluent to the edge of the cover slip. Be careful not to make bubbles.

4. **Counting** Allow to stand for 5min. Focus the counting chamber under the microscope with low power lens first and then switch to high power lens. If the cell concentration was too high, dilute and count again. The average of the two counting chamber is necessary to reduce the experimental error.

5. **Cleaning** After counting, rinse the blood counting chamber with 75% ethanol and water to ensure thorough cleaning. Don't use any tough implement to clean the surface of blood counting chamber.

(2) Viable plate technique:

1. **Labeling** Label 9 tubes containing 4.5ml sterile water with 10^{-1} to 10^{-9} and label 9 plates with 10^{-7}, 10^{-8}, 10^{-9} respectively (3 plates for every dilution).

2. **Diluting** Serial dilution is achieved by adding quantitative *Escherichia coli* suspension to 4.5ml water - containing tubes. 0.5ml of *Escherichia coli* suspension (with a sterile pipette) is first-

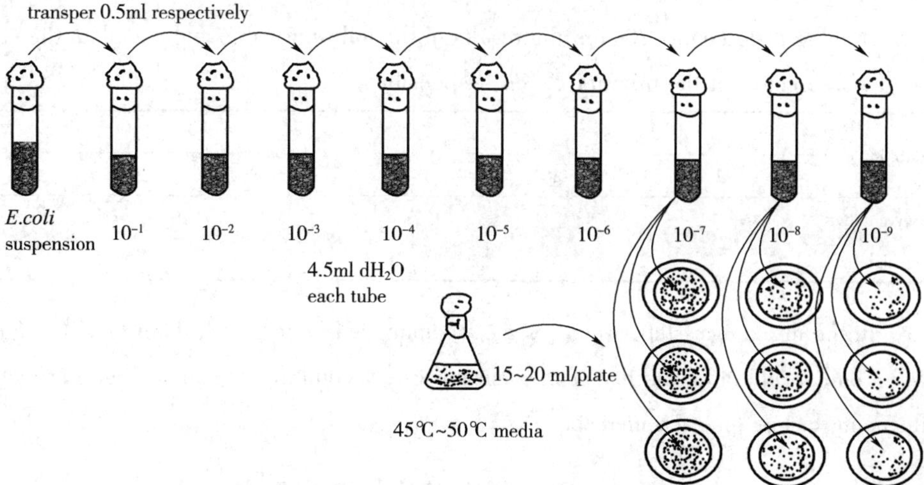

Fig. **18 – 3** Diagram of Viable count tachnique

ly added to the 10^{-1} tube to make the 10^{-1} dilution. After mixing adequately, transfer 0. 5ml of the suspension from the 10^{-1} tube to the 10^{-2} tube with another sterile pipette and the dilutability is 10^{-2}. The whole dilution procedure is shown in fig. 18 – 3. If the sample was solid, 10g of sample could be added to a 250ml flask containing 90ml sterile water and then shake for 20 mins followed by standing for 30sec. The dilutability is also 10^{-1}. The other dilutions could be achieved by the same method mentioned above.

3. Preparing mixed agar plates Using a sterile pipette, transfer 0. 5ml of the 10^{-7} *E. coli* suspension to each labeled (10^{-7}) plate respectively. Then pour about 15 ~ 20ml of medium at 45℃ ~ 50 ℃ into the plate and mix gently and immediately. After solidification, incubate the agar plate upside down at 37 ℃ for 48h.

This step can also be done with the spread plate technique: The preparation of sterile nutrient agar plates needs to be done first. After solidification, add 0. 5ml of bacteria suspension (10^{-7}、10^{-8}、10^{-9}) onto the surface of the corresponding agar plate. Use sterile spreaders to spread uniformly (one spreader should be used only for one dilution). After standing for 20 minutes for penetration, incubate the plates at 37 ℃ for 48h upside down.

4. Counting after incubation, count the number of colonies of the same dilutability and calculate the average value. Then calculate the concentration of microorganisms in the original suspension according to the following formula:

Total viable number/ml = the average of colonies (same dilutability) × dilution ratio × 2

Results and Discussion

(1) Direct microscopic counting: Record the results in the following table and calculate the concentration of the total count in the original yeast suspension.

	Cell number in each square						Average in a smaller square	Dilution ratio	Cell concentration (/ml)
	1	2	3	4	5	Average			
First counting									
Second counting									
Average									

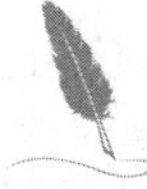

(2) Viable plate count: Record the results in the following table and calculate the concentration of the viable count in the original *E. coli* suspension.

Dilutability	10^{-8}											
	1	2	3	average	1	2	3	average	1	2	3	Average
Colony number												
Viablecell number /ml												

(3) In the mixed agar step, why does the medium need to be cooled down to 45℃ ~50 ℃?

(4) Compare the applicability of microscopic direct counting and plate counting method. List the influencing factors for each method.

实验十九　细菌的生长曲线测定

扫码“学一学”

【实验目的】

(1) 掌握光电比浊计数法测定细菌生长曲线的方法。

(2) 了解光电比浊计数法的原理和细菌生长曲线的特点。

【实验原理】

在微生物学的研究和生产实践中，为了及时掌握发酵培养过程中的微生物生长情况，需要定时测定培养液中微生物的数量，以便对培养条件进行适当控制，获得最佳的培养物。细菌的生长一般指群体的生长，常常具有一定的规律性。描述细菌在液体培养基中生长规律的曲线叫生长曲线。将一定量的细菌接种到一定体积的液体培养基中，在适宜的条件下进行培养，以培养时间为横坐标，以菌数的对数为纵坐标进行作图即得到生长曲线。典型的生长曲线可分为延迟期、对数生长期、稳定期和衰亡期四个时期。

细菌在液体培养基中生长时，由于原生质含量的增加，会引起培养物混浊度的增高。细菌悬液的混浊度和透光度成反比、与光密度成正比，透光度或光密度可借助光电比浊计精确测出，因此可用光电比浊计测定细胞悬液的光密度（OD 值），表示该菌在特定实验条件下细菌的相对数目，进而反映出其相对生长量。本法的优点是操作简便迅速，可连续测定并及时看到结果，但缺点是无法区分死菌和活菌。可采用上一实验中的活菌平板计数法对实验中各培养时间的细菌悬液进行测数，以大肠埃希菌悬液光密度值为横坐标，以活菌数目为纵坐标，可绘制一条标准曲线。这样便可在测定任意培养时间菌悬液的光密度值后，在标准曲线上查出活菌总数。该方法较稀释平板菌落计数法节省时间，已经广泛应用在工业生产上。

本实验将以大肠埃希菌为例，讲述比浊法测定生长曲线的操作过程。

【实验材料】

1. 菌种　大肠埃希菌（*Escherichia coli*）16 ~18 小时斜面培养物。

2. 培养基与试剂　牛肉膏蛋白胨液体培养基，无菌生理盐水。

3. 仪器　721 型分光光度计，摇床。

4. 其他　三角瓶，试管，1ml 无菌移液管。

【实验方法】

1. 菌种准备　以无菌操作技术将大肠埃希菌接入装有 100ml 牛肉膏蛋白胨液体培养基

的三角瓶中，37℃，180r/min，振荡培养18小时。

2. 接种与培养　取预先编号的17支分别装有10ml牛肉膏蛋白胨液体培养基的大试管，采用无菌操作技术，用移液管向其中16支试管（编号0～16）准确加入大肠埃希菌悬液0.2ml，轻轻振荡混匀，将第17支试管设为空白对照组（不加大肠埃希菌悬液），用于调仪器零点。迅速拿出1号管于分光光度计上测定OD_{600}，此为零时的读数。除零点试管外，将接种后的剩余16支试管置于摇床上，37℃，180r/min，振荡培养。

3. 比浊测定　按照实验结果表格中所列培养时间定时取样测定OD_{600}，取样时需摇匀样品，测得的光密度值应在0.1～0.65（如超出范围，可将大肠埃希菌培养液进行适当稀释），每次都要以没有接种的空白对照组液体培养基调零点，依次进行OD值的测定。

4. 绘制生长曲线　以光密度（OD值）为纵坐标，培养时间为横坐标，绘制大肠埃希菌的生长曲线。

【结果与讨论】

（1）将测定的OD值填入表19－1中，并绘制大肠埃希菌的生长曲线。

表19－1　OD值

培养时间（h）	0	0.5	1	1.5	2	2.5	3	4
试管编号	1	2	3	4	5	6	7	8
OD_{600}								
培养时间（h）	5	6	8	10	12	14	16	18
试管编号	9	10	11	12	13	14	15	16
OD_{600}								

（2）如果用平板活菌计数法制作生长曲线，你认为两个曲线有什么不同？

EXPERIMENT 19　Bacteria Growth Curve

Purposes

(1) To grasp the procedures of turbidimetry to measure the growth curve of bacteria.

(2) To understand the principle of turbidity measurement and the features of bacterial growth curve.

Principles

In the microbial research and manufacture, cellular growth condition is always of great practical value. Measurement of microbial biomass is one of the parameters used to assess the cultivation conditions. When inoculating quantitative bacteria into quantitative liquid medium, they grow in a closed system. The growth curve can be gained by plotting incubation time versus logarithm of viable cell count. A typical growth curve can be described as four phases including lag phase, log phase, stationary phase and death phase.

In liquid medium, the turbidity of culture would increase with the protoplasm's increasing. The concentration of cells in bacteria suspension is in proportion to the optical density, but in inverse proportion to the transmittance in given range. So optical density (OD) of the bacteria suspension can be used to determine the relative number of bacteria at specific experimental conditions to reflect the relative growth. The advantage of this method is the easy and rapid operation but it

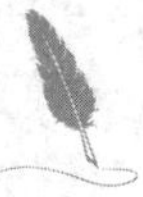

cannot distinguish between dead and living cells. Viable plate count from the previous experiment offers an opportunity to draw a standard curve of OD versus viable count. This method has already been applied in the industry.

This experiment illustrates the procedure of making a growth curve of *E. coli* with turbidimetry.

Materials and Apparatus

1. **Specimens** 16 ~ 18h slant cultures of *E. coli*.

2. **Cultures and Reagents** nutrient broth medium, sterile saline.

3. **Apparatus** 721 – spectrophotometer, table concentrator.

4. **Others** flask, tube, 1ml sterile pipette.

Procedures

1. **Preparation of cell suspension** Inoculate the flask containing 100ml nutrient broth with *E. coli* (on the agar slant) and then incubate at 180rpm, 37℃ for 18h.

2. **Inoculation and incubation** Prepare 17 pre – labeled tubes containing 10ml of nutrient broth. Add 0. 2ml of *E. coli* suspension to 16 tubes respectively, and mix gently. Leave the 17th tube only containing 10ml of nutrient broth as the blank control. Measure OD_{600} of No. 1 tube at time zero. Incubate the other 16 tubes at 37 ℃ with 180rpm.

3. **Measurement of OD_{600} value** Take out the tubes and mix well according to the incubation time listed in the result table and measure OD_{600} value of each tube using the sterile broth medium as a blank. The inoculum can be diluted with the medium when necessary to keep the OD_{600} value in the range of 0. 10 ~ 0. 65.

4. **Plotting the growth curve** Plot the growth curve of *E. coli* with OD values as ordinate and incubation time as abscissa.

Results and Discussion

(1) Record the OD values in the following table and plots the growth curve of *E. coli*.

Incubation time (h)	0	0. 5	1	1. 5	2	2. 5	3	4
Tuber number	1	2	3	4	5	6	7	8
OD_{600}								
Incubation time (h)	5	6	8	10	12	14	16	18
Tube number	9	10	11	12	13	14	15	16
OD_{600}								

扫码“练一练”

(2) What is the difference between the two growth curves obtained from OD value and viable count?

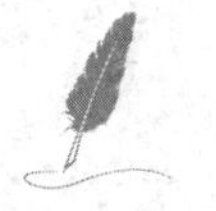

第三部分　细菌的生理生化反应

异养型微生物依赖于周围环境的有机物生长，而许多有机物由于相对分子质量太大、结构过于复杂，不能被微生物吸收利用。有些微生物可以分泌水解性酶类到细胞外，在体外将大分子有机物分解为它们的结构单元或亚基，再加以吸收利用。不同类型的异养微生物可以水解的有机物是不同的，借此可以对微生物进行分类鉴定。

实验二十　淀粉水解和明胶液化试验

扫码"学一学"

【实验目的】

了解不同的微生物对淀粉（多糖）和明胶（蛋白质）的分解能力，说明微生物具有分泌不同酶的特性。

【实验原理】

淀粉是葡萄糖的多聚物，微生物对淀粉的利用依赖于分泌到细胞外的淀粉酶，淀粉首先被分解成糊精，再进一步分解成麦芽糖和葡萄糖：

淀粉→糊精→麦芽糖→葡萄糖

淀粉和碘可进行反应生成蓝色的化合物，而淀粉的水解产物：糊精、麦芽糖和葡萄糖却不会生成蓝色化合物，据此可以用碘试剂来判断细菌是否具有分解淀粉的能力。

蛋白质是氨基酸的多聚物，蛋白质如明胶的水解过程为：

明胶→朊蛋白→蛋白胨→多肽→氨基酸

明胶酶是有些微生物分泌的一种蛋白酶，催化蛋白质分解。明胶液化试验用于判断微生物是否具有分解蛋白质的能力。将待检微生物穿刺接种于明胶培养基，经过培养，如细菌分解明胶就会发生明胶液化现象。

【实验材料】

1. **细菌**　枯草杆菌、金黄色葡萄球菌和大肠埃希菌斜面培养物。
2. **试剂**　淀粉琼脂平板，碘试剂，明胶高层培养基。
3. **其他**　接种环，接种针。

【实验方法】

1. 淀粉水解试验

（1）将淀粉琼脂平板分成三个区，并在底部做好标记。

（2）使用无菌操作，在各区划线接种适宜的培养物，倒置培养。

（3）置37℃恒温箱中培养48小时后，在平板上滴加碘液，无菌处平板呈蓝黑色。若细菌生长线周围变成透亮的无色，则为淀粉试验阳性（+），说明该菌能够产生淀粉酶，将淀粉水解；若细菌生长线四周仍为蓝黑色，表明淀粉不被水解，淀粉水解试验为阴性（-）。

2. 明胶液化试验

（1）取明胶高层培养基三支，通过穿刺接种法，一支接种大肠埃希菌，另一支接种枯

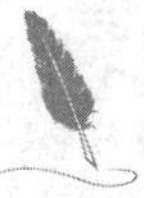

草杆菌，余下一支为对照。

（2）置37℃恒温箱中培养24～48小时。

（3）将试管置于冰箱或冰浴中30～60分钟。

（4）观察结果，明胶培养基呈液化状态者为阳性（+）；无液化现象发生者则为阴性（-）。

【结果与讨论】

（1）淀粉水解试验结果（表20-1）

表20-1　淀粉水解试验结果

细菌	枯草杆菌	金黄色葡萄球菌
淀粉水解		
对照		

（2）明胶液化试验结果（表20-2）

表20-2　明胶液化试验结果

细菌	枯草杆菌	大肠埃希菌
明胶液化		
对照		

（3）什么是水解？它在本试验中的作用是什么？

（4）碳水化合物、脂肪及蛋白质各自的结构单元是什么？

PART THREE　Biochemical Activities of Bacteria

Heterotrophic microorganisms are dependent on organic molecules in their environment. Many types of organic molecules are too large and complex to be absorbed by the cells. The cells can use these molecules by digesting them to their component subunits with the extracellular hydrolytic enzymes secreted into the environment and transporting these subunits across the membrane into the cells. Different types of heterotrophic microorganisms are different in their hydrolyzing abilities. The tests you will perform in this exercise are often valuable in identifying microbial species or strains.

EXERIMENT 20　Hydrolysis of Starch and Protein

Purpose

1. To understand the extracellular hydrolysis of starch and gelatin.

2. To understand that microbes have the ability to secrete enzymes to hydrolyze the macromolecules in the surrounding environment.

Principle

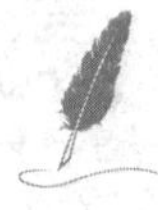

The starch is a polymer of glucose; starch hydrolysis by bacteria depends on the extracellular enzymes called amylases. The starch molecule is first hydrolyzed to smaller polysaccharide molecules which are called dextrins. The dextrin is then hydrolyzed to maltose which is further hydrolyzed to glucose, the end product of the digestive process:

Starch→dextrin→maltose→glucose

Iodine interacts with starch and produces a dark blue complex. The hydrolytic products of starch— dextrin, maltose and glucose—do not interact with iodine in this manner. Therefore we can use an iodine solution to determine whether a given bacterial stain is capable of hydrolyzing starch.

Protein molecules are composed of amino acid subunits. Hydrolysis of a large protein molecule such asgelatin proceeds through smaller and smaller amino acid chains and finally to amino acids:

Gelatin→proteoses→peptones →peptides→amino acids

Gelatinase, which is produced by many microorganisms, catalyzes the hydrolysis of the gelatin; the measurement of gelatin hydrolysis is a measure of the activity of this enzyme. The hydrolysis of gelatin produces soluble carbohydrates that are readily metabolized as a source of carbon and energy.

Materials and Apparatus

1. Culture Broth cultures of: *Escherichia coli*, *Bacillus subtilis* and *Staphylococcus aureus*.

2. Reagents Starch agar plate, Iodine solution, sterile nutrient broth tubes supplemented with 12% gelatin.

3. Apparatus Inoculating loop, inoculating needle.

Procedures

1. Starch Hydrolysis

(1) Mark the bottom of the starch agar plate into three sectors.

(2) Inoculate each sector with the appropriate culture, making a wavy line. Invert the plate and place it in the designated area.

(3) After 48h, flood the surface of the plate with iodine solution. Note that the surface of the agar is not occupied by bacterial colony becomes dark blue. A clear zone appearing around the bacterial colony indicates hydrolysis of starch. If the surrounding area of bacterial colony is dark blue, no hydrolysis occurs.

(4) Record the results and discussion in the table.

2. Gelatin Hydrolysis

(1) Inoculate one nutrient broth – gelatin tube with each microorganism. Leave one tube uninoculated as a control. Label the tubes.

(2) Incubate at 37℃ for 24 ~48h.

(3) Place the tubes in a refrigerator or an ice bath for 30 ~60min.

(4) Check each of the tubes for liquificaion. If solid, the reaction is negative, indicating the lack of gelatin hydrolysis.

(5) Record your results and discussion.

Results and Discussion

(1) Results of Starch Hydrolysis.

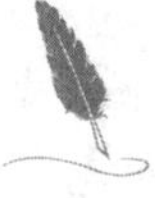

Bacteria	*Bacillus subtilis*	*Staphylococcus aureus*
starch		
control		

（2）Results of Gelatin Hydrolysis.

Bacteria	*Bacillus subtilis*	*Escherichia coli*
gelatin		
control		

（3）What is hydrolysis? What role does hydrolysis play in the tests you performed in this experiment?

（4）For carbohydrates, fats and proteins, what are their respective subunits?

扫码“学一学”

实验二十一　糖发酵试验

【实验目的】

（1）了解微生物利用单糖（如葡萄糖）和双糖（如乳糖、蔗糖）的能力。

（2）了解不同的微生物具有利用不同碳源的酶系。

【实验原理】

微生物具有不同的利用各种碳源的能力，其原理在于不同微生物具有不同的酶系。微生物利用碳源能力和结果的不同可用于微生物的鉴定。

溴甲酚紫是一种酸碱指示剂，在 pH 中性时为紫色，碱性时为深红色，而在酸性时呈现黄色。试验时，在各试验管中加一倒置小管，称为杜氏管（Durham tube），分装入试验用培养基，高压灭菌，培养基被压进杜氏管，并赶走管内气体，随后滞留在管内的气体是由微生物在生长过程中产生的。当溴甲酚紫的颜色由紫色变为黄色时，表明微生物利用碳源产生了酸性物质。

微生物在进行碳源代谢时可以产生不同的代谢产物。有些产物为酸性物质——如醋酸、甲酸以及乳酸等。酸性物质的积累有时会超出培养基的缓冲范围，导致 pH 下降，溴甲酚紫的颜色由紫色转为黄色。在产酸过程中，有时伴随气体的产生，这可以在杜氏管中的气泡反应出来；若碳源代谢的终产物为中性化合物，既无颜色变化也无气体产生，表明此时的代谢较为复杂。

【实验材料】

1. **细菌**　大肠埃希菌和伤寒杆菌培养物。

2. **试剂**　蛋白胨水培养基，葡萄糖，乳糖，麦芽糖，甘露醇，蔗糖，溴甲酚紫指示剂。

3. **其他**　接种环，试管，杜氏小管。

【实验方法】

（1）在试验管上标记好试验用菌的名称。

（2）使用无菌操作，将试验用菌接入各个试管，第六管为对照，不接种。

（3）将试验管置于培养箱中，直立放置培养。

（4）48 小时后和 5 天后检查培养状况。

（5）记录试验结果：－表示无反应或结果复杂；＋表示产酸不产气；⊕表示产酸产气；

B 表示产生碱性物质。

【结果与讨论】

（1）将实验结果填入表 21－1。

表 21－1　实验结果

生化反应	细菌	现象与结果					原理
		葡萄糖	乳糖	麦芽糖	甘露糖	蔗糖	
糖发酵试验	大肠埃希菌						
	伤寒杆菌						

（2）本试验中对照管有什么意义？

EXERIMENT 21　Utilization of Carbohydrates

Purpose

（1）To understand how to test the ability of bacterial species to use the monosaccharide sugar glucose and the disaccharide sugars lactose and sucrose.

（2）To understand that different microorganisms have different enzymes to use carbohydrates.

Principle

Organisms differ in their abilities to utilize different carbohydrates. The underlying reason is that they have different enzymes to use carbohydrates. These differences are useful in the characterization of microorganisms.

Bromocresol purple is a pH indicator that appears red at neutral pH, deep red at basic pH, and yellow at acidic pH. Each tube contains an inverted vial, the Durham tube. Such a broth tube is prepared by dispensing the medium into the tube. The pressure of autoclaving forces the medium into the vial, which displaces the trapped air. Subsequent gas production in the medium by a bacterial strain can be detected, because some of the gas is trapped in the vial and displaces the medium. Acid production is indicated by a change in color from red to yellow.

Organisms may produce a variety of end products in carbohydrate metabolism. Some of these products are acids, for example, acetic, formic, and lactic acids. If acids accumulate in sufficient quantity to overcome the buffers present in the medium, the pH is lowered. A change in color from red to yellow indicates this alteration in pH. Acid production may or may not be accompanied by gas production. If acid and gas are produced, the medium turns yellow and gas accumulates in the inverted vial. In some cases the end products of carbohydrate metabolism are neutral, there will be no change in the color and no accumulation of the gas in the vial. The only indication of growth is turbidity.

Materials and Apparatus

1. Culture　Broth cultures of *Escherichia coli* and *Salmonella typhi.*

2. Regent　Carbohydrates broth, glucose, lactose, maltose, mannitol, sucrose, bromocresol puple.

3. Apparatus　Inoculating loop, ten tubes of bromocresol purple carbohydrates broth containing Durham tubes.

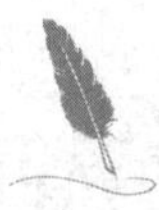

Procedures

(1) Mark each set of 5 tubes with the names of your 2 cultures (5 tubes of each culture).

(2) Using aseptic technique, inoculate each of the 5 tubes. As control, the sixth tube in each case is not inoculated.

(3) Place the tubes in the assigned location, make sure they are in an upright position.

(4) Examine the tubes after 48h and again after 5 days.

(5) Record the results and discussion on the data sheet. Use the following abbreviations:

- (for "no reaction"): purple tube.

+ (for "acidic"): yellow tube, no gas production.

⊕ (for "acid and gas"): yellow tube, gas production.

B (for "basic"): darker red color than control.

Results and Discussion

(1) Describe the results of utilization of carbohydrates.

Carbohydrates	glucose	lactose	maltose	mannitol	Sucrose
E. coli					
S. typhi					

(2) Why is it important to maintain control tubes for the tests performed in this experiment?

扫码“学一学”

实验二十二　IMViC 试验

【实验目的】

1. 掌握微生物鉴定中常用的几种生化反应原理及结果判断方法。

2. 熟悉微生物生化反应中各种培养基的设计和用途。

【实验原理】

IMViC 是以下四个试验的缩写：吲哚试验（indole production，I）、甲基红试验（methyl red test，M）、V－P 试验（Voges－Proskauer test，V）和枸橼酸盐利用试验（citrate utilization test，C），字母“i”是为了发音的需要加入的。

IMViC 试验常用于革兰阴性的肠道细菌检测中。如产气杆菌和大肠埃希菌在许多测试中反应很相似，极其容易混淆。IMViC 则可以区分产气杆菌属和大肠埃希菌属的微生物。

1. 吲哚试验　色氨酸几乎存在于所有蛋白质中，有些细菌可以将色氨酸分解为吲哚，吲哚在培养基中的积累可以由寇氏试剂（Kovacs' reagent）检测出来。试验操作必须在 48h 内完成，否则吲哚进一步代谢，会导致假阴性的结果。

寇氏试剂包含盐酸、异戊醇和对二甲基氨基苯甲醛三种成分，每种试剂均有其作用：醇用于浓缩分散在培养基中的吲哚；对二甲基氨基苯甲醛可以和吲哚反应形成红色的化合物，该反应必须在酸性条件下完成，盐酸的作用就是制造酸性环境。一旦指示剂的颜色变为红色，就表明吲哚试验为阳性（+）。

2. 甲基红试验　大肠埃希菌和产气杆菌利用葡萄糖时有所不同，大肠埃希菌接种到诸如 MRVP 培养基中时，将产生一些酸性物质，导致 pH 下降。而产气杆菌利用葡萄糖时则产生中性物质，培养基的 pH 没有显著变化。

3. V－P 试验　产气杆菌利用葡萄糖时产生的中性物质之一就是乙酰甲基甲醇，大肠埃希菌并不产生此物质。V－P 试验可用于特异性地检测乙酰甲基甲醇。V－P 试验和甲基红试验一起，是检测大肠埃希菌和产气杆菌的最有效的方法。

4. 枸橼酸盐利用试验　另一个可以区分大肠埃希菌和产气杆菌的培养基是枸橼酸盐琼脂。若以枸橼酸盐作为唯一的碳源制备培养基，大肠埃希菌不能在上面生长，而产气杆菌却可以生长得特别好。而且产气杆菌代谢产生的终产物为碱性，最终导致培养基 pH 的显著上升。指示剂溴百里酚蓝（bromthymol blue）可以检测到这一变化，pH 中性时溴百里酚蓝为绿色，当 pH 达到 7.6 时，颜色转为深蓝。除此之外，枸橼酸盐利用试验也可以用于某些肠道致病菌的检查。大多数的沙门菌可以利用枸橼酸盐，但是伤寒沙门菌和所有志贺菌却不利用。

【实验材料】

1. 细菌　大肠埃希菌培养物，产气杆菌培养物，普通变形杆菌培养物。

2. 试剂　寇氏试剂，蛋白胨－水－磷酸盐培养基，甲基红试剂，6% α－萘酚，40% KOH 溶液，西蒙枸橼酸盐琼脂斜面，醋酸营养琼脂高层。

3. 其他　接种环等。

【实验方法】

1. 吲哚试验

（1）在 2 支装有试验用培养基的试管上标记好试验菌名称，另一管作为对照。

（2）按照无菌操作，接种于试验菌培养基中。

（3）37℃培养 48 小时后，取出试验管，每管加入 10 滴寇氏试剂，在手掌中搓动试管，使管内液体混合均匀，置于试管架上 5 分钟后，观察，寇氏试剂由黄色转为红色表示有吲哚存在，为试验阳性（＋）。

（4）记录试验结果。

扫码“看一看”

2. 甲基红试验

（1）在 2 支装有试验用培养基的试管上标记好试验菌名称，另一管作为对照。

（2）按照无菌操作，接种于试验菌培养基中。

（3）37℃培养 48 小时后，取出试验管。取两个空试管，每管加入 5ml 培养基（此时无须无菌操作）。再加入 5 滴甲基红试剂，若甲基红试剂由黄色转为红色表示培养基为酸性，为试验阳性（＋）。

（4）记录试验结果。

3. V－P 试验

（1）在 2 支装有试验用培养基的试管上标记好试验菌名称，另一管作为对照。

（2）按照无菌操作，接种于试验菌培养基中。

（3）37℃培养 48 小时后，取出试验管。加入 0.5ml α－萘酚溶液以及 0.5ml 40% KOH，静置 5 分钟，若管内颜色转为红色为 V－P 试验阳性（＋），如果所有试管均无红色产生，应稍微加热后，再看试验结果。

（4）记录试验结果。

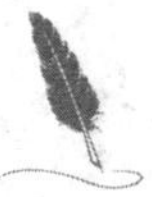

4. 枸橼酸盐利用试验

（1）在 3 支装有试验用西蒙氏培养基的试管上标记好试验菌名称，另一管作为对照。

（2）按照无菌操作，接种于试验菌培养基中。

（3）37℃培养48h后，取出试验管，观察，若管内颜色转为深蓝色为枸橼酸盐利用试验阳性（+），若试管仍为绿色，为试验阴性（-）。

（4）记录试验结果。

【结果与讨论】

（1）IMViC试验结果（表22-1）

表22-1 IMViC试验结果

IMViC项目	吲哚试验	甲基红试验	V-P试验	枸缘酸盐利用
大肠杆菌				
产气杆菌				

注：+为试验阳性；-为试验阴性。

（2）说明寇氏试剂的主要成分以及各自的作用。

（3）说明MRVP培养基的主要成分，各自的功能是什么？字母MRVP代表什么？

（4）在V-P试验中利用何种细菌代谢的中间物进行检测？它来源于何种底物的代谢产物？

（5）在西蒙枸橼酸盐斜面加入5g/L的葡萄糖，会改变该培养基的作用吗？

EXERIMENT 22　IMViC Series

Purpose

（1）To grasp the principle of biochemical tests and the judgment of these tests.

（2）To be familiar with the design and purpose of test media.

Principle

The acronym IMViC refers to a series of four tests: indole production（I）, the methyl red test（M）, the Voges－Proskauer test for the production of acetyl－methylcarbinol（V）, and the citrate utilization test.（The“i”in IMViC is included merely for ease of pronunciation）. The IMViC series is valuable for the information it can provide, but it is especially useful in differentiating gram-negative enteric bacteria. For example, *Enterobacter aerogenes* is often confused with *Escherichia coli* because of their similar reactions to various tests. This confusion sometimes arises in analyzing the bacterial content of water. The IMViC series may be run to make a distinction between members of the genus *Escherichia* and members of the genus *Enterobacter*.

1. Indole production The amino acid tryptophan is almost present in all proteins. Some bacterial can degrade tryptophan to indole. Indole accumulates in the medium, where it can be detected with Kovacs' reagent. It is important to perform the test within 48 hours, because after this time indole begins to be metabolized and the test often yields false negative results and discussion.

Kovacs' reagent contains three ingredients: hydrochloric acid, isoamyl alcohol, and para－dimethyl－amina－benzaldehyde. Each ingredient plays a critical role in the test for indole. The alcohol concentrates indole that is dispersed throughout the medium. Para－dimethyl－amina－ben-

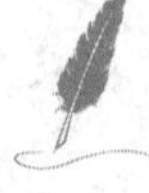

zaldehyde reacts with indole to form a red complex. Finally, this reaction occurs only at a low pH, which explains the function of hydrochloric acid. Thus a positive indole test involving Kovacs' reagent is indicated by a color change from yellow to red.

2. The Methyl Red Test *Escherichia* and *Enterobacter* differ in their utilization of glucose. If *Eschericia* is inoculated into a medium containing glucose, such as MRVP broth, several acids are produced. As a result, there is a marked decline in pH. By contrast, *Enterobacter* does not produce acids in its metabolism of glucose. Instead, the end products are neutral and there is no significant change in pH.

3. The Voges – Proskauer Test One of the neutral substances produced by *Enterobacter* in its metabolism of glucose is acetyl – methylcarbinol. *Escherichia* does not produce this substance. The Voges – Proskauer test is specific for acetyl – methylcarbinol. Together with the methyl red test, it is most useful in distinguishing *E. coli* from *E. aerogenes*.

4. Citrate Utilization An additional medium that can be used to differentiate between *Escherichia* and *Enterobocter* is citrate agar. If citrate (a salt of citric acid) is the sole carbon source in a medium, *Eschichia* can not grow. By contrast, *Enterobacter* grows quite well on citrate. Furthermore, the end products of *Enterobacter*'s citrate metabolism are basic and raise the pH of the medium significantly. Incorporation of the pH indicator bromthymol blue provides a ready means of measuring the rise in pH. (Bromthymol blue is green at a neutral pH but changes to a deep blue at pH 7.6). In addition to its value in distinguishing *Escherichia* and *Enterobacter*, the citrate utilization test may be used to differentiate among certain intestinal pathogens. Most members of the genus *Salmonella* utilize citrate, but *S. typhi* and all members of the genus *Shigella* do not.

Materials and apparatus

1. Culture Broth cultures of *Escherichia coli* and *Enterobacter aerogenes*.

2. Reagent Bottle of kovacs' reagent, tubes of tryptone broth, tubes of MRVP broth, Methyl red indicator, Bottle of alpha naphthol, Bottle of potassium hydroxide (KOH) solution, Simmons' citrate agar slants.

3. Apparatus Inoculating loop.

Procedures

1. Indole production

(1) Mark 2 of the tryptone broth tubes with the names of your 2 cultures.

(2) Using aseptic technique, inoculate the tubes and place them in the appropriate location for incubation. The third tube, which serves as a control, is also incubated.

(3) Take out the tubes 48h after incubation, and add 10 drops of Kovacs' reagent to each tube. Rotate the tubes between your palms to mix the contents. Place them in a test tube rack and let them stand for 5min. (Kovacs' reagent rises to the top). A change in the color of Kovacs' reagent from yellow to red indicates the presence of indole.

(4) Record your results and discussions.

2. The Methyl Red Test

(1) Mark 2 of the MRVP broth tubes with the names of two cultures.

(2) Using aseptic techniques inoculate the tubes and place them in the appropriate location for

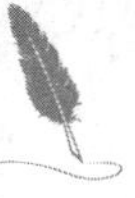

incubation. The third tube, which serves as a control, is also incubated.

(3) Take out the tubes 48 hours after incubation. Mark 2 empty tubes, and pour 5 ml of the medium from each culture into the empty tube. Because the medium is "spent", you need not make this transfer aseptically. However, take care not to spill any of the culture medium. Do not discard the remainder of the spent medium; you will use it in the Voges – Proskauer test. Add 5 drops of methyl red indicator to each of the 2 tubes that you just poured. If the pH of the medium is acidic, the color of the reagent will remain red. If the pH of the medium is neutral or basic, the color will change to yellow.

(4) Record your results and discussion.

3. The Voges – Proskauer Test

(1) Mark 2 of the MRVP broth tubes with the names of two cultures.

(2) Using aseptic techniques inoculate the tubes and place them in the appropriate location for incubation. The third tube, which serves as a control, is also incubated.

(3) Remove the tubes from inculcation after 48 hours. Add 0. 5 ml of alpha naphthol and 0. 5 ml of potassium hydroxide solution to each of the original culture tubes (now containing 5 ml of spent medium). Allow the tubes to stand for 5 minutes. A red color indicates the production of acetyl – methylcarbinol. Note: If none of the tubes shows a red color after 5 minutes, subject the *E. aerogenes* tube to mild heating, which enhances formation of color. Subject the other tubes to the same degree of heating.

(4) Record your results and discussion.

4. Citrate Utilization

(1) Mark 3 of the Simmons' citrate agar tubes with the names of your 3 cultures.

(2) Using aseptic technique, inoculate the tubes by the stab technique and incubate them at 37℃. The third tube serves as a control; stab the agar with a sterile needle.

(3) After 48h, remove the tubes from the incubator and observe the color. A blue color indicates the ability to utilize citrate as a carbon source. A green color indicates the inability to utilize citrate as a carbon source.

(4) Record your results and discussion.

Results and Discussion

(1) Record the results of IMViC on the data sheet.

IMViC	Indole	Methyl Red	Voges – Proskauer	Citrate Utilization
E. coli				
E. aerogenes				

(2) Name the key ingredients in Kovacs' reagent. What is the special role of each ingredient?

(3) Name two key ingredients in MRVP broth. What is the function of each these ingredients? What do the letters MRVP represent?

(4) What compound is the Voges – Proskauer test designed to detect in a growth medium? What substrate is metabolized to produce this compound?

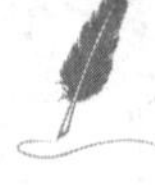

(5) Suppose you add 5 grams of glucose per liter to Simmons' citrate agar. Would this change

make any difference in the function of this medium?

扫码"学一学"

实验二十三　硫化氢产生试验和触酶试验

【实验目的】

（1）掌握微生物鉴定中常用的几种酶催化的反应原理及结果判断方法。

（2）熟悉微生物生化反应中各种培养基的设计和用途。

【实验原理】

硫化氢（Hydrogen sulfide，H_2S）是某些微生物在分解半胱氨酸等含硫氨基酸时脱硫产生的。硫化氢的产生是半胱氨酸转化为丙酮酸和氨这一系列反应的第一步，可以由醋酸铅检测出来，硫化氢遇到醋酸铅，可以形成黑色的沉淀。

触酶催化过氧化氢分解为水和氧，大多数需氧微生物可进行该过程。触酶的功能是将代谢过程产生的毒性的过氧化氢除去，以保护细胞不被伤害。当过氧化氢加入到微生物或菌体上，将有氧气气泡产生，以此证明触酶的存在。

【实验材料】

1. **细菌**　大肠杆菌培养物，普通变形杆菌培养物，枯草杆菌培养物，梭杆菌培养物。

2. **试剂**　醋酸铅营养琼脂高层，过氧化氢溶液（3%～10%）。

3. **其他**　接种针，灭菌牙签，灭菌枪头，载玻片，体视镜等。

【实验方法】

1. 硫化氢产生试验

（1）使用接种针，按照无菌操作，将细菌接入醋酸铅琼脂高层。一支穿刺接种甲型副伤寒杆菌，另一支穿刺接种乙型副伤寒杆菌，注明菌名。

（2）置37℃恒温箱中培养24～48小时。

（3）培养结束后，观察结果时，有黑褐色硫化铅者为阳性（+），无此现象者为阴性（-）。

（4）记录实验结果。

2. 触酶试验

（1）使用接种环或无菌牙签将枯草杆菌和梭杆菌平板或斜面上的菌体取下。

（2）将菌体涂于载玻片上。

（3）用移液枪将一滴过氧化氢溶液加于菌体之上。

（4）观察有无气泡产生，若有，则为触酶试验阳性。有时产生气泡较小，观察较困难，可使用体视镜辅助观察。

（5）记录实验结果。

【结果与讨论】

（1）将硫化氢产生试验结果填入表23-1。

试验菌	现象	结果	原理
甲型副伤寒杆菌			
乙型副伤寒杆菌			

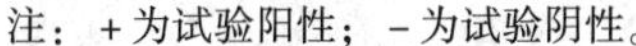

注：+为试验阳性；-为试验阴性。

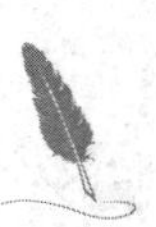

（2）将触酶试验结果填入表 23－2。

表 23－2　触媒试验结果

试验菌	现象	结果	原理
枯草杆菌			
梭杆菌			

EXERIMENT 23　Hydrogen sulfide Production and Catalase Test

Purpose

1. To grasp the principle of enzyme tests and the judgment of these tests.

2. To be familiar with the design and purpose of test media.

Principle

Hydrogen sulfide（H_2S）is produced from cysteine by certain bacteria that synthesize the enzyme cysteine desulfurase. The production of H_2S takes place in the first step of a series of reactions in which cysteine is converted to pyruvic acid and ammonia. The production of hydrogen sulfide can be detected by including lead acetate in the medium; when H_2S reacts with lead, a black precipitate（PbS）forms.

Catalase is an enzyme that catalyzes the decomposition of hydrogen peroxide（H_2O_2）to water and gaseous oxygen. Most aerobic microorganisms possess catalase. The function of catalase is to remove toxic hydrogen peroxide that forms during the oxidation－reduction reactions that are coupled with oxygen in respiratory metabolism. The presence of catalase is important for aerobic growth because it prevents the accumulation of toxic metabolites that would otherwise kill the cell. The presence of catalase is demonstrated when hydrogen peroxide is added to a colony or loopful of bacteria and bubbles of oxygen are released from the surface.

Materials and Apparatus

1. Culture　Broth cultures of *Salmonella paratyphi A and Salmonella paratyphi B.*

2. Reagent　Butt tubes of lead acetate－nutrient agar; hydrogen peroxide（3～10% solution）.

3. Apparatus　Inoculating loop; sterile wooden applicator sticks or toothpicks; Pasteur pipette; Microscope slide; binocular（dissecting）microscope.

Procedures

1. Hydrogen sulfide production

（1）With the inoculating needle, aseptically transfer each culture to a tube of lead acetate nutrient agar medium. Stab the agar butt with the inoculating needle to inoculate the subsurface regions of the agar.

（2）Incubate the tube with *Salmonella paratyphi A and Salmonella paratyphi B* at 37 ℃ for 24～48 hours.

（3）Observe the tubes after incubation. The presence of a black precipitate along the line of inoculation indicates the production of hydrogen sulfide.

(4) Record your results and discussion.

2. Catalase test

(1) Aseptically pick up some bacterial culture from the colony or slant growth with a sterile wooden applicator stick or toothpick.

(2) Deposit the mass of bacterial cells adhering to the stick or toothpick onto a clean glass microscope slide.

(3) Pipette a drop of hydrogen peroxide onto the mass of bacterial cells adhering to the loop.

(4) Observe the drop of hydrogen peroxide to see if bubbles evolve. The production of gaseous bubbles indicates the presence of catalase. It is sometimes difficult to see the bubbles when they are small. In these cases a binocular (dissecting) stereomicroscope is used.

(5) Record your results.

Results and Discussion

Record the results on the data sheet.

(1) H_2S production test

Bacteria	Result	Principle
Salmonella paratyphi A		
Salmonella paratyphi B		

(2) Catalase test

Bacteria	Result	Principle
B. subtilis		
Clostridium sp.		

扫码“练一练”

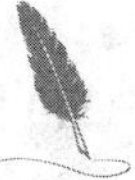

第四部分　病毒学实验

作为一类非细胞型微生物，病毒仅由核酸和蛋白质组成，具有严格细胞内寄生性，必须在易感的活细胞内才能增殖。病毒的分离与培养，对病毒感染性疾病的疫苗制备、感染机制研究、以及临床诊断与治疗方法的开发等均具有重要意义，是病毒学研究的基础。常用的病毒人工培养方法有动物接种、鸡胚培养与组织（细胞）培养三种。本部分共包括两方面内容：流感病毒的培养方法与效价测定——介绍了流感病毒的鸡胚接种方法和血凝效价测定；烈性噬菌体的分离培养与生长曲线测定——介绍了大肠杆菌烈性噬菌体的分离培养、效价测定、以及一步生长曲线的绘制。

实验二十四　流感病毒的培养与检测

扫码“学一学”

【实验目的】

（1）掌握采用鸡胚接种法培养流感病毒。

（2）了解检测流感病毒的血凝试验法。

【实验原理】

鸡胚培养为病毒常用的培养方法之一，该法操作简便、成本低廉，可用于黏病毒、痘病毒、疱疹病毒、脑炎病毒等多种病毒的培养。鸡胚有四个部位可用于接种，即绒毛尿囊膜、尿囊腔、羊膜腔和卵黄囊，如图 24－1 所示。流感病毒的培养常采用尿囊腔接种法或羊膜腔接种法（本实验以尿囊腔接种法为例）。

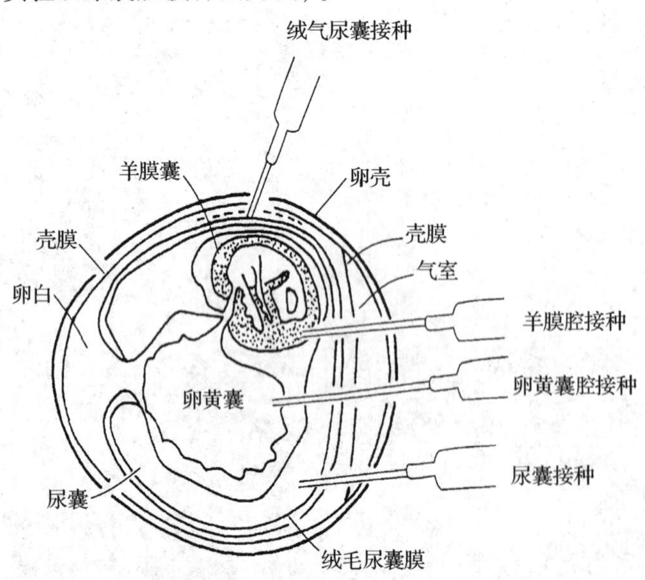

图 24－1　鸡胚的结构和接种途径

血凝试验是检测流感病毒的常用方法。由于流感病毒包膜上有血凝素（hemagglutinin，HA）分子，能与禽类及多种哺乳动物红细胞膜上的血凝素受体结合，使得红细胞凝集，故

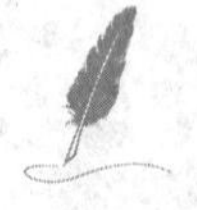

称为血凝试验。通过血凝试验可测定血凝效价，从而反映尿囊液中流感病毒的滴度。

扫码“看一看”

【实验材料】

1. 病毒与鸡胚　流感病毒或其他黏病毒（10^{-8}稀释）溶液，10～12日龄鸡胚。

2. 试剂　无菌石蜡，无菌生理盐水，0.5%鸡红细胞悬液。

3. 其他　蛋座，检卵灯，镊子，碘酒和酒精棉球，砂轮，1ml的无菌注射器，6号针头，无菌试管，20孔反应板，刻度吸管等。

【实验方法】

1. 尿囊腔接种

（1）准备鸡胚。孵育前的鸡卵先用清水以毛刷清洗，再用干布擦干，放入孵箱内进行孵育（37℃，相对湿度45%～60%），鸡卵每日翻动1～2次。孵至第4日，用检卵灯观察鸡胚发育情况。未受精卵，只见模糊的卵黄黑影，不见鸡胚的形迹，这些鸡卵剔出不用。活胚可看到清晰的血管和鸡胚的暗影，有些还可以看见胚动，随后每日观察一次，胚动呆滞、没有运动的或血管昏暗模糊者，即可能已死或将死的鸡胚，要随时加以淘汰。

（2）在选取的10～12日龄活鸡胚上用铅笔画出气室、鸡胚及大血管的位置，先用碘酒再用酒精棉球消毒气室部蛋壳，用砂轮在胚胎位置的尿囊腔与气室交界处磨一小口，定为注射入口，勿损伤蛋膜。

（3）用注射器抽取病毒稀释液，在注射口使针头与卵壳成30°角插入0.5cm深度，注入0.1～0.2ml，注射完后用熔化的石蜡封口。

（4）置35℃孵箱培养3～4天，再移置4℃冰箱过夜或4～6小时。将气室朝上放置，使鸡胚血液凝固，避免收获时流出的血球同尿囊液中的病毒发生凝集，造成病毒滴度的下降。

（5）收获时，先用碘酒再用酒精棉球消毒气室部位蛋壳，用无菌镊子除去气室蛋壳，再用无菌眼科镊子去除气室部壳膜，用毛细吸管通过绒毛尿囊膜进入尿囊腔，吸取尿囊液，放入小瓶或试管内冰冻保存，并做无菌试验。

2. 血凝试验（表24－1）

（1）在20孔反应板上编号（1～9孔，第10孔作对照孔）。

（2）用1ml吸管于各孔加入生理盐水0.25ml。

（3）第1孔加入1:5稀释的尿囊液0.25ml，混匀即成1:10。从1号孔取0.25ml放入第2号孔中，混匀后再取0.25ml至第3号孔，如此依次稀释到第9号孔为止。每稀释一个浓度换用吸管，最后从第9孔中弃去0.25ml，即第10孔为不加尿囊液阴性对照。

（4）在各孔加入0.5%鸡血球悬液0.25ml，摇匀，室温下静置30～60分钟后，观察结果。

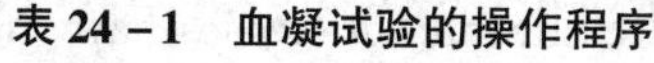

表24－1　血凝试验的操作程序

孔号	1	2	3	4	5	6	7	8	9	10
生理盐水（ml）	0.25	0.25	0.25	0.25	0.25	0.25	0.25	0.25	0.25	0.25
尿囊液（ml）	0.25	↘	↘	↘	↘	↘	↘	↘	↘	↘弃
初始病毒稀释度	1:10	1:20	1:40	1:80	1:160	1:320	1:640	1:1280	1:2560	去0.25
0.5%鸡红细胞（ml）	0.25	0.25	0.25	0.25	0.25	0.25	0.25	0.25	0.25	0.25
最终病毒稀释度	1:20	1:40	1:80	1:160	1:320	1:640	1:1280	1:2560	1:5120	-

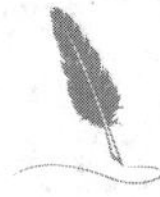

（5）结果判断见表 24－2。

表 24－2　血凝试验结果判断标准

孔底所见	结果
凝集的血球颗粒在底部铺开成网状，无血球下滑，即 100% 血细胞凝集	＋＋＋＋
基本同上，但边缘不齐整，絮状凝集略有下沉趋向，75% 血细胞凝集	＋＋＋
孔底中央血球呈一环状，四周有絮状小块，50% 以上血细胞凝集	＋＋
血球于孔底呈一小团，边缘不光滑，四周有小凝集块，25% 以上血细胞凝集	＋
血球于孔底呈一小圆点，边缘光滑整齐，血细胞无凝集现象	－

出现"＋＋"（50%）血球凝集现象者，其最高稀释度即为流感病毒的血凝效价。如图 24－2 所示，A4 孔即为血凝效价判定点，因此其最终稀释度 1∶160 为血凝效价。

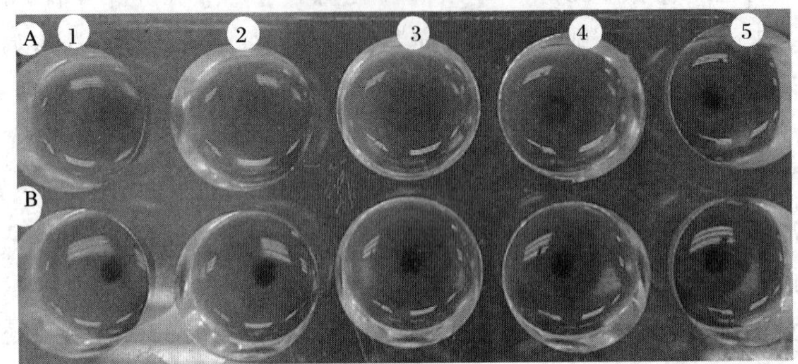

图 24－2　血凝试验的结果

【结果与讨论】

（1）血凝实验的原理是什么？

（2）血凝试验结果记录（表 24－3）。

表 24－3　血凝试验结果

孔号	A1	A2	A3	A4	A5
结果					
孔号	B1	B2	B3	B4	B5
结果					

（3）鸡胚尿囊液中有无流感病毒增殖？病毒的血凝效价是多少？

PART FOUR　The Experiments of Virus

Viruses are non－cellular microorganisms, composed of nucleic acids and proteins. Proliferation of these intracellular parasitic organism depends on its susceptible living host cells. As the basis for viral research, the isolation and cultivation of viruses have great significance in the vaccine developments, infection mechanisms, clinical diagnosis and treatment methods of viral infectious diseases. The common virus isolation and culture methods including chick embryo inoculation, animal inoculation, and tissue (cell) culture. There are two sections in this part. Virus culture method and hemagglutination titer test of influenza virus are introduced in the first section. Isolation, cultivation, titration and the drawing of one－step growth curve for *Escherichia coli* bacteriophage are introduced in the second section.

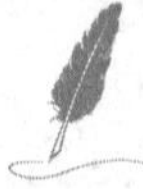

Experiment 24　Culture and Detection of Influenza Virus

Purpose

(1) To grasp the culture method of influenza virus in chick embryo.

(2) To understand the method of detecting influenza virus by hemagglutination test.

Principle

Chick embryo is commonly used to culture and propagate virus including visco - virus, pox virus, herpes virus and encephalitis virus *etc*, due to the simplicity and low cost. Four different parts of chick embryo including chorioallantoic membrane, urinary allantoic cavity, amniotic cavity and yolk sac can be inoculated with virus. Urinary allantoic and amniotic cavities are often used for the adaptation and propagation of influenza virus. Here, we use urinary allantoic inoculation in this experiment. A 10 ~ 12 dpc (days post coitum) embryonated egg is diagrammed in fig. 24 - 1, showing the important structures involved in virus culture. The time and area of embryo injection and inoculation vary according to the type of virus.

Visco - viruses (including influenza viruse) can associate with red blood cells and in many cases cause agglutination of these cells. It is called hemagglutination (HA) test. This test furnishes a relatively simple, fast, convenient and fairly quantitative way for virus detection, identification and titration.

Materials and Apparatus

1. Virus and chick embryo　the influenza virus or other visco - virus (10^{-8} dilution) solution, 10 ~ 12 dpc chick embryos.

2. Reagents　sterile paraffin, sterile saline, 0.5% chicken red blood cell suspension.

3. Others　egg holders, eggs candlers, tweezers, iodine and alcohol cotton balls, grinding wheel, 1 ml sterile syringes, 6 - gauge needles, sterile test - tube, 20 - hole reaction plate, calibrated pipette.

Procedures

1. Chick Embryo Inoculation (Urine Allantoic Cavity)

(1) Preparation of eggs: it is necessary that the 10 ~ 12 dpc fertile eggs are incubated at 37℃ in a humid atmosphere (relative humidity: 45% ~ 60%). Also, the eggs should be turned once a day for proper embryo development.

(2) After the desired incubation period, candle the egg and determine the viability of the embryo (does it move?) and the position of the air sac.

Place the egg on a firm surface. Swab a small area with 70% alcohol immediately below the air sac. Then gently puncture the eggshell with a grinding wheel. Be careful not to penetrate the chorioallantoic membrane (CAM).

In order to obtain virus for subsequent work, and attempt to obtain an endpoint of infection, diluted influenza virus should be used for inoculation, as provided.

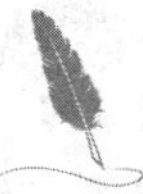

(3) Draw 0.2ml of virus solution into a 1ml syringe fitted with a 6 - gauge needle. Expel any

air bubbles.

Carefully insert the needle through the hole in the shell below the air sac and go through the CAM about 0. 5cm, directing it slightly toward the air sac.

Inject exactly 0. 1 ~ 0. 2ml by twisting the barrel of the syringe inward.

Carefully remove the needle and seal the holes with small pieces of plastic tape, label each egg.

(4) Place the egg at 35℃ and incubate for 72 ~ 96 hours.

Retrieve your eggs from the incubator. Chill by placing them in the refrigerator overnight (or for at least 4 ~ 6 hours before step 5).

(5) Place the egg in a holder contained in a porcelain pan.

Break the shell over the air sac by penetrating it with the point of a pair of forceps. Carefully peel back the shell over the air sac.

Tear the shell membrane and allantois. Insert a Pasteur pipette equipped with a rubber bulb into the allantoic cavity, be careful not to rupture any blood vessels.

Aspirate 2 ~ 3ml of fluid and transfer to a sterile tube.

Empty embryo and remaining allantoic fluid into a petri dish and further tear the allantoic membrane to encourage bleeding. Allow to sitting at room temperature for 10min then observing for clumping of erythrocytes. If virus is present a positive test may be observed.

Discard the embryo into appropriate container.

2. Hemagglutination (HA) Test

(1) Add 250μl of PBS to each of the wells in the first two rows of the plastic microtitre plate (A1 ~ A5 and B1 ~ B5). Use the 10th well of B5 for the negative controls (no allantoic fluid).

(2) Add 250μl of 5 – fold diluted influenza – containing allantoic fluid (AF) to A1 and mix gently. With a fresh pipette tip, transfer 250μl to A2 and mix gently. Repeat this procedure for the whole row, discarding 250μl from the last well in the series (B1 ~ B4).

(3) Using a clean pipette tip, add 250μl of RBCs to each well, including the negative controls (resuspend the cells before using). Work from right to left (starting with the negative controls and finishing with the lowest virus dilution).

(4) Mix the cell suspensions by tapping the plate gently and incubate at room temperature for 30 ~ 60min.

(5) Read and record the titration

In wells with enough amount of influenza viruses, all the RBCs have agglutinated (i. e. they are linked together in a 3 – dimensional matrix, see Fig. 24 – 2). In wells where the concentration of influenza virus has been diluted below the critical point (CP), the cells settle at the bottom of the well to form a "button".

The minimum amount of virus that causes about 50% of the RBCs hemagglutinating in a well is known as one hemagglutinating unit (HAU). As shown in the fig. 24 – 2, the well of A4 is the determination point of hemagglutination titer, and the virus titer in the allantoic fluid of chick embryo is 1:160.

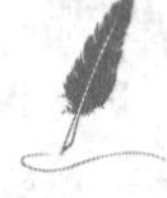

Results and Discussion

(1) What is the principle of hemagglutination test?

(2) Result of hemagglutination test:

No. of the hole	A1	A2	A3	A4	A5
result					
No. of the hole	B1	B2	B3	B4	B5
result					

(3) Is there any influenza virus reproducing in in allantoic fluid of the chick embryo? And how high is the hemagglutination titer of the virus?

实验二十五　污水中大肠埃希菌噬菌体的分离、培养和效价测定

扫码“学一学”

【实验目的】

(1) 掌握污水大肠埃希菌噬菌体分离纯化原理。

(2) 掌握噬菌体效价的测定方法。

(3) 了解噬菌体的培养特征。

【实验原理】

噬菌体是感染细菌、放线菌和真菌的病毒。噬菌体广泛存在于自然界，凡是有细菌的场所，就有其特异的噬菌体存在。例如河水、阴沟污水和粪便是各种肠道细菌尤其是大肠埃希菌的栖息地，故可分离到大肠埃希菌的噬菌体。

基本原理：①噬菌体对宿主具有高度特异性，可以利用其宿主作为敏感菌株在液体或固体培养基中培养它们；②在固体培养基中，可利用噬菌斑进行噬菌体分离纯化。

在融化的培养基中，将噬菌体和敏感细菌混合，将其倾注到底层肉汤固体培养基上，噬菌体侵入宿主细菌细胞后进行复制而导致细胞裂解，释放出噬菌体，进而感染更多的敏感菌，释放更多的新的噬菌体。在有宿主菌生长的琼脂平板上，噬菌体可裂解宿主菌而形成透明的肉眼可见的空斑，即噬菌斑（plaque）。而宿主菌未被裂解之处呈现浑浊现象。

噬菌斑形状、大小、边缘以及透明度等特征均随噬菌体的种类而异，故不仅可用于噬菌体的检出和定量，还可用于噬菌体的分离和鉴定。可以采用肉汤澄清法和噬菌斑形成法，来测定待测样品中噬菌体的存在和效价。

肉汤澄清方法：以能够引起宿主菌裂解的噬菌体溶液的最高稀释度表示。

噬菌斑形成单位测定法：一般采用琼脂叠层法或双层琼脂平板法（agar layer method）测定噬菌体效价。由于含有特异宿主细菌的平板上，噬菌体可繁殖并裂解细菌产生肉眼可见的噬菌斑，因此可以进行噬菌体计数。理论上一个噬菌斑是由一个噬菌体感染宿主形成，但也有些噬菌斑是由几个噬菌体颗粒感染相应的宿主形成，所以，为了准确表达噬菌体的浓度，一般不用噬菌体的绝对数量，而是用噬菌斑形成单位表示。

噬菌体的效价是指1ml培养液中所含活噬菌体的数量，以噬菌斑形成单位/ml（plaque forming units，PFU/ml）表示。

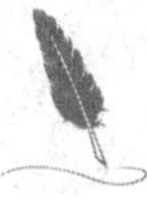

例如，稀释度为10^{-3}时，在0.1ml噬菌体试样中有65个噬菌斑，则该噬菌体原悬液的

效价为：

$$\frac{65}{0.1\times10^{-3}}=6.5\times10^{5}\ (\text{PFU/ml})$$

【实验材料】

1. **菌种** 大肠埃希菌 18～24 小时斜面培养物。

2. **噬菌体样品** 阴沟污水或池塘污水。

3. **培养基**

（1）上层半固体培养基；

（2）肉汤琼脂培养基（底层培养基，含琼脂 1.4%～1.6%）；

（3）肉汤液体培养基；

（4）三倍浓缩的肉汤培养基；

（5）5 支小试管（内装 0.9ml 无菌肉汤液体培养基），肉汤琼脂平板（10ml 培养基/皿）5 个，含 3ml 半固体琼脂培养基的试管 5 支。

4. **仪器** 离心机，细菌过滤器，真空泵，抽滤装置，水浴锅。

5. **其他** 无菌涂布棒，无菌吸管，无菌培养皿，三角瓶等。

【实验方法】

1. 噬菌体的分离与纯化

（1）培养敏感菌：取经活化的大肠埃希菌斜面 1 支，从中挑取 1 环菌接种至肉汤液体培养基中，培养至对数期，使菌悬液在 600nm 的 OD 值约为 0.6。

（2）增殖噬菌体样品：① 取 1ml 上述敏感菌培养液于装有 50ml 三倍浓缩肉汤琼脂培养基的三角瓶中，37℃振荡培养 4～6 小时。

② 培养后向其中加入 100ml 污水，37℃继续培养 12～14 小时。

（3）获得噬菌体悬液（或裂解液）：

① 将上述增殖的混合培养液于 2500～3000 r/min 离心 20 分钟，得上清液。

② 取上清液用细菌过滤器过滤，装置如图 25－1，收集滤液。

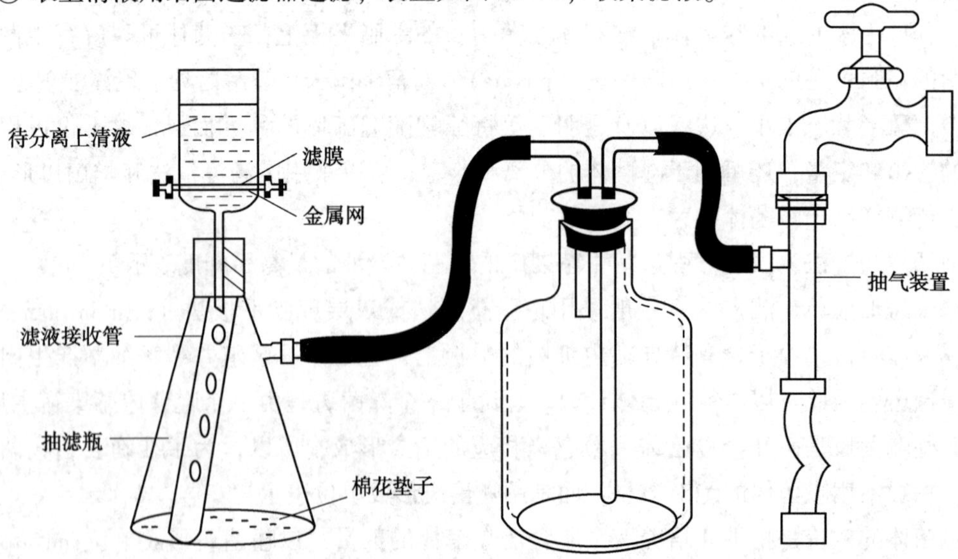

图 25－1 负压抽滤装置

③ 取少量滤液接种到10ml营养肉汤培养基中，37℃培养过夜，同时以另一瓶未接种的营养肉汤培养基为阴性对照。如果培养液经培养未变浑浊，表明滤液已无菌。

（4）噬菌体的检出

①试管法：于幼龄的细菌液体培养物（4～6小时）内加上述过滤液一滴，37℃培养30～60分钟，如液体由浑浊变澄清，证明有噬菌体存在。

②固体平板法：

a. 取三只无菌培养皿，分别倒入融化并冷却到50℃左右的肉汤琼脂培养基，待凝固（图25－2）。

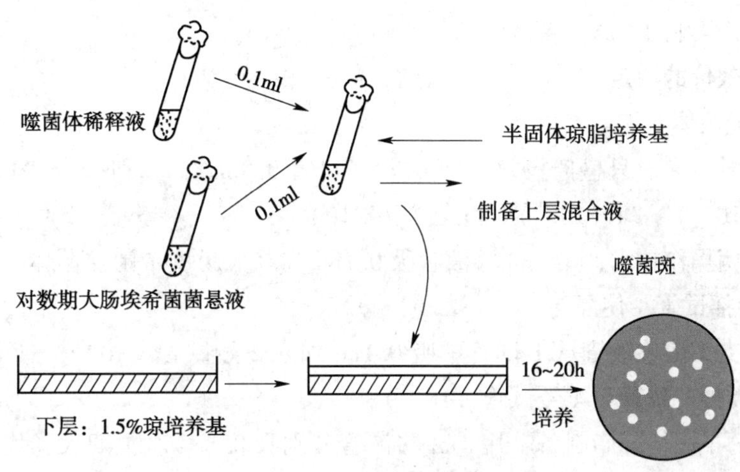

图25－2　双层琼脂平板法分离噬菌体

b. 涂布接种：在上述底层培养基表面，分别加入数滴培养至对数期的大肠埃希菌菌液，涂匀。

c. 取2只涂布接种的平板，在平板上分别分散滴加5～8滴噬菌体裂解液。第3只平板滴加无菌生理盐水作为对照。

d. 培养：将上述三只平板于37℃，倒置培养18～20小时。

结果判定：若平板上出现噬菌斑，而对照组无噬菌斑，则表明该滤液中一定含有大肠埃希菌噬菌体。

（5）噬菌体的分离

① 标记试管：将4只盛肉汤培养基试管，分别编号“1（10^{-1}）”～“4（10^{-4}）”。

② 噬菌体样品的稀释：采用无菌操作技术，用1ml移液管吸0.1ml大肠埃希菌噬菌体悬液（前面步骤3制备），注入1号试管中，旋摇试管，使混匀。用另一支无菌移液管从1号管中吸0.1ml加入2号管中，旋摇试管，使混匀，依次稀释为10^{-1}、10^{-2}、10^{-3}、10^{-4}等4个稀释度。

③ 含敏感菌半固体制备：用移液管分别吸0.1ml对数期大肠埃希菌液，加入4支半固体培养基试管中，放置在50℃水浴锅保存。

④ 倒底层琼脂平板：取无菌平皿4只，每皿倒入10ml肉汤琼脂培养基（底层培养基），并在皿底依次表明10^{-1}、10^{-2}、10^{-3}、10^{-4}稀释度。

⑤ 制备噬菌体和敏感菌的混合液：操作从标记4（10^{-4}）的肉汤试管开始。采用无菌操作，吸取0.1ml 10^{-4}的噬菌体稀释液，加到含有敏感菌的半固体培养基试管中，立即搓试管充分混匀，并倒在标注对应稀释度（10^{-4}）的底层琼脂平板表面，平置待凝。然后，

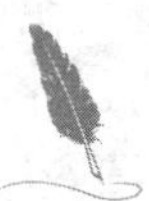

用同一个移液管吸取0.1ml标记3（10^{-3}）的噬菌体稀释液，加到含有敏感菌的半固体培养基试管中，立即搓试管充分混匀，并倒在标注对应稀释度（10^{-3}）的底层琼脂平板表面，平置待凝。其他平皿的操作方法雷同。

⑥ 培养：将上述平皿于37℃倒置培养至噬菌斑出现。

（6）噬菌体的纯化：初步分离的噬菌体往往不纯，噬菌斑的大小、形态常不一致，所以还需要进行噬菌体的纯化。

用接种针挑取典型的噬菌斑，接种至含有大肠埃希菌的肉汤培养基中，37℃培养18～24小时，以增殖噬菌体。然后重复上述分离步骤，直至平板上出现的噬菌斑形态、大小一致，则表明已获得纯的大肠埃希菌噬菌体。

2. 噬菌体效价的测定

（1）稀释噬菌体：

① 试管编号：取5只盛肉汤培养基试管（每管0.9ml），分别编号“1（10^{-3}）”“2（10^{-4}）”“3（10^{-5}）”“4（10^{-6}）”和“5”（对照）。

② 采用无菌操作技术，用1ml移液管吸0.1ml 10^{-2}大肠埃希菌噬菌体，注入1号试管（10^{-3}）中，旋摇试管，使混匀。

③ 用另一支无菌移液管从1试管中吸0.1ml加入2号试管（10^{-4}）管中，旋摇试管，使混匀，依次类推，稀释至4号试管（10^{-6}）。

（2）接种的半固体琼脂制备：用1ml移液管分别吸0.1ml对数期大肠埃希菌液，各加入5支半固体琼脂试管中，放置在50℃水浴保存。

（3）倒底层琼脂平板：取无菌平皿5只，每皿倒入10ml肉汤琼脂培养基（底层培养基），并在皿底依次表明10^{-3}、10^{-4}、10^{-5}、10^{-6}和对照组。

（4）制备噬菌体和敏感菌的混合液：操作从标记“5（对照）”的肉汤试管开始。采用无菌操作，吸取0.1ml 5号试管的稀释液，加到含有敏感菌的半固体琼脂试管中，立即搓试管充分混匀，并倒在标注对应稀释度的底层琼脂平板表面，平置待凝。然后，用同一个移液管吸取0.1ml标记“4（10^{-6}）”的噬菌体稀释液，加到含有敏感菌的半固体琼脂试管中，立即搓试管充分混匀，并倒在标注对应稀释度“4（10^{-6}）”的底层琼脂平板表面，平置待凝。其他平皿的操作方法雷同。

（5）培养：将上述平皿于37℃倒置培养至噬菌斑出现（约6～8h）。

（6）观察噬菌斑：将每一稀释度的噬菌斑数目记录于实验报告表格内，选取噬菌斑数目在25～250个的平板，计算每毫升未稀释的原液的噬菌体数（效价）。

【结果与讨论】

（1）在噬菌斑法测定效价过程中，选择一个噬菌斑数在25～250个的平板，绘图描述实验结果。

（2）将平板中各稀释度的噬菌斑记录于表25－1，计算噬菌体的效价。

表25－1　各稀释度的噬菌斑

噬菌体稀释度	1（10^{-3}）	2（10^{-4}）	3（10^{-5}）	4（10^{-3}）	5（blank control）
噬菌斑数					
效价					

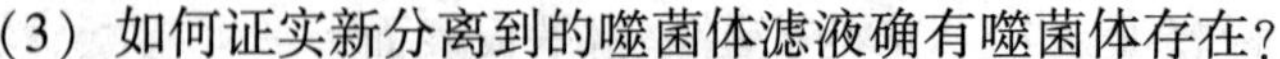

（3）如何证实新分离到的噬菌体滤液确有噬菌体存在？

（4）测定噬菌体的效价时，哪些操作决定测定准确性？

（5）哪些因素影响噬菌斑的大小？

EXPERIMENT 25　Isolation, Cultivation and Titration of *Escherichia coli* phage from Sewage

Purposes

（1）To grasp the principle of isolating and purifying *Escherichia coli* phage from sewage.

（2）To grasp the assay method of determining the titer of bacteriophage sample.

（3）To understand the cultural characteristics of phage.

Principles

Bacteriophage is the virus which infects bacteria, actinomycetes and fungi. It widely exists in nature. All the places where bacteria exist, there is specific bacteriophage. Some particular environments, such as water, sewage, feces, are the habitats where various intestinal bacteria exist, especially *Escherichia coli*. Phages can be separated from them.

The principle：①Bacteriophage is highly host - specific. Bacteriophage can be grown in liquid or solid cultures of specific bacteria. ②When solid media are used, the plaque forming method allows isolation of bacteriophage.

Host bacteria and bacteriophages are mixed together in melted agar, which is then poured onto a Petri dish containing hardened nutrient agar. Each bacteriophage that infects a bacterium multiplies, releasing several hundred progeny phages. The progeny phages infect neaby bacteria, and more new phages are produced. All those bacteria in the area surrounding the original bacteriophage are destroyed, leaving a clear zone, or a plaque, against a confluent "lawn" of bacteria. The lawn of bacteria is produced by the growth of uninfected bacteria.

Different types of bacteriophage have different characteristics such as the shape, size, edge, transparency and so on. Plaques can be used not only for detection and quantification, but also for separation and identification of the bacteriophage.

The titer assay includes broth clearing assay and plaque forming method.

In the broth clearing assay, the end point is the highest dilution (smallest amount of viruses) producing lysis of bacteria and clearing of the broth. The titer, or concentration, that result in a recognizable effect is the reciprocal of the endpoint.

In the plaque forming method, agar overlay method is usually used. The titer is determined by counting plaques. Each plaque theoretically corresponds to a single infective virus in the initial suspension. Some plaques may arise from more than one virus particles, and some virus particles may not be infectious. Therefore, the titer is determined by counting the number of plaque - forming units (PFU).

The titer, plaque - forming units per milliliter, equals the number of plaques divided by the volume of suspension plated multiplying with the dilution factor.

For example, 65 plaques with 0.1ml suspension plated at a 1：10^3 dilution equals to

$$\frac{65}{0.1 \times 10^{-3}} = 6.5 \times 10^5 \text{PFU/ml}$$

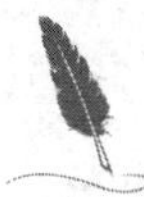

(note: When counting the number of plaque – forming units, choose the plates with 10 to 100 plaques/plate)

Materials and Apparatus

1. Strains *Escherichia coli* slant culture for 18 ~ 24h.

2. Bacteriophage samples Sewage as source.

3. Media and Reagents

(1) Semi – solid agar tube (or upper medium, 3ml/tube).

(2) Nutrient broth agar medium (substratum or bottom medium, containing 1.4 % ~ 1.6 % agar).

(3) Nutrient broth.

(4) 3 ×nutrient broth medium.

(5) 4 sterile tubes (with 0.9ml sterile broth medium), 5 plates with nutrient broth agar medium (10ml each plate), 4 semi – solid agar tubes (3ml/tube).

4. Apparatus Centrifuge, bacterial filter, vacuum pump, sterile membrane filter assemblies (0.45μm), water bath.

5. Others Sterile glass spreader, sterile pipette, sterile petri dish, erlenmeyer flask, *etc.*

Procedures

1. Isolation and purification of Bacteriophage

(1) Incubation of sensitive bacteria

Take an activated *Escherichia coli* slant, inoculate one loopful of *E. coli* to nutrient broth and incubate to logarithmic phase, allowing the OD_{600nm} value to reach about 0.6.

(2) Proliferation of phage samples

① Take 1ml of sensitive bacteria inoculum to erlenmeyer flask with 50ml of 3 ×nutrient broth medium, incubate at 37℃ for 4 ~ 6h with shaking.

② After incubation, add 100 ml sewage to the above proliferated solution, incubate for another 12 ~ 14h.

(3) Preparation of bacteriophage suspension (or bacteriophage lysate)

① The mixed proliferation cultures are centrifuged at 2500 ~ 3000 r/min for 20 min, collect the supernatant.

② Filtrate the supernatant through a membrane filter (Fig. 25 – 1). Decant the clear liquid into a screw capped tube.

③Sterility test: Add a small amount of filtrate to 10 ml nutrient broth, incubate at 37℃ overnight, another bottle of nutrient broth is used as the negative control. If the cultured solution is clear, the filtrate is sterile.

(4) Detection of Bacteriophage

1) Broth – Clearing Assay: Add a drop of the filtrate into the nutrient broth inoculum (4 ~ 6h), incubate at 37 ℃ for 30 ~ 60min. It would prove the presence of phage if the turbid liquid became clear.

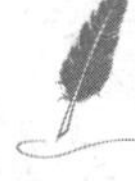

2) Plaque – Forming Assay

① Pouring plate: Take 3 sterile Petri dishes, pour nutrient broth medium (about 50 ℃) onto the dishes with aseptic technique (15 ~ 20ml each dish), allow to cool down (Fig. 25 – 2).

② Add a few drops of the sensitive bacteria incubation onto the surface of the plate (made by the last step) and spread it.

③ Drop 5 ~ 8 drops of the bacteriophage lysate on the surface of the 2 plates mentioned above. As a blank control, the third plate is added with sterile saline.

④ Incubate all plates in an inverted position at 37 ℃ for 18 ~ 20h.

Analysis of the results: If the plaque appears on the plates, and at the same time no plaque appear on the blank control, it indicates that the filtrate contains *E. coli* phage.

(5) Isolation of bacteriophage

① Labeling: Label the broth tubes from "1 (10^{-1})" to "4 (10^{-4})".

② Serial dilutions of bacteriophage: Aseptically add 1ml of phage suspension (from step 3) to tube1. Mix by carefully aspirating up and down three times with the pipette. Using a different pipette, transfer 1 ml to the second tube, mix well. Continue until the fourth tube.

③ Semi – solid agar tube with *E. coli*: Using a pipette, add 0. 1ml *E. coli* to the semi – solid tubes and place them back in the 50℃ water bath.

④ Pouring the substratum agar plate: Prepare 4 sterile petri dishes, label them with the dilution 10^{-1} ~ 10^{-4}. Melt the nutrient agar media (as the substratum) and cool down to 50℃ ~ 55 ℃, add 10 ml of the agar media to each dish and wait to cool down.

⑤ Prepare the mixture of bacteriophages and their sensitive bacteria: Using a pipette, start with broth tube 4 and aseptically transfer 0. 1 ml from tube 4 to a semi – solid agar tube, mix by swirling, and quickly pour the inoculated semi – solid evenly over the surface of petri plate 4. Then, using the same pipette, transfer 0. 1 ml from tube 3 to a semi – solid tube, mix and pour over plate 3. Continue until you have completed tube 1.

⑥ Incubation: Incubate all plates in an inverted position at 37℃ until plaques develop.

(6) Purification of Bacteriophage

The initial isolated phage is always impure, such as the size and the uneven shape of the plaque, *etc.* So it is necessary to purify the bacteriophage.

Pick the typical plaque with an inoculating needle and inoculate to *E. coli* nutrient broth, then incubate at 37 ℃ for18 ~ 24 h. Repeat the isolation process until the sizes and morphologies of the isolated plaques are uniform.

2. Titer Detection of Bacteriophage

(1) Serial dilutions of bacteriophage

① Label the broth tubes (0. 9 ml/tube) "1 (10^{-3})" "2 (10^{-4})" "3 (10^{-5})" "4 (10^{-6})" and "5" (blank control).

② Aseptically add 0. 1ml *E. coli* phage suspension (10^{-2}) to tube1 (10^{-3}). Mix carefully by aspirating up and down with the pipette.

③ Using a different pipette, transfer 1ml from tube 1 to the second tube, mix well. Continue until the fourth tube (10^{-6}).

(2) Inoculated semi – solid agar medium

Using a pipette, add 0. 1ml *E. coli* to the semi – solid agar tubes and place them back in the

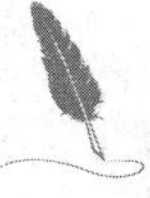

water bath.

(3) Pouring the substratum agar plate

Prepare 5 sterile Petri dishes, label them with the dilution 10^3 ~ 10^{-6} and blank control. Melt the nutrient agar media (as the substratum) and cool down to 50℃ ~55 ℃, add 10ml of the agar media to each plate and wait to cool down.

(4) The mixtures of bacteriophage and their sensitive bacteria

Using a pipette, start with broth tube 5 and aseptically transfer 0. 1 ml from tube 5 to a semi – solid agar tube . Mix by swirling, and quickly pour the inoculated semi – solid agar evenly over the surface of Petri plate 5. Then, using the same pipette, transfer 0. 1ml from tube 4 to a semi – solid agar tube, mix and pour over plate 4. Continue until you have completed tube 1.

(5) Incubation

Incubate all plates in an inverted position at 37 ℃until plaques develop (about 6 ~8h) .

Observe the plaques on the plates. Record your results. Select a plate with 25 ~ 250 plagues. Count the number of plaques, and calculate the number of plaque – forming units (PFU) per milliliter.

Results and discussion

(1) With Plaque – forming Assay, choose one plate with 25 ~ 250 plaques, draw what you have observed.

(2) Fill the table with the number of plaques /plate, and calculate the PFU/ml.

Dilution	1 (10^{-3})	2 (10^{-4})	3 (10^{-5})	4 (10^{-6})	5 (blank control)
the number of plaques					
PFU/ml					

(3) How to confirm that the newly isolated phage filtrate indeed contains phages ?

(4) Which step determines the accuracy of titer determination?

(5) What are the factors affecting the plaque' s size?

实验二十六　噬菌体一步生长曲线的测定

扫码"学一学"

【实验目的】

了解噬菌体一步生长曲线测定的基本方法。

【实验原理】

定量描述烈性噬菌体生长规律的实验曲线，称为一步生长曲线。用噬菌体的稀释液感染高浓度宿主细胞，控制每个细胞所吸附的噬菌体最多只有一个（通常噬菌体和宿主的混合比例为1：10，以避免几个噬菌体同时浸染一个宿主细胞）。经数分钟吸附后，高倍稀释噬菌体和宿主细胞共培养物，以建立同步感染。培养期间，每隔数分钟取样，连续测定噬菌体效价。以感染时间为横坐标，噬菌体效价为纵坐标，绘制噬菌体特征曲线，即一步生长曲线。一步生长曲线分为三个时期，其中噬菌体核酸侵入宿主细胞后至第一个成熟子代噬菌体装配完成前的时期称为潜伏期，宿主细胞迅速裂解、溶液中噬菌体急剧增多的时期为裂解期，宿主细胞全部裂解，溶液中噬菌体效价达到最高点的时期则为平稳期。

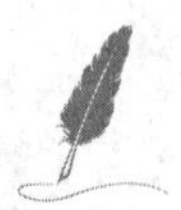

一步生长曲线最初为研究噬菌体的复制而建立，现已推广到动植物病毒复制研究中。一步生长曲线的测定，有助于了解病毒在宿主细胞内的增殖情况和病毒感染的动力学，为病毒提纯时间和培养繁殖的最佳收获时间提供了依据，同时也被广泛应用于病毒感染机理研究以及病毒性疾病的防治研究中。

【实验材料】

1. **细菌和噬菌体**　大肠埃希菌培养液（5×10^8CFU/ml），噬菌体悬液（2×10^8phage/ml）。

2. **试剂和培养基**　半固体营养琼脂高层（3ml），营养琼脂平板，营养肉汤培养（9.9ml/管），营养肉汤培养（9.0ml/管）。

3. **其他**　涂布棒，灭菌小试管，灭菌枪头，50℃水浴锅等。

【实验方法】

（1）将装有半固体高层的试管，做好标记，在水浴上熔化管内培养基，50℃保温。

（2）取2.2ml过夜培养的检测用大肠埃希菌，无菌操作接入稀释的噬菌体悬液1ml，记录时间 $t=0$。

（3）37℃孵育，5分钟后，高速离心5分钟，弃上清，沉淀用9.9ml营养肉汤重悬。

（4）将0.1ml悬液加入9.9ml营养肉汤（稀释100倍），以此出发，再作10^{-3}、10^{-4}、10^{-5}稀释。

（5）37℃孵育10^{-3}和10^{-4}稀释度的试管。

（6）$t=20$分钟时，各取0.1ml培养液，分别与步骤（1）准备的半固体培养基混匀，倾注于固体平板。

（7）每隔5分钟，重复上述步骤一次，一直到 $t=40$ 分钟。

（8）平板于37℃培养24～48小时。

（9）检查噬菌斑数，计算每个取样点的噬菌体数。

（10）绘制生长曲线图。

【结果与讨论】

（1）将平板中各稀释度的噬菌斑记录于表26-1，并计算噬菌体的效价。

表26-1　各稀释度的噬菌斑

时间（min）	20	25	30	35	40
噬菌斑数					
样品中噬菌体数					

（2）为何不能绘制 t_0 至 t_{20} 的曲线图？

（3）为什么噬菌体的生长曲线称为一步生长曲线？

Experiment 26　One-Step Growth Curve of Bacteriophage

Purpose

To understand the method of plotting one-step growth curve of bacteriophage.

Principle

The one-step growth curve is a common experimental procedure for studying replication of the

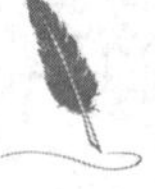

lytic bacteriophage. At first, lytic bacteriophages are co – incubated with its host bacteria for adsorption. In order to ensure that each host cell is infected with no more than one bacteriophage, the mixing ratio of the bacteriophage and the host is usually 1 : 10. Several minutes later, synchronous infections will be established by high dilution of the co – incubated cultures. During the culture period, the titers of bacteriophage were continuously measured every few minutes. With the infection time as abscissa, and the bacteriophage titer as ordinate, the characteristic curve of bacteriophage was drawn as one – step growth curve. The one – step growth curve can be divided into three stages. The period from the invasion of phage nucleic acid into host cells to the completion of the first mature phage particle assembly is called the incubation period. Rapid lysis of host cells and sharp increase of phages would happen in the lysis period. In stable period, all host cells are lysed and the titer of bacteriophage reaches the maximum. Besides bacteriophages, the one – step growth curves have also been used in the research about replications of animal and plant virus.

The one – step growth curve can be used to guide optimal purification and harvest time of virus, and is also widely used in the studies about the mechanisms, disease prevention and treatment of viral infection.

Materials and Apparatus

1. Cultures cultures of *Escherichia coli* (5×10^8 CFU/ml), suspension of bacteriophage titer (2×10^8 phage/ml).

2. Regent 10 × strength trypticase soy broth, trypticase soy agar plates, soft agar tubes (TSA: 5 ml/tube), semisolid agar in tubes (3ml), nutrient agar plates, nutrient broth tubes, nutrient broth tubes.

3. Apparatus 250ml erlenmeyer flasks, sterile pipettes, graduated cylinders, water bath at 50℃, vortex mixer, and centrifuge.

Procedures

(1) Semisolid agar in tubes will be melted and labeled, then be returned into the water bath at 50℃.

(2) Add 1ml of the phage suspension to 2.2ml of *E. coli* culture. Record the time as t_0.

(3) Incubate at 37℃. After 5 minutes centrifuge the tubes in a clinical centrifuge for 5 minutes at the highest speed setting. Discard the supernatant and resuspend the pellet in 9.9ml of nutrient broth.

(4) Prepare a 100 – fold dilution by taking 0.1ml resuspension and adding it to 9.9ml of nutrient broth (10^{-2} dilution). Take the 10^{-2} dilution 1.0ml to 9.0ml sterile nutrient broth (10^{-3} dilution) and 0.1ml to 9.9ml sterile nutrient broth (10^{-4} dilution). Prepare an additional dilution by taking 1.0ml from the 10^{-4} dilution broth and transferring it to 9.0 ml of sterile nutrient broth (10^{-5} dilution).

(5) Incubate the 10^{-3} and 10^{-4} dilutions at 37℃.

(6) At t = 20 minutes, transfer 0.1ml suspension from the 10^{-3} and 10^{-4} dilutions to separate tubes of semisolid agar. Mix each tube and pour onto separate agar plates, separately.

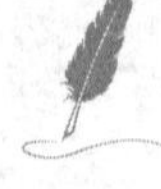

(7) At 5 – minute intervals, until t = 40, repeated step (6).

(8) Incubate the plate at 37℃ for 24 ~ 48h.

(9) After incubation, count the number of plaques (clear zones) in the lawn of confluent bacterial growth. Use the number of plaques and the dilution factors to calculate the concentration of bacteriophage at each sampling time.

(10) Plot the concentration of bacteriophage against time.

Results and Discussion

(1) Plot of the concentration of bacteriophage against time.

Time (min)	20	25	30	35	40
Number of plaque Number of phage					

扫码“练一练”

(2) Why can't you recover bacteriophage between t_0 and t_{20}?

(3) Why is the growth curve of bacteriophage called one-step growth curve?

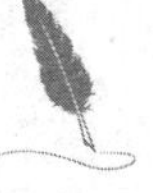

第五部分　微生物遗传学实验

扫码“学一学”

遗传和变异是微生物的基本特性。微生物的变异现象有很多，一些变异只是表型的改变，而遗传物质的改变称为突变，突变可遗传给子代。抗药性是对药物敏感的微生物获得了对药物的抗性。突变可以自发产生或用诱变剂诱发产生。由于化学物质对微生物的诱变作用，反映了其对哺乳动物潜在的致癌作用，所以 Ames 试验通过检测细菌的回复突变来测试化学物质的诱变性。在原核生物中已知有三种遗传交换机制，DNA 转移都是从供体菌到受体菌。① 转化，供体菌释放的游离 DNA 被受体菌吸收；② 转导，供体菌 DNA 转移由噬菌体介导，转移至受体菌；③ 接合，DNA 转移需要供体菌和受体菌细胞直接接触和接合型质粒。在细菌的分类鉴定工作中，16S rRNA 基因序列分析已成为广泛应用的分子鉴定技术。

实验二十七　微生物的遗传与变异现象

【实验目的】

（1）熟悉细菌的菌落变异现象。

（2）熟悉菌体的形态变异现象。

【实验原理】

遗传和变异是微生物的基本特性。细菌的变异现象有很多，包括菌落和细胞形态变异，荚膜、芽孢、鞭毛等结构变异，以及生化变异如毒力和抗药性变异等。一些变异只是表型的改变，而一些变异是遗传物质的改变（称为突变）。只有后者可传递给子代。

【实验材料】

1. 菌种　普通变形杆菌 18～24 小时斜面培养物，黏质沙雷氏菌 18～24 小时斜面培养物，金黄色葡萄球菌 24 小时肉汤培养物，光滑型、粗糙型大肠埃希菌琼脂斜面 18～24 小时培养物，鼠疫杆菌（无毒株）琼脂斜面 18～24 小时培养物。

2. 培养基　普通琼脂培养基，0.1% 石炭酸琼脂培养基，3%～6% NaCl 血琼脂斜面，L 型培养基（牛肉浸液 800ml，蛋白胨 20g，NaCl 50g，琼脂 8g，pH7.4）。高压蒸汽灭菌，等温度降至 50℃左右时，加入无菌人血浆 200ml 后倾注平板。

3. 试剂　青霉素溶液，革兰染液，细胞壁染液。

4. 器材　接种环，低浓度青霉素药物纸片（40μg/片），镊子，涂布棒，无菌平皿，37℃和 25℃培养箱。

【实验方法】

1. 鞭毛变异　普通变形杆菌通常可产生鞭毛，但当某些化学药品存在时，鞭毛生长受到抑制，菌落产生变异。取变异的菌落再分离，去除化学药品影响时，其产鞭毛的特性又得以恢复。

（1）分别在普通琼脂平板和 0.1% 石炭酸琼脂平板的中央接种普通变形杆菌。

（2）37℃培养24h后观察菌落有无迁徙现象。

（3）将菌落再分别接种至普通琼脂平板，37℃培养24小时后观察菌落有无迁徙现象。

2. 色素变异　有些细菌产生色素常与培养温度相关，例如黏质沙雷氏菌在25℃培养时能产生深红色的灵杆菌素而使菌落显色，但在37℃培养时却形成无色菌落。取37℃培养的无色菌落再分离于25℃培养，其产生色素的特性又得以恢复。

（1）菌悬液制备：用约4ml无菌生理盐水刮洗下斜面上的黏质沙雷氏菌的菌苔，制备成均匀分散的菌悬液。

（2）划线分离：用接种环取满环菌液，在预先制备的普通琼脂平板表面分区划线分离接种，使最后一区出现较多单菌落的分布处。

（3）培养与观察：将接种后的一块平板于25℃培养，另一平板于37℃培养，各培养48h，观察并记录在不同培养温度下，黏质沙雷氏菌的菌落产生色素的情况。

（4）复查产色素试验：在37℃培养的平板上挑取不产生红色色素或产生色素不明显的单菌落上的少许菌体，再次划线分离接种于新鲜普通琼脂平板，并于25℃培养48小时。观察能否再现色素分泌的特性。

3. 光滑型与粗糙型菌落变异　细菌菌体抗原称为“O”抗原，细胞壁中脂多糖为群特异性抗原，“O”抗原特异性由脂多糖末端重复结构的多糖残基侧链决定。具有“O”抗原的细菌菌落呈光滑型（S）；丢失多糖侧链的细菌菌落呈粗糙型（R）。在一定条件下，细菌菌落可由光滑型（smooth，S）转变为粗糙型（rough，R），即为S－R变异。平板上光滑型菌落表面光滑、边缘整齐、湿润；粗糙型菌落表面粗糙、边缘不整齐、干皱。S－R变异是一种全面的变异，不仅菌落形态不同，其生化反应能力、抗原性及致病性等也往往发生改变，例如R型菌的致病性明显降低。

（1）分别接种光滑型和粗糙型大肠埃希菌于两个普通平板上。

（2）37℃孵育18～24小时后，观察两型大肠埃希菌的菌落特性。

4. 形态变异　鼠疫杆菌培养在含高盐的培养基中时，可出现大小不等的多形态。

（1）接种鼠疫杆菌（无毒株）于3%～6% NaCl血琼脂斜面，28℃～30℃培养3日。

（2）取出涂片、革兰染色，与未变异株作对比观察。

5. 细菌L型变异　细菌在有些水解酶（如溶菌酶）或某些抗生素（如青霉素）的作用下，肽聚糖的合成受阻导致细胞壁受损，成为细胞壁缺陷型细菌，称为L型细菌。由于其细胞壁缺陷，在低渗环境中，菌体会裂解死亡，但在高渗含血清的培养基中仍能生长，形成油煎蛋样的细小菌落。

（1）在L型培养基上加入0.05ml金黄色葡萄球菌培养物，然后以涂布棒均匀涂布，待平板稍干后，取青霉素药物纸片1张贴于平板中央，置37℃培养，次日观察有无抑菌圈。

（2）每隔一天用放大镜或在低倍镜下观察抑菌圈内有无油煎蛋样小菌落出现。

（3）选取油煎蛋样菌落和抑菌圈外细菌分别进行涂片，做革兰染色和细胞壁染色后，镜检。抑菌圈内出现油煎蛋样小菌落，经染色后可见细菌呈多形性，经细胞壁染色后，看不清细胞壁结构，与原来的菌对比区别明显。

【结果与讨论】

（1）鞭毛变异实验结果（表27－1）。

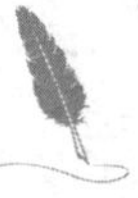

表 27－1　鞭毛变异实验结果

细菌名称	培养基	生长状况
普通变形杆菌		

（2）色素变异实验结果（表 27－2）。

表 27－2　色素变异实验结果

细菌名称	培养温度	色素产生状况
黏质沙雷菌	25℃	
	37℃	

（3）光滑型与粗糙型菌落变异实验结果（表 27－3）。

表 27－3　光滑型与粗糙型菌落变异实验结果

细菌名称	菌株分型	菌落形态
大肠埃希氏菌	光滑型	
	粗糙型	

（4）形态变异实验结果（表 27－4）。

表 27－4　形态变异实验结果

细菌名称	培养基	菌体形态
鼠疫杆菌（无毒株）		

（5）细菌 L 型变异实验结果（表 27－5）。

表 27－5　细菌 L 型变异实验结果

细菌名称	培养基	菌落形态	菌体形态
金黄色葡萄球菌			

PART FIVE　Experiments for Microbial Genetics

Heredity and variation are common properties of microorganisms. Many phenomena of microbial variation can be observed. Some variations are just phenotypic change while some variations are genetic change called mutation which can be transferred to progeny. Mutations may occur spontaneously or induced by mutagen. Antimicrobial drug resistance is the acquired ability of a microorganism to resist the effects of an antimicrobial drug to which it is normally susceptible. Since some mutagens can cause cancer in animals, the Ames test makes practical use of detecting revertants in large populations of mutant bacteria to test the mutagenicity of potentially hazardous chemicals. Three mechanisms of genetic exchange in prokaryotes are known, in which DNA transfer typically occurs from donor to recipient: ① transformation, in which free DNA released from donor is taken

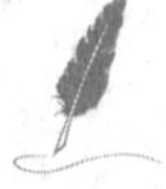

up by recipient; ② transduction, in which donor DNA transfer is mediated by a bacteriophage; ③ conjugation, in which DNA transfer requires cell – to – cell contact and a conjugative plasmid in the donor cell. 16S rRNA gene sequencing has become prevalent in bacterial identification as a molecular identification technique.

EXPERIMENT 27 Heredity and Variation of Microorganism

Purpose

(1) To be familiar with the variations in colonies of microorganisms.

(2) To be familiar with the variations in morphology of microorganisms.

Principle

Heredity and variation are common properties of microorganisms. There are many phenomena of bacterial variation including colonial or cellular morphological variation, structural variation in capsule, spore and flagella, biochemical variation such as virulence and drug resistance. Some variations are just phenotypic change, but some are genetic changes (called mutation) that can be transferred to progeny.

Materials and Apparatus

1. Strains 18 ~ 24h nutrient agar cultures of *Proteus vulgaris*, *Serratia marcescens*, *Escherichia coli* (S type and R type), *Yersinia pestis* (non – toxic strain), 24h nutrient broth culture of *Staphylococcus aureus*.

2. Media Nutrient agar, nutrient agar containing 0.1% phenol, 3% ~6% NaCl blood agar, L media.

3. Reagents Penicillin, Gram's dye, cell wall dye.

4. Apparatus Inoculating loop, sterile filter paper disc (containing 40μg penicillin/disc), tweezer, spreading rod, sterile petri dish, 37℃ and 25℃ incubator.

Procedures

1. Flagella Variation *Proteus vulgaris* usually have flagella. But the flagella growth can be inhibited with the presence of certain chemicals, causing changes in the colony. The production of flagella can resume when chemicals removal.

(1) Inoculate *Proteus vulgaris* using inoculating loop in the center of the plates.

(2) Incubate at 37℃ for 24h. Examine the motility of the colonies.

(3) Transfer some biomass from the colony onto nutrient agar plate containing 0.1% phenol. Incubate at 37℃ for 24h. Examine the motility of the colonies.

2. Pigment Variation The production of pigment by some bacteria is often associated with temperature. *Serratia marcescens* can produce red pigment and form red colonies when cultured at 25℃, but form colorless colonies when cultured at 37℃. The characteristics of pigment production can resume when cultured at 37℃ again.

(1) Preparation of bacteria suspension: Add about 4ml sterile saline to the slant. Wash and scratch the lawn to prepare uniformly dispersed suspension of bacteria.

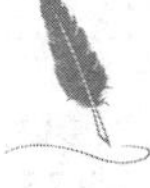

(2) Streak - plate: Transfer a loopful of the bacteria suspension and streak on the plate to let single colonies could be distributed in the last area.

(3) Incubation and observation: Incubate the plate at 25℃ and 37℃ separately for 48h. Observe and record the pigment production of the colonies under different temperature.

(4) Review the production of the pigment: Transfer some material from the colorless colonies at 37℃ and streak on nutrient agar plate. Incubate at 25℃ for 48h. Observe the reproduction of pigment.

3. S - R Colony Variation Bacterial cell antigen is known as the "O" antigen. Cell wall lipopolysaccharide is a group - specific antigen and the specificity is determined by polysaccharide side chain residues on terminal repeat. The colony is smooth (S) with "O" antigen and rough (R) with loss of polysaccharide side chains. Under certain conditions, bacterial colonies may change from a smooth - type (smooth, S) into a rough - type (rough, R), which is called S - R colony variation. Smooth - type colonies are surface smooth, edge neat and humid. Rough - type colonies are surface rough, edge irregular and dry - wrinkled. S - R variation is a comprehensive variation not only in colony morphologies but also in biological and chemical response capabilities, antigenicity and pathogenicity. For example, R - type bacteria have decreased pathogenicity.

(1) Inoculate S - type and R - type on the nutrient agar plate separately.

(2) Observe the characteristics of the colonies after 18 ~ 24h incubation.

4. Morphology Variation *Yersinia pestis* can form many different sizes and morphologies when cultured at high - salt medium.

(1) Inoculate *Yersinia pestis* (non - toxic strain) at 3% ~ 6% NaCl blood agar slant and incubate at 28℃ ~ 30℃ for 3d.

(2) Smear and stain with Gram's dyes. Observe the size and morphology and compare with the normal strain.

5. Bacterial L - type Variation Bacterial peptidoglycan synthesis will be inhibited and cell wall will be damaged under the effect of some hydrolases (such as lysozyme) or certain antibiotics (such as penicillin). The cell wall deficient bacteria, known as L - type, will lyse and die in low - permeability environment due to its cell wall defects. L - type can still grow and form oil - fried egg - like small colonies in hypertonic medium containing serum.

(1) Pipette 0.05ml of the *Staphylococcus aureus* culture onto L - medium plate and spread the culture over the surface of the plate using the sterile glass spreader. Let the plate dry. Place a filter paper disc containing penicillin at the center of the plate. Incubate at 37 ℃. Observe whether the inhibition zone appears on the next day.

(2) Observe whether oil - fried egg - like small colonies appear inside the inhibition zone every other day with a magnifying glass or microscope at low magnification.

(3) Select the oil - fried egg - like colonies and the colonies outside the inhibition zone to smear and stain with Gram's dye and cell wall dye. Observe under microscope. The bacteria from oil - fried egg - like small colonies inside the inhibition zone are poly - morphological and the cell wall can not be clearly observed after staining, which are very different from the original strain.

Results and Discussion

(1) The results of flagella variation.

Strain	Medium	Description of growth
Proteus vulgaris		

(2) The results of pigment variation.

Strain	Temperature	Pigment
Serratia marcescens	25℃	
	37℃	

(3) The results of S－R colony variation.

Strain	Type	Colony
E. coli	S	
	R	

(4) The results of morphology variation.

Strain	Medium	Morphology
Yersinia pestis (non－toxic strain)		

(5) The results of bacterial L－type variation.

Strain	Medium	Colony	Morphology
Staphylococcus aureus			

实验二十八 微生物的抗药性变异

扫码“学一学”

【实验目的】

(1) 熟悉细菌的抗药性变异现象。

(2) 熟悉青霉素酶的简易测定方法。

(3) 了解用梯度平板法分离抗药性突变株。

【实验原理】

微生物以低频率发生抗药性突变，突变株在含抗生素的培养基上生长，而正常细菌被抑制，因而突变株虽然很少但很容易被检出。抗药突变株的抗药机制包括：①产生改变抗生素结构的酶，例如对青霉素的抗性。②改变细胞膜的通透性，例如对红霉素的抗性。③改变抗生素的作用靶位，例如对链霉素的抗性，链霉素干扰核糖体的翻译过程。

抗药突变株对抗生素具有相对的抵抗力。多剂抗药株显示对几种不同作用机制的药物具有抗药性。

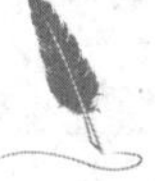

金黄色葡萄球菌青霉素抗药株可产生青霉素酶。该酶水解 β－内酰胺环，使青霉素分解为青霉噻唑酸，该酸可被碘氧化，淀粉（遇碘显蓝色）可作为指示剂，即在抗药株的菌

落周围因碘被消耗而显出无色透明圈（图 28－1）。

梯度平板法是筛选抗药性突变株的一种有效简便的方法，例如抗链霉素金黄色葡萄球菌突变株的分离，如图 28－2 制备双层平板，底层平板倾斜且不含药物，将含药的上层培养基倒在底层上，就会形成药物的含量梯度。将敏感菌涂布在平板上，在高链霉素含量区长出的菌落可能就是抗链霉素突变株。

【实验材料】

1. **菌种** 金黄色葡萄球菌青霉素敏感株和抗药株的 18～24 小时斜面培养物，金黄色葡萄球菌 24h 肉汤培养物。

2. **培养基** 普通琼脂培养基。

3. **试剂** 青霉素溶液（5U/ml），1ml 青霉素 G 钾盐溶液（20000U/ml），5ml 淀粉琼脂（含淀粉 0.5%，琼脂 0.8%），碘液（0.08mol I_2 溶于 3.2mol/L KI 溶液），链霉素溶液（0.1mg/ml）。

4. **器材** 接种环，无菌滤纸片，镊子，涂布棒，无菌平皿，37℃培养箱。

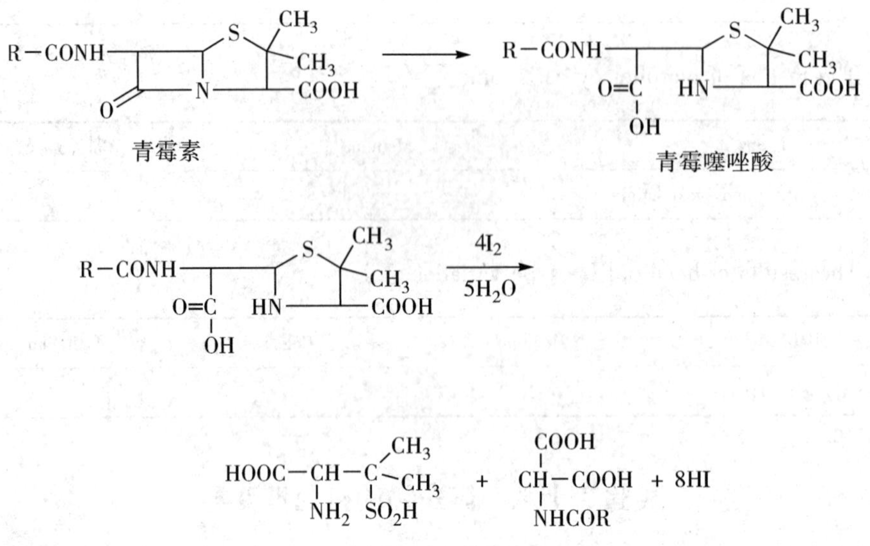

青霉素 → 青霉噻唑酸

青霉噻唑酸 $\xrightarrow[5H_2O]{4I_2}$ 青霉胺酸 + $CH(COOH)(NHCOR)COOH$ + 8HI

图 28－1 青霉素酶测定原理

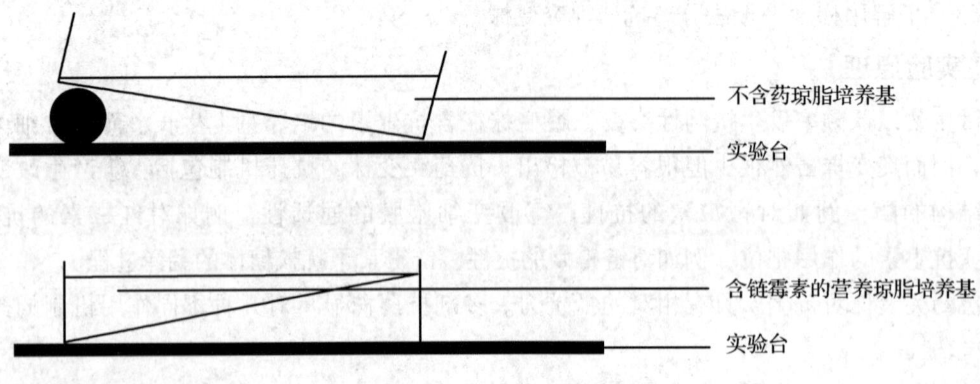

图 28－2 梯度平板的制备

【实验方法】

1. 抗药性变异

（1）将金黄色葡萄球菌青霉素敏感株和抗药株分别密集涂布于琼脂平板表面的一半。

（2）用镊子取滤纸片两片，用青霉素溶液（5U/ml）浸湿并分别置于上述平板上。

（3）37℃培养 24 小时，观察滤纸片周围有无抑菌圈形成。

2. 青霉素酶的简易测定法（碘淀粉平板法）

扫码“看一看”

（1）将金黄色葡萄球菌青霉素敏感株和抗药株分别密集涂布于琼脂平板表面的两处（约 1cm^2）。

（2）37℃培养 24 小时，敏感株和抗药株生长。

（3）将淀粉琼脂加热融化并恒温于 50℃水浴，加入 1.0ml 青霉素 G 钾盐溶液（20000U/ml），混匀后即刻倾注于上述培养好的平板上，铺平待凝。

（4）用滴管吸取碘液铺满平板表面，吸去多余的碘液，倒置于 37℃培养箱，10～15 分钟后观察抗药菌周围出现无色透明圈。

3. 梯度平板法分离抗药株

（1）融化 2 支 10ml 营养琼脂，冷却并维持在约 50℃。

（2）将一支铅笔垫在平皿下的一端。无菌操作将融化的营养琼脂倒入平皿覆盖整个底层，待凝成斜面。

（3）平板凝固后，取出铅笔将平板放平。

（4）在第二支融化的营养琼脂试管中加入 0.1ml 链霉素，用手搓匀，无菌操作将其倒在倾斜的底层平板上，待凝，成链霉素梯度平板。

（5）吸取 0.2ml 金黄色葡萄球菌培养物于梯度平板，用涂布棒涂布均匀。

（6）37℃倒置培养 48 小时。

（7）培养后，选择 1～2 个生长在中间链霉素含量的菌落，向平板上高浓度的方向划线。

（8）37℃倒置培养 48 小时。

（9）观察划线后的菌落生长情况，在高链霉素含量区域出现的菌落可能是链霉素抗药株。

【结果与讨论】

（1）抗药性变异实验结果。

表 28－1　抗药性变异实验结果

细菌名称	培养基	生长状况
金黄色葡萄球菌（青霉素敏感株）		
金黄色葡萄球菌（青霉素耐药株）		

（2）青霉素酶测定实验结果（表 28-2）。

表 28－2　青霉素酶测定实验结果

细菌名称	实验结果
金黄色葡萄球菌（青霉素敏感株）	
金黄色葡萄球菌（青霉素耐药株）	

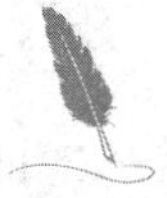

（3）梯度平板法分离抗药菌实验结果。

(4) 细菌抗药性机制是怎样的?

(5) 分离抗药突变株为什么可以用梯度平板法?

(6) 是链霉素导致了抗链霉素突变的产生吗? 为什么?

(7) 为什么近年来抗药菌在增加?

EXPERIMENT 28 Drug Resistant Variation

Purpose

(1) To be familiar with variations in drug resistance of bacteria.

(2) To be familiar with a simple method to determine penicillinase.

(3) To understand how to isolate a drug resistant mutant by gradient – plate technique.

Principle

Mutations resistant to antibiotics such as streptomycin occur at a very low ratio in the microbial cell population. However, these rare strains can be easily detected because they grow at the antibiotic concentrations that inhibit the growth of normal bacteria.

In a drug resistant organism, the mutated gene enables the cell to circumvent the antimicrobial effect of the drug by a variety of mechanisms, including: ①The production of an enzyme that alters the chemical structure of the antibiotic, as in penicillin resistance. ②A change in the selective permeability of the cell membrane, as in erythromycin resistance. ③A modification of the target site of antibiotics, as in the resistance to streptomycin, which interferes with the translation process at the ribosomes.

A drug resistant mutant has relative resistance to antimicrobial agents. A multiple drug resistant strain shows resistance to multiple drugs that have different mechanisms.

Penicillin – resistant strain of *Staphylococcus aureus* can produce penicillinase. The enzyme hydrolyzes the β – lactam ring of penicillin to penicilloic acid which can be oxidized by I_2. Starch is used to indicate the presence of I_2 because it can form a blue complex with I_2. I_2 will be exhausted and a clear and colorless area appears around the colony of drug resistant strain.

The gradient – plate is an effective and convenient technique in isolating drug – resistant mutant from a prototrophic (wild type, drug – sensitive) culture. This requires preparation of a double – layer agar plate as illustrated in Fig. 28 – 2. the bottom slanted nutrient agar layer lacks streptomycin. When poured the melted agar containing streptomycin over the bottom slanted layer a drug concentration gradient in the surface layer will produce. Following a spread – plate inoculation of the drug – sensitive culture and incubation, the appearance of colonies in a region of high streptomycin concentration is indicative of streptomycin – resistant mutants.

Materials and Apparatus

1. Strains 18 ~ 24h nutrient agar slant cultures of *Staphylococcus aureus* penicillin sensitive strain and penicillin resistant strain, 24h nutrient broth culture of *Staphylococcus aureus*.

2. Media nutrient agar.

3. Reagents Penicillin solution (5U/ml), sterile filter paper discs, starch agar (5ml, starch 0. 5% , agar 0. 8%), penicillin G potassium solution (20000 U/ml), I_2 solution (dissolve 0. 08mol of I_2 into KI solution of 3. 2mol/L), streptomycin solution (0. 1 mg/ml) .

4. Apparatus inoculating loop, sterile filter paper disc, tweezer, spreading rod, sterile petri dish, and incubator.

Procedures

1. Drug – Resistant Mutation (drug sensitivity test)

(1) Spread the cultures of sensitive and resistant strains on 1/2 of the plate surface, respectively.

(2) Place two filter paper discs containing penicillin on the area of sensitive and resistant strains, respectively.

(3) Incubate at 37℃ for 24h. Examine the plate for bacterial growth.

2. Determination of Penicillinase (I_2 – starch plate method)

(1) Inoculate the sensitive and resistant strains on the plate, respectively. The area is about $1cm^2$.

(2) Incubate at 37℃ for 24h.

(3) Melt the starch agar and maintain in 50℃ water bath. Add 1. 0ml penicillin G potassium solution (20000 U/ml) into starch agar tube, mix quickly and pour on the incubated plate.

(4) After cooling, pipette I_2 solution on the surface of all the plate. Move away the surplus I_2 solution. Incubate the plate inverted at 37℃ for 10 ~ 15min. Examine the clear and colorless area around the colony of resistant strain.

3. Isolation of a Streptomycin – Resistant Mutant

(1) Melt two 10ml nutrient agar tubes. Cool and maintain at about 50℃.

(2) Place a pencil under one end of a sterile petri dish. Pour aseptically a tube of melted nutrient agar into the plate to cover the entire bottom surface, and allow it to solidify in the slanted position.

(3) After the agar has hardened, remove the pencil and place the plate flat on the table.

(4) Add 0. 1ml of the streptomycin solution to a second tube of melted nutrient agar. Mix by rotating the tube between the palms of your hands. Aseptically pour the mixture on the surface of the gradient – plate and allow it to harden.

(5) Pipette 0. 2ml of the *Staphylococcus aureus* culture onto the agar surface. Spread the culture over the surface of the plate using the sterile glass spreader.

(6) Incubate at 37℃ for 48h in an inverted position.

(7) Following incubation, select one or two isolated colonies present in the middle of the streptomycin concentration gradient. Streak the selected colonies toward the high – concentration end of the plate using a sterile inoculating loop.

(8) Incubate the plate at 37℃ for 48h in an inverted position.

(9) Observe the line of growth from the streaked colonies into the area of high streptomycin concentration. Growth in this area is indicative of streptomycin resistant mutants.

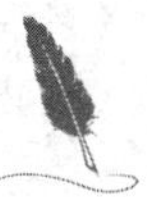

Results and Discussion

(1) The results of drug – resistant mutation.

Strains	Medium	Description of growth
Staphylococcus aureus (penicillin sensitive)		
Staphylococcus aureus (penicillin resistant)		

(2) The results of determination of penicillinase (I_2 - starch plate method).

Strains	Description of results
Staphylococcus aureus (penicillin sensitive)	
Staphylococcus aureus (penicillin resistant)	

(3) The results of isolation of a streptomycin - resistant mutant.

(4) What are the underlying mechanisms for antibiotic resistance?

(5) Why can gradient - plate be used to isolate mutants?

(6) Does streptomycin in the medium cause the mutations? Explain.

(7) Why has there been an increase in drug resistant bacterial strains in recent years?

实验二十九　组氨酸营养缺陷型菌株的诱变和筛选

扫码“学一学”

【实验目的】

(1) 熟悉诱发突变和理化诱变剂的诱变作用。

(2) 了解营养缺陷型的浓缩和检出方法以及生长谱鉴定方法。

【实验原理】

突变是DNA核苷酸序列的稳定可遗传的改变。突变的发生有两条途径，自发和诱发。自发突变是在没有外来因素的作用下在细胞中以极低的频率发生。而诱发突变是微生物暴露在诱变剂中产生的。诱变剂是能够提高突变频率的物理或化学因素。

营养缺陷型是丧失合成某一物质（如氨基酸、维生素、核苷酸等）的能力而必须从环境中获得该物质的突变细菌，它们在基本培养基上不能生长，必须补充某些物质才能生长。能够在基本培养基上生长的菌株称为原养型。筛选营养缺陷型菌株主要经过如下四个步骤：诱变处理、营养缺陷型浓缩、营养缺陷型检出、生长谱鉴定。

浓缩营养缺陷型的方法有青霉素浓缩法、菌丝过滤法、差别杀菌法、饥饿法等，这些方法适用于不同的微生物。细菌的缺陷型筛选可用青霉素浓缩法，酵母菌和霉菌的缺陷型筛选可以用制霉菌素代替青霉素。放线菌和霉菌可用菌丝过滤法，它们的野生型孢子能在基本培养基中萌发并长成菌丝，缺陷型的孢子不能长成菌丝。所以把经诱变处理的孢子悬浮在基本培养液中振荡培养，在培养过程中过滤几次，每次培养时间不宜过长，这样才能充分浓缩。

营养缺陷型的检出一般有四种方法：随机筛选法（逐个点种法）、影印法、夹层培养法和限量补给法。逐个点种法，简便易行，但效率较低。

营养缺陷型的生长谱鉴定一般分两步，第一步先确定为哪一大类（氨基酸、维生素或核苷酸等）缺陷型，第二步再具体鉴定为哪种营养要求。

本实验采用化学诱变，用烷化剂硫酸二乙酯（DES）处理大肠埃希菌以获得营养缺陷型。采用青霉素浓缩法和逐个点种法进行营养缺陷型的浓缩和检出。本实验不进行大类测定，主要鉴定氨基酸缺陷型。由于氨基酸有20种，故将它们排列组合成几大组，可直接用氨基酸混合粉末点种，也可制成滤纸片贴于平板上。

【实验材料】

1. **菌种**　大肠埃希菌K12S。

2. **培养基**　肉汤液体培养基，完全培养基（肉汤固体培养基），无N基本液体培养基，2N基本液体培养基，50×Vogel盐溶液（即50倍浓度），平板用基本培养基。

3. **试剂**　硫酸二乙酯，0.1mol/L pH 7.1磷酸缓冲液，生理盐水，20% $Na_2S_2O_3$溶液，青霉素，混合六组氨基酸（表29－1）。

表29－1　混合六组氨基酸

类别	氨基酸					
Ⅰ	赖	精	甲硫	胱	亮	异亮
Ⅱ	缬	精	苯丙	酪	色	组
Ⅲ	苏	甲硫	苯丙	谷	谷氨酰胺	脯
Ⅳ	羟脯	胱	酪	谷	天冬	天冬酰胺
Ⅴ	丙	亮	色	谷氨酰胺	天冬	甘
Ⅵ	丝	异亮	组	脯	天冬酰胺	甘

4. **器材**　恒温水浴，离心机，摇床，锥形瓶，离心管，试管，吸管，吸球，平皿，牙签等。

【实验方法】

1. 诱变

（1）取一环过夜活化的斜面菌，接种于盛有10ml肉汤培养基的锥形瓶中，37℃摇育5小时。

（2）将菌液转移至离心管，3500r/min离心10分钟，倾去上清液，混旋器混匀沉淀，加pH 7.1磷酸缓冲液10ml，放置37℃水浴中备用。

（3）取存放于37℃水浴中的备用菌液2ml，加入含8ml磷酸缓冲液的锥形瓶中，混匀，加0.1ml硫酸二乙酯，迅速摇匀，立即放入37℃，100 r/min作用20分钟。

（4）将处理过的菌液，加入0.3ml 20% 硫代硫酸钠溶液以终止反应。离心集菌，菌体沉淀打匀，加入10ml肉汤培养基，取1ml用生理盐水作10倍系列稀释至10^{-4}～10^{-5}（以每只平板50～100个菌落为宜，故稀释度应视具体情况变动）；其余菌液于37℃培养2～3h使表型表达。

（5）从10^{-4}、10^{-5}的稀释管中，分别吸取0.1ml，加入铺有15ml完全培养基的底层平板上，倾注约5ml融化并冷至50℃左右的完全培养基，迅速摇匀待凝。每稀释度做2块平板。

（6）37℃孵箱培养48小时，活菌计数。平板冰箱保存，以备营养缺陷型检出用。

（7）对照处理：步骤同诱变处理，诱变剂用磷酸缓冲液代替，最后稀释至10^{-5}～10^{-6}，37℃培养24小时，活菌计数。

2. 营养缺陷型的浓缩

（1）取5ml表型表达过的菌液于灭菌离心管，3500r/min离心10分钟。倒去上清液，沉淀打匀，加入生理盐水，离心洗涤3次，加生理盐水到原体积。

（2）吸取经离心洗涤的菌液0.1ml，于5ml无N基本培养液中，37℃培养12小时。

（3）按1∶1加入2N基本培养液5ml，称取青霉素钠盐，使青霉素在菌液中的最终浓度约为1000 U/ml，再放入37℃培养。

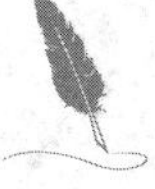

（4）分别于培养12小时、16小时、24小时取样，各取0.1ml菌液倒在两个灭菌培养皿中，再分别倒入融化并冷却到50℃的基本及完全培养基，摇匀铺平待凝，放入37℃培养（培养皿上分别注明取样时间）。

3. 营养缺陷型的检出

（1）制备平板用基本培养基和完全固体培养基平板。

（2）选用经诱变、浓缩处理后长出单个菌落的若干平板，用灭菌牙签轻轻地随机取单个菌落上少量菌，先划叉点种于基本培养基，随之点种于完全培养基平板的相应位置，依次点种，每个平板可点种50个细菌。37℃培养24小时。

（3）选取在基本培养基平板上不长、完全培养基平板上生长的菌落，再在基本培养基和完全培养基上划线复证，经培养后，基本培养基上仍不生长者，可疑为营养缺陷型。

（4）将这些可疑营养缺陷型，接种于完全培养基斜面上保存，以备生长谱鉴定。

4. 营养缺陷型生长谱鉴定

（1）将可疑的营养缺陷型菌株斜面，取一环接种于装有5ml肉汤的离心管内，37℃摇育14～16h。

（2）离心，3500r/min、10分钟，倾去上清，打匀沉淀，加生理盐水5ml，离心、洗涤2次，最后加生理盐水至原体积。

（3）吸取菌液1ml，加于已铺有固体基本培养基平板上，然后再倒入融化冷却至50℃的基本培养基约5ml，摇匀，放平待凝。也可以将菌液加入装有5ml已融化的基本培养基的试管中，迅速摇匀，即刻倾注底层平板上，铺平。

（4）在凝固的平板底上用红笔划分6区，用灭菌牙签分别挑取极少量各组混合氨基酸（每换一组必须换一根牙签），加入平板的相应位置上。

（5）37℃培养24～36小时，观察生长圈，根据表29-1，可初步确定为哪种氨基酸缺陷型。

（6）进一步确证：将此菌按同法制成双层固体基本培养基平板，用牙签挑取该种氨基酸粉末少许，点于平板中间，经培养后，在该氨基酸周围出现明显生长圈。

【结果与讨论】

（1）诱变作用结果记录（表29-2）

表29-2　诱变作用结果

试验组	稀释度	加菌液量（ml/皿）	平均菌落数（个/皿）	菌数（个/ml）	死亡率（%）
对照	10^{-5}				
	10^{-6}				
诱变处理	10^{-4}				
	10^{-5}				

（2）生长谱鉴定结果记录（表29-3）。

表29-3　生长谱鉴定结果

菌株编号	生长组别	营养要求

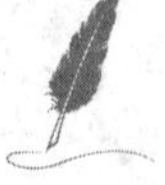

（3）用化学诱变剂处理细菌，为什么要用缓冲液来制备菌悬液？

（4）为什么诱变处理要在充分振荡的条件下进行？

（5）营养缺陷型的浓缩有哪些常用方法？

（6）用逐个点种法筛选营养缺陷型时，为什么要先点种在基本培养基平板上，然后再点种在完全培养基平板上？

EXPREIMENT 29　Mutagenesis and Isolation of *his*⁻ Auxotroph

Purpose

（1）To be familiar with how to induce mutations through mutagenesis with mutagen.

（2）To understand how to detect and isolate auxotroph and how to identify auxanograms of auxotroph.

Principle

A mutation is the result of a stable, heritable change in the nucleotide sequence of DNA. Mutations may occur in one of two ways, spontaneous or induced. Spontaneous mutations arise at a very low rate in all cells and develop in the absence of any external agent. Induced mutations, on the other hand, are results of exposure of the microorganism to mutagen. Mutagen is physical or chemical agent that can raise mutation rate.

An auxotroph is a mutated bacterium that lacks the ability to synthesize an essential nutrient such as amino acids, vitamins and nucleotides and must obtain it from its surroundings. That is, the mutant can grow on medium containing the nutrient supply, but not on minimal medium. Microbial strains that can grow on minimal medium are called prototrophs.

There are four main procedures to acquire an auxotroph: mutagensis, enrichment, detection and isolation, auxanograms identification.

The methods to eliminate prototroph and enrich auxotroph include penicillin enrichment method, filtration enrichment method, selective bactericidal method and starvation method and so on. They can be used to enrich different microorganisms. To enrich auxotroph of bacteria penicillin method can be used. Mycostatin is used instead of penicillin in the case of yeast and mold. Filtration method is used to enrich auxotroph of actinomycetes and mold. The prototroph spores of actinomycetes and mold can germinate to hyphae while the auxotroph spores not. Incubate the spores after mutagensis in minimal broth for a short period, during which the culture is filtrate for several times. By this way, the auxotroph will be enriched fully.

The usual methods for detection and isolation of auxotroph include random isolation (one by one isolation), replica plating, layer plating and limited supply method. The random method is easy to do but its efficiency is low.

The auxanogram identification of auxotroph includes two steps. The first is to define which nutrient (amino acids, vitamins or nucleotides) the auxotroph cannot synthesize. The second is to define which specific amino acid or others is required for its growth.

In this experiment, DES, one kind of alkylating agent, will be used to induce mutation in *Escherichia coli* to acquire auxotroph. Penicillin enrichment and random isolation method will be

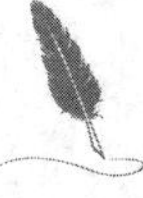

used to enrich and isolate auxotroph. In auxanogram identification, amino acid auxotroph is the focus in this experiment. Twenty types of amino acids are divided into six groups and drop the mixture powder directly or place the mixture filter paper on the plate.

Materials and Apparatus

1. Strains *E. coli* K12S.

2. Media nutrient broth, nutrient broth agar (complete medium, CM), minimal broth without N source, minimal broth containing two – fold N source, 50 ×Vogel salt solution (*i. e.* enriched 50 – fold), minimal agar (minimal medium, MM) used in plate.

3. Reagents Diethyl sulfate (DES), 0. 1 mol/L pH 7. 1 phosphate buffer (PBS), normal saline (NS), 20% $Na_2S_2O_3$ solution, penicillin, mixture of amino acids (see the table below) .

Group	Amino acids					
Ⅰ	Lys	Arg	Met	Cys	Leu	Ile
Ⅱ	Val	Arg	Phe	Lys	Trp	His
Ⅲ	Thr	Met	Phe	Glu	Gln	Pro
Ⅳ	Hyp	Cystine	Tyr	Glu	Asp	Asn
Ⅴ	Ala	Leu	Trp	Gln	Asp	gly
Ⅵ	Ser	Ile	His	Pro	Asn	Gly

4. Apparatus Water bath, centrifuge, rotator, flask, centrifuge tube, tube, pipette, petri dish, toothpick.

Procedures

1. Mutagenesis

(1) Transfer a loopful of overnight agar slant culture and inoculate it to a flask containing 10 ml broth. Incubate the flask with shaking at 37℃ for 5h.

(2) Transfer the suspension to a centrifuge tube. Centrifuge at 3500 rpm for 10min. Discard the supernatant and resuspend the cells in 10 ml of PBS. Store in 37℃ water bath.

(3) Transfer 2ml of the suspension in 37℃ water bath to a flask containing 8ml of PBS and mix well. Add 0. 1ml DES to the flask and mix quickly by rotating and incubate in 37 ℃ water bath with shaking at 100 rpm for 20min.

(4) Add 0. 3ml $Na_2S_2O_3$ solution (20%) into the flask to stop the mutagenesis. Centrifuge and harvest the cells. Resuspend the cells in 10 ml nutrient broth. Transfer 1ml and dilute serially at 10 – fold with NS to 10^{-4} and 10^{-5} (The dilution degree may be changed to make 50 ~ 100 colonies grow on every plate) . Incubate the rest culture at 37℃ for 2 ~ 3h to let the phenotype express.

(5) Transfer 0. 1ml from the 10^{-4} and 10^{-5} tubes to the plates containing 15ml nutrient agar bottom. Pour 5ml of nutrient agar that has been already melted and cooled to about 50 ℃ onto the bottom plate and mix quickly. Let it solidify. Make 2 plates for each dilution degree.

(6) Incubate all the plates at 37℃ for 48h. Count the colonies.

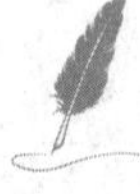

(7) Add 0. 1ml PBS instead of DES to the control flask. The dilution degrees are 10^{-5} and 10^{-6}. Incubate at 37 ℃ for 24h and count the colonies. The other steps are same as to the mutagen-

esis case.

2. Enrichment of Auxotroph

(1) Transfer 5ml culture after phenotype expression to a centrifuge tube. Centrifuge at 3500 rpm for 10 min. Discard the supernatant. Wash and centrifuge the cells with NS for 3 times. Then re-suspend the cells to the original volume.

(2) Transfer 0.1ml of suspension to 5ml of minimal broth without N source. Incubate at 37 ℃ for 12h.

(3) Add 5 ml minimal broth containing 2 - fold N source to the culture (V/V = 1: 1). Add penicillin sodium to the culture to a concentration of approx. 1000 U/ml. Incubate at 37 ℃.

(4) Take samples at the 12h, 16h, 24h. Transfer 0.1ml to 2 petri dishes and pour MM and CM that are melted and cooled to about 50 ℃, respectively. Mix well rapidly and let them harden. Mark the sample time on the plates and incubate at 37 ℃.

3. Detection and Isolation of Auxotroph

(1) Prepare MM and CM plates.

(2) Select the plates on which the colonies are single after mutagenesis and enrichment. Transfer randomly the single colony by stabbing the colony with the sterile toothpick. Streak a cross on the surface of MM plate and then on the same area of CM plate. Inoculate in turn. There are about 50 inoculation crosses on every plate. Incubate at 37℃ for 24h.

(3) Select the colony that can grow on the CM plate but can't grow on the MM plate. Streak again on the MM and CM plates. The colony that can still grow on CM plate but not on MM plate may be auxotroph.

(4) Inoculate the suspicious auxotroph to CM agar slant and store for auxanogram identification.

4. Auxanogram Identification of Auxotroph

(1) Transfer a loopful the suspicious auxotroph CM agar slant culture to a centrifuge tube containing 5 ml broth and incubate with shaking at 37℃ for 14 ~ 16h.

(2) Centrifuge at 3500 rpm for 10min. Discard the supernatant. Wash and centrifuge the cells for 2 times with NS. Then add NS to 5ml.

(3) Transfer 1ml of the suspension to the bottom of MM plate and pour about 5 ml of MM that is melted and cooled to about 50℃. Mix well rapidly and allow it to harden. The suspension can also be transferred to a tube containing 5ml of MM that is melted and cooled to about 50℃. Mix well rapidly and pour it down onto the plate and allow it to harden.

(4) Divide the plate into 6 areas on the bottom surface using a red wax pencil. Pick the mixture powder of amino acids of the 6 groups using toothpick and put it on the corresponding area (one toothpick for each group only).

(5) Incubate at 37℃ for 24 to 36h. Examine the growth circles and identify which amino acid the auxotroph cannot synthesize.

(6) For further identification: Make the double - layer plate containing the auxotroph by the above method. Pick the amino acid powder onto the center of the plate. After incubation, the growth circle surrounding the amino acid will be obvious.

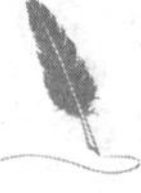

Results and Discussion

(1) The results of mutagenesis.

Group	Dilution degree	Culture (ml/dish)	Average number of colonies/plate	Number of bacteria/ml	Mortality (%)
Control	10^{-}				
	10^{-}				
Mutagenesis	10^{-}				
	10^{-}				

(2) The results of auxanogram identification.

Strain No.	Group No. of amino acid	Amino acid requirement

(3) When treating the bacteria with chemical mutagen, PBS should be used to prepare the bacterial suspension, why?

(4) Why should the mutagenesis be conducted under the shaking condition?

(5) What are the methods for auxotroph enrichment?

(6) When isolating auxotroph using random isolation method, the colony is first inoculated on MM plate and then on CM plate, why?

实验三十　鼠伤寒沙门菌/微粒系统检测化学诱变剂

扫码“学一学”

【实验目的】

了解 Ames 试验的基本原理和方法。

【实验原理】

Ames 等人用鼠伤寒沙门菌的组氨酸营养缺陷型突变株，观察其在测试物作用下，回复突变为原养型而建立了化学诱变剂的检测系统。所用的菌株是几种不同的组氨酸突变型的标准测试菌株，它们除了组氨酸突变（*his*$^{-}$）外，还有 DNA 切除修复系统的缺失突变（Δ*uvrB*）和细菌表面脂多糖屏障突变（*rfa*）。

由于化学物质对微生物的诱变作用，反映了它对哺乳动物的潜在的致癌作用，所以可用此系统来检测一些化学物质的诱变性。该法简便、快速、有一定可靠性，是检测农药、药物、食品添加剂以及工厂、实验室和环境中的一些化学物质诱变性的好方法。

【实验材料】

1. **菌种**　TA97 移码突变（*rfa* Δ*uvrB* *hisD*6610，R 因子：抗氨苄青霉素 Ap^r），TA98 移码突变（*rfa* Δ*uvrB* *hisD*3052，R 因子：抗氨苄青霉素 Ap^r），TA100 碱基置换（*rfa* Δ*uvrB* *hisG*46，R 因子：抗氨苄青霉素 Ap^r），TA102 赭石型突变（*rfa* Ap^r *hisG*428，R 因子：抗氨苄青霉素 Ap^r和抗四环素 Tc^r）。

2. **培养基**　50 × Vogel 盐溶液（即 50 倍浓度），平板用基本培养基，上层半固体培养基，肉汤液体培养基，固体完全培养基。

3. 试剂

(1) 药物：氨苄青霉素溶液（8mg/ml），四环素溶液（8mg/ml），结晶紫溶液（0.1%），正定霉素溶液，亚硝基胍溶液，丝裂霉素C溶液，2-氨基芴溶液。

(2) 大鼠肝匀浆（S-9部分），NADP（辅酶Ⅱ）和G-6-P（葡萄糖-6-磷酸钠盐）使用液。

4. 器材　水浴，15W紫外灯，摇床，培养箱，镊子，培养皿，锥形瓶，吸管，试管等。

【实验方法】

（一）菌株遗传标记的鉴定

1. 组氨酸需要

(1) 制备含生物素3μmol/L和同时含生物素3μmol/L及组氨酸260μmol/L的平板用基本培养基平板各一个。

(2) 将过夜培养的各菌株培养物分别取一环先于含生物素平板上划一道，然后在含生物素和组氨酸平板上划一道。

(3) 平板于37℃培养过夜，检查2种平板上各株菌的生长情况。

2. *rfa* 突变

(1) 测试菌过夜培养物0.1ml，加入装有3ml，恒温于45℃的半固体培养基试管内，摇匀，迅速倾倒于铺有固体完全培养基底层平板上，使上层琼脂均匀分布，待凝。

(2) 用灭菌镊子取无菌滤纸片，在结晶紫溶液中浸湿后，放置在上述平板中央，37℃培养过夜，观察滤纸片周围有无出现抑菌圈。

3. Δ*uvr*B 突变

(1) 制备固体完全培养基平板一个。

(2) 分别取各测试菌液一环，平行划线于平板表面。平板一半用黑纸遮盖，另一半置于15W紫外灯下，距离33cm，照射8秒。避光，放置37℃培养24小时。具有Δ*uvr*B缺陷的菌株，对紫外线敏感，故只有未照射的一边平板上生长。

4. R因子菌株（抗氨苄青霉素试验）

(1) 制备固体完全培养基平板一个。

(2) 取一环氨苄青霉素溶液在平板上涂一条带。

(3) 待药液干后，将各测试菌液分别垂直于药液带接种一条，待干后，37℃培养24小时，观察在氨苄青霉素带的周围是否有生长抑制区。

（二）诱变剂测试

1. 点试法

(1) 灭菌培养皿，倒入融化并冷至50℃左右的平板用基本培养基约15ml作为底层，铺平待凝。

(2) 吸取0.1ml测试菌的新鲜过夜培养物于装有3ml上层半固体培养基试管中，摇匀，迅速倾注底层平板上，铺平待凝。

(3) 分别将蘸有化学诱变剂NTG（1mg/ml）、正定霉素（20mg/ml）和丝裂霉素C（2.5mg/ml）的滤纸片，放入各平板中央。37℃培养48小时，观察结果。

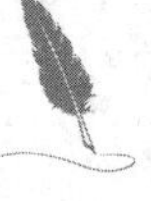

2. 平板掺入法

（1）制备底层平板用基本培养基平板 2 个。

（2）装有 2ml 上层半固体培养基试管内，加 0.1ml 菌液，摇匀，倾注于底层平板上作对照。

（3）吸取 0.1ml 菌液和 0.1ml 待检物于同一小试管内，混匀（也可放置 37℃，振荡作用 20 分钟，使充分接触），随后加入 2ml 上层半固体培养基，摇匀，迅速铺平于底层平板上。37℃培养 48 小时，计数。如回复突变数为阴性对照（自发回复突变数）2 倍以上，即为阳性。各菌株自发回复突变菌落数正常范围如表 30－1。

表 30－1　各菌株自发回复突变菌落数正常范围

菌株	TA97	TA98	TA100	TA102
自发回变菌落数	90～180	30～50	120～200	240～320

基本方法同平板掺入法，只是在上层培养基中还需要加入 S－9 混合液 0.2ml，该混合液必须现用现配，把低温储存的 S－9 置室温下融化，每 2ml 加入 10ml 的 NADP 和 G－6－P 使用液。混合液置冰浴中，用后多余部分弃去，下次实验时重配。

【结果与讨论】

（1）菌株遗传标记鉴定（描述现象）（表 30－2）。

表 30-2　菌株遗传标记鉴定

鉴定 菌株	组氨酸	结晶紫	紫外线	R 因子
TA97				
TA98				
TA100				
TA102				

（2）点试法　以图表示各部位的含义，写出菌株及诱变剂。

（3）平板掺入法　完成表 30－3。

表 30－3　平板掺入法结果

测试物名称	浓度（mg/ml）	测试菌	测试物菌落数/皿	自发回变菌落数/皿
正定霉素	2	TA97		
正定霉素	2	TA98		
NTG	0.1	TA100		
丝裂霉素	0.005	TA102		
2－氨基芴（加 S－9 混合液检测）	0.4	TA97		
		TA98		
		TA100		
		TA102		

结论：

（4）Ames 试验中加入 S－9 的目的是什么？

（5）Ames 试验中组氨酸－生物素溶液的作用是什么？

（6）用细菌系统替代哺乳动物系统检测化学致癌剂的优点和缺点各是什么？

（7）滤纸片周围可观察到抑菌圈。你能解释原因吗？如果出现这种情况，你怎样判断

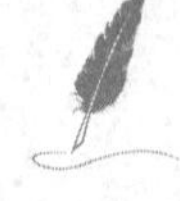

该化合物是否致突变？

EXPERIMENT 30　Ames Test: A Bacterial Test System for Detecting Mutagens and Carcinogens

Purpose

To understand how to screen for potential chemical carcinogens using a bacterial test system.

Principle

Various chemical compounds such as industrial pollutants, pesticides, food additives, hair dyes, cigarette smoke, increase the rate of mutations. It is important to identify such mutagens because they present a potential health risk. Additionally, the carcinogenic (cancer - causing) potential of many compounds to which we are exposed in our environment is highly correlated with their ability to induce mutation. From a genetic aspect there is strong evidence linking carcinogenicity to mutagenicity. Research indicates that approximately 90% of the chemicals proved to be carcinogens are mutagens. They cause cancer by inducing mutations in somatic cells.

Because it is easy to handle large bacterial populations, the mutagenic potential of various chemicals can be demonstrated most easily by using bacterial cell systems. Despite the fact that mammalian cell structure and human enzymatic pathways differ from those in bacteria, the chemical nature of DNA is common to all organisms. This permits the use of bacterial test systems for the rapid detection of possible mutagens and therefore possible carcinogens.

The Ames test, developed by Bruce Ames in the 1970s and still widely used nowadays, is a simple and inexpensive procedure that uses a bacterial test organism to screen for mutagens. Ames test is a mutational reversion assay employing several special strains of *Salmonella typhimurium*, each of which has a different mutation in the histidine biosynthesis operon. The test organism is a histidine - negative (his^-) and biotin - negative (bio^-) auxotroph that will not grow on a medium deficient in histidine unless a back mutation to his^+ (histidine - positive) has occurred. The bacteria also have mutational alterations in their cell walls (*rfa*) that make them more permeable to test substances. To further increase assay sensitivity, the strains are defective in the ability to carry out excision repair of DNA and have plasmid genes that enhance error - prone DNA repair ($\Delta uvrB$).

The Ames test generally requires the addition of a liver homogenate, S - 9, to make this bacterial system more comparable to a mammalian test system. Because many compounds must be activated before they demonstrate carcinogenicity, the reliability of the Ames *Salmonella* test is enhanced by the use of a liver enzyme system which may convert inactive substances to carcinogenic forms as sometimes occurs in animal metabolism.

In the Ames test the strains are plated with the substance being tested and the appearance of visible colonies followed. To ensure that DNA replication can take place in the presence of the potential mutagen, the bacteria and test substance are mixed in dilute molten top agar to which a trace of histidine has been added. This molten mix is then poured on top of minimal agar plates and incubated for 2 to 3 days at 37℃. All of the histidine auxotrophs will grow for the first few hours in the presence of the test compound until the histidine is depleted. Once the histidine supply is exhaus-

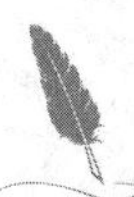

ted, only revertants that have mutationally regained the ability to synthesize histidine will grow. The visible colonies need to be counted and compared to controls in order to estimate the relative mutagenicity of the compound; the more colonies, the greater the mutagenicity.

Materials and Apparatus

1. Strain *Salmonella typhimurium*, TA97, TA98, TA100, TA102.

2. Media Minimal medium, Top agar medium, Nutrient agar, Nutrient broth.

3. Reagent Sterile biotin – histidine solution, ampicillin solution (8mg/ml), tetracycline solution (8mg/ml), crystal violet solution (0.1%), daunomycin solution, NTG solution, 2 – nitrofluorene solution, MMC solution, S9 fraction, NADP and G – 6 – P solution.

4. Apparatus UV lamp, water bath, sterile pipette, tube.

Procedures

1. Identifying the Genetic Marker of Test Strains

1.1 Histidine – require test

(1) Prepare minimal agar plates containing biotin (3μmol/L) and minimal agar plates containing biotin (3μmol/L) and histidine (260μmol/L).

(2) Using sterile inoculating loop, transfer a loopful of overnight broth culture and streak out on the surface of the plates to form a line. Streak the plate of biotin first, then the plate containing both biotin and histidine.

(3) Incubate at 37℃ for 48h in an inverted position.

(4) After incubation, examine the growth on the two types of plates.

1.2 *rfa* mutation test

(1) Prepare nutrient agar plate.

(2) Melt tubes of 3ml top agar in a hot – water bath and maintain the molten agar at 45℃.

(3) Add 0.1ml overnight broth culture to the tube and mix quickly by rotating it between your palms.

(4) Pour the top agar cultures onto the nutrient agar plates and allow them to solidify.

(5) Using sterile tweezers, dip filter paper discs into crystal violet and place them in the center of the plates, respectively.

(6) Incubate at 37℃ overnight.

(7) Examine the inhibition zone surrounding the disc.

1.3 Δ*uvr B* mutation test

(1) Prepare nutrient agar plate.

(2) Transfer a loopful of culture and streak out on the surface of nutrient agar plate to form a line. Shelter 1/2 plate with black paper and expose another 1/2 plate under the UV lamp at a distance of 33 cm for 8s.

(3) Incubate at 37℃ for 24h in an inverted position, keeping from light.

(4) After incubation, examine the growth on the plate.

1.4 R – plasmid

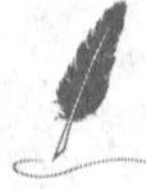

(1) Prepare nutrient agar plate.

(2) Transfer a loopful of ampicillin solution and draw a band on the plate and allow it to dry.

(3) Inoculate the cultures vertically to the drug band to form lines.

(4) Incubate at 37℃ for 24h in an inverted position.

(5) Observe the growth and examine the inhibition zone surrounding the drug band.

2. Mutagen Test

2.1 Spot method

(1) Prepare minimal agar plates.

(2) Melt tubes of 3ml top agar in a hot – water bath and maintain the molten agar at 45℃.

(3) Add 0.1ml overnight broth culture to the tube and mix quickly by rotating it between your palms.

(4) Pour the mixture onto the nutrient agar plate and allow it to solidify.

(5) Using sterile tweezers, dip filter paper discs into the chemical mutagens and place them in the center of the plates, respectively.

(6) Incubate at 37℃ for 48h.

(7) Observe the area around each disc for revertant colonies. Scattered colonies of revertant mutants will appear on the surface of the plate. A positive result is indicated by a relatively high concentration of colonies surrounding the disc.

2.2 Plate method

(1) Prepare minimal agar plates.

(2) Melt tubes of 2ml top agar in a hot – water bath and maintain the molten agar at 45℃.

(3) Add 0.1ml overnight broth culture to the tube and mix quickly by rotating it between your palms. Pour the mixture onto the nutrient agar plate and allow it to solidify. This plate is negative control. The spontaneous revertant ranges are: TA97: 90 ~ 180, TA98: 30 ~ 50, TA100: 120 ~ 200, TA102: 240 ~ 320.

(4) Transfer 0.1ml of culture and 0.1ml chemical mutagens to a tube. Mix and place on the rotator at 37℃ for 20min.

(5) Add the mixture to the top agar tube and mix quickly by rotating it between your palms. Pour the mixture onto the nutrient agar plate and allow it to solidify.

(6) Incubate at 37℃ for 48h. After incubation, count the colonies of revertant.

2.3 Adding S – 9 method

The method is almost the same as plate method above. The only difference is to add 0.2ml S – 9 mixture to top agar tube. S – 9 mixture must be freshly prepared.

Results and Discussion

(1) The results of identifying the genetic marker of test strains.

Identification / Strain	Histidine	*rfa* mutation	Δ*uvrB*	R – plasmid
TA97				
TA98				
TA100				
TA102				

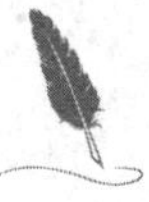

(2) The results of spot test: illustrate each site of the plate and record the strain and mutagen.

(3) The results of plate method.

Test chemical	Concentration (mg/ml)	Strain	Number of induced mutations/plate	Number of spontaneous mutations/plate
Daunomycin	2	TA97		
Daunomycin	2	TA98		
NTG	0.1	TA100		
MMC	0.005	TA102		
2-AF (Add S-9 mixture)	0.4	TA97		
		TA98		
		TA100		
		TA102		

(4) What is the purpose of adding S-9 in Ames test?

(5) What is the function of the biotin-histidine solution in Ames test?

(6) What are the advantages and disadvantages of utilizing bacterial systems instead of mammalian systems to test for chemical carcinogenicity?

(7) An inhibition zone may be observed surrounding the filter paper disc. Can you explain the reason? If this happens, what would you do to determine whether or not the compound was mutagenic?

实验三十一　抗药质粒接合传递试验

扫码“学一学”

【实验目的】

熟悉抗药质粒接合传递的基本原理和方法。

【实验原理】

供体菌痢疾杆菌 D15，对四环素、链霉素和氯霉素抗药，是多剂抗药菌，由抗药质粒编码。受体菌大肠埃希菌 K12W1485F^-，对利福平抗药，由染色体编码。供、受体菌在一定条件下混合，随之接合，接合子在含选择性标记氯霉素（或链霉素或四环素）和利福平的 EMB 培养基上生长，形成具有紫黑色金属光泽的菌落，证明供体菌抗药质粒转移至受体菌。而二亲本在上述含药平板上均不生长。接合子可进一步通过药敏试验和电泳检测抗药质粒的存在来证明。

【实验材料】

1. 菌种

(1) 供体菌　痢疾杆菌 D15（R 因子为氯霉素、四环素、链霉素抗药）。

(2) 受体菌　大肠埃希菌 K12W1485 F^-（利福平抗药）。

2. 培养基　肉汤培养基，EMB 培养基。

3. 试剂　氯霉素（3mg/ml），利福平（3mg/ml）。

4. 器材　无菌吸管，小试管，平皿等。

【实验方法】

1. 活化 将二亲本分别接种肉汤培养基斜面，37℃培养过夜。然后分别取少量菌转种于盛有1ml肉汤试管内，37℃培养5～6小时。

2. 接合传递

（1）用吸管吸取1ml肉汤，置于无菌小试管内，同时加入供、受体菌培养物各0.1ml，混匀。37℃培养2h使之接合。

（2）制备EMB含药平板：吸取氯霉素溶液0.15ml于平皿中，倾注15ml融化并冷至50℃左右的EMB培养基，迅速摇匀，待凝，氯霉素作用浓度为30μg/ml。吸取利福平溶液0.25ml于平皿中，倾注15ml融化并冷至50℃左右的EMB培养基，迅速摇匀，待凝，利福平作用浓度为50μg/ml。吸取氯霉素溶液0.15ml和利福平溶液0.25ml于同一平皿中，倾注15ml融化并冷至50℃左右的EMB培养基，迅速摇匀，待凝。

（3）将EMB含药平板背面，用红笔划分三个区域，吸取0.1ml混合菌液涂布于其中一大区域，另两区域分别用接种环取一环接种供、受体菌，作为对照，37℃培养过夜。

（4）在不含药的EMB平板上划分三个区域，分别接种二亲本和混合菌，培养过夜。

（5）观察供、受体菌和接合子的生长情况，注意观察菌落色泽。

【结果与讨论】

（1）观察平板上细菌的生长状况，特别是菌落的色泽，记录实验结果（表31－1）。

表31－1 实验结果

菌株 / EMB	D15	W1485	接合子
含利福平平板			
含氯霉素平板			
含氯霉素及利福平平板			
无药平板			

（2）怎样判定抗药基因是质粒编码还是染色体编码？

（3）本实验中怎样选择接合子？

（4）实验中形成了多少双重抗药菌的菌落？发生了多少质粒转移？质粒转移是否会随着培养时间的延长而增加，为什么？

（5）本实验中利福平抗性会从大肠埃希菌转移到痢疾杆菌吗？为什么？

EXPERIMENT 31 Bacterial Conjugation: The Transfer of Antibiotic－Resistant Plasmids

Purpose

To be familiar with the principles and methods of the transfer of antibiotic－resistant plasmids through conjugation.

Principle

Plasmids that can affect the conjugation between individual bacteria are termed conjugative plasmids. These plasmids carry genes that code for the ability to transfer themselves from the donor host bac-

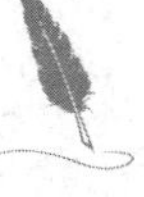

terium to a suitable recipient bacterium by conjugation. The donor strain is *Shigella dysenterlae* D15, which is a multiple drug resistant strain that is resistant to chloramphenicol (CM), tetracycline and streptomycin. Its resistance determinant is located on a conjugative plasmid. The recipient strain is *E. coli* K12W1485 that carries a chromosomal gene for rifampin (Rif) resistance. Mix the two strains and let conjugation occur. On the EMB plate containing both chloramphenicol (streptomycin or tetracycline) and rifampin the conjugant will form purple – black metallic sheen colonies. Neither the donor nor the recipient can grow on this plate. The conjugant can be detected by drug – sensitivity test and its R plasmid can be detected by electrophoresis.

Materials and Apparatus

1. Strains donor strain: *Shigella dysenterlae* D15 (R plasmid: resistant to chloramphenicol, tetracycline and streptomycin). recipient strain: *E. coli* K12W1485 (resistant to rifampin).

2. Media nutrient broth, EMB agar.

3. Drug chloramphenicol (CM) solution (3mg/ml), rifampin (Rif) solution (3mg/ml).

4. Apparatus petri dish, tube, pipette, glass spreader.

Procedures

1. Activation Inoculate the donor and recipient strains to nutrient agar slant and incubate at 37℃ overnight, respectively. Then inoculate them to 1ml broth tubes and incubate at 37℃ for 5 ~ 6h, respectively.

2. Prepare the EMB plates

(1) Prepare EMB agar plate without drug: pour 15ml of EMB agar that has been already cooled to about 50℃ into the petri dish bottom and mix quickly. Let agar solidify.

(2) Prepare EMB agar plate containing 30μg CM per ml: Transfer 0. 15ml of CM solution and pour 15ml EMB agar.

(3) Prepare EMB agar plate containing 50μg Rif per ml: Transfer 0. 25ml of Rif solution and pour 15ml EMB agar.

(4) Prepare EMB agar plate containing CM (30μg/ml) and Rif (50μg/ml): Transfer 0. 15ml of CM solution and 0. 25ml of Rif solution and pour 15ml EMB agar.

Divide the plates into three areas by drawing lines on the back of the plates.

3. Conjugation

(1) Prepare the mating mixture by aseptically transferring 0. 1ml of a broth culture of donor and recipient strains respectively into 1ml of sterile broth. Mix and incubate at 37℃ for 2h.

(2) Transfer a drop of donor culture to one area and a drop of recipient culture to another area of the plates.

(3) Remove the mating mixture from the incubator and transfer 0. 1ml to the third area of the plates. Carefully spread it over the area using the glass spreader.

(4) Incubate invertedly at 37℃ overnight.

Results and Discussion

(1) Examine all plates for bacterial growth especially the color of the colonies and record the results in the report.

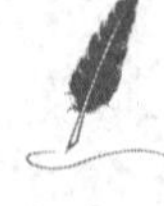

Plate	D15	W1485	Conjugant
CM			
Rif			
CM + Rif			
No drug			

(2) How to distinguish bacterial drug - resistance encoded by plasmid or by chromosomal gene?

(3) How to select conjugant in this exercise?

(4) How many colonies with double resistance were formed? About how many plasmid transfers took place? Does this number increase with incubation time? Why or Why not?

(5) Is it possible that rifampin resistance transfers from *E. coli* W1485 to D15? Why?

实验三十二 抗药质粒 DNA 的分离及检测和转化

扫码“学一学”

【实验目的】

(1) 熟悉质粒 DNA 分离的常用方法和基本原理。

(2) 了解琼脂糖凝胶电泳技术检测质粒 DNA 的基本方法。

(3) 熟悉用质粒转化细菌的基本方法和原理。

【实验原理】

质粒是染色体外的遗传因子，是共价闭合环状的双链 DNA 分子，能够在细胞质中独立自主地进行复制，并稳定地遗传给子代细胞，赋予细胞以某些性质和功能。本实验用的大肠埃希菌携带 pBR322 抗药质粒，使该菌对四环素和氨苄青霉素抗药。根据质粒的抗药性较容易检出和鉴定。pBR322 是遗传工程中常用的基因载体。

分离质粒 DNA 的方法很多，都是利用质粒与染色体 DNA 在特性和构型上的不同而进行的，包含三个基本步骤：①培养菌体和扩增质粒。②收获和裂解菌体。③纯化质粒 DNA。本实验采用煮沸分离法，利用溶菌酶和表面活性剂等的作用，破坏细胞壁中的糖肽层，同时使细胞膜崩解，从而达到菌体的充分裂解，此时细菌染色体可以形成卷曲状折叠结构，附着在细胞膜碎片上，随后通过沸水浴快速作用，使蛋白质迅速凝固并将染色体包裹，经离心呈胶状沉淀物而去除，质粒 DNA 存在于上清液中，加入冷无水乙醇，在 -20℃ 放置 30min，可使 DNA 析出。所获质粒 DNA 可用于转化及酶切等。

质粒 DNA 的检测一般采用琼脂糖凝胶电泳。DNA 分子在高于其等电点的 pH 溶液中带负电荷，在电场中向正极移动。DNA 分子在电场中，通过凝胶介质而泳动，除电荷效应外，凝胶介质还有分子筛效应。泳动速度与分子大小及构象有关。相对分子质量相同而构型不同的质粒 DNA 电泳迁移位置明显不同。为了检测 DNA，一般用溴乙锭（EB），其原理是 EB 可插入 DNA 双螺旋结构的两个碱基之间，它和核酸形成一种荧光络合物，在 254nm 波长紫外光照射下，呈现橙红色的荧光。

转化是将供体 DNA 分子，引入受体细胞，以传递遗传信息的一种手段。目前转化常用于微生物遗传学、分子遗传学及基因工程等方面。转化时受体细胞需处于感受态，一般用氯化钙处理处于对数早期受体菌，使获得感受态。此时细胞膜的通透性发生变化，DNA 分子易进入细胞，实现了遗传信息转移。这种被供体 DNA 所转化的受体细胞叫做转化子。本实验用 pBR322 质粒 DNA 转化大肠埃希菌 K12 802，使获得的转化子对四环素和氨苄青霉素抗药。

【实验材料】

1. **菌种** 大肠埃希菌 C600（pBR322），大肠埃希菌 K12 802。

2. **培养基** LB 培养基，M9 培养液，固体完全培养基。

3. **试剂** STET 液，溶菌酶液，TE 液，电泳液，0.7% 琼脂糖，溴酚蓝 - 甘油溶液，EB 溶液（10μg/ml），60mmol/L $CaCl_2$，4mg/ml 氨苄青霉素溶液，5mg/ml 四环素溶液，生理盐水，无水乙醇。

4. **器材** 无菌牙签，离心管，台式高速离心机，电泳仪，电泳槽，毛细管，254nm 紫外分析仪，恒温水浴，摇床，离心机，吸管，试管，平皿，涂布棒等。

【实验方法】

1. 质粒 DNA 的分离

（1）取新鲜培养过夜的活化斜面菌约 1mm^3 菌量，磨匀于含 100μl 的 STET 液的小离心管内。加溶菌酶液 8μl，室温放置 5 分钟。放入 100℃的沸水浴中，作用 60s。随即迅速放入 0℃的冰水浴中 5 分钟。

（2）8000r/min 离心 5 分钟。用无菌牙签挑出胶状沉淀物，弃去。

（3）加入预冷的无水乙醇约 100μl，混匀，－20℃放置 30 分钟，10000r/min 离心 5 分钟。

（4）倾去乙醇，即得 DNA，加入 20μl TE 液使 DNA 溶解，即可用电泳检测。

2. 质粒 DNA 的检测

（1）琼脂糖凝胶制备：称取 0.7g 琼脂糖置于锥形瓶中，加入电泳液 100ml，盖上棉塞，121℃10 分钟，融化备用。

（2）凝胶板制备：先将融化的琼脂糖凝胶用毛细管吸取少量滴加在玻璃板四周，封边。再将冷却至 50℃的琼脂糖凝胶迅速倒入，使成厚约 3mm 的凝胶层。室温放置 1 小时，待胶液全部凝结后，轻轻拔出试样及挡板。电泳槽内倒入电泳液。

（3）加样：吸取 40μl pBR322 质粒 DNA，与 10μl 溴酚蓝 - 甘油液混匀，加入样品槽内，该染料在电泳过程中作为前沿指示剂。

（4）电泳：接通电源，使电压恒定为 80V，使溴酚蓝液向正极移动。

（5）注意观察，指示剂前沿走至所需距离时，停止电泳。取出凝胶板于 254nm 的紫外灯下观察。

（6）画出点样孔、染色体、质粒带、RNA 及溴酚蓝位置（本法染色体去除较彻底，可能看不见染色体带）。

3. 细菌转化

（1）取一环斜面菌，接种于含 5ml M9 培养液的试管内，37℃振荡培养过夜。

（2）吸取 0.5ml 菌液，加入含 5ml 新鲜 M9 培养液的锥形瓶中，37℃摇育 2 小时，离心集菌，3500r/min，15 分钟。用预冷的灭菌生理盐水洗涤一次，沉淀物加 0.5ml 预冷的 60mmol/L $CaCl_2$ 溶液混匀，即得感受态菌液。

（3）吸取感受态菌液0.1ml加入0.1ml已稀释的DNA（根据预试验结果），冰浴放置30分钟，随即放入42℃水浴约4分钟，再冰浴1小时。

（4）加入2倍体积（约0.4ml）M9培养液，37℃表型表达3小时。

（5）适当稀释，取某稀释度0.1ml涂布于含氨苄青霉素（终浓度20μg/ml）和四环素（终浓度25μg/ml）的完全固体培养基上。同时取不加DNA的菌液及DNA，在相应平板上作对照实验，37℃培养过夜。

【结果与讨论】

（1）转化实验结果（表32-1）。

表32-1　转化实验结果

培养基 / 实验组	完全培养基上生长情况（含氨苄青霉素和四环素）
受体菌	
质粒DNA	
转化组	

（2）怎样制备感受态的大肠埃希菌？

（3）本实验中若省略表型表达结果会有不同吗？为什么？

（4）在进行正式转化实验前需测定受体菌的生长曲线，为什么？

EXPERIMENT 32　Isolation and Characterization of Plasmid DNA and Transformation

Purpose

(1) To be familiar with isolating plasmid DNA.

(2) To understand how to characterize the plasmid DNA by gel electrophoresis.

(3) To be familiar with how to form recombinant bacterial cells by transformation.

Principle

Some microorganisms contain plasmids, which are relatively small extra－chromosomal genetic elements. Plasmids are covalently closed and circular (CCC) DNA molecules that permit the cell to store additional genetic information beyond that is encoded on the chromosome. In general, plasmids contain genetic information for specialized features rather than for the essential metabolic activities of the microorganism. Plasmids can replicate themselves and many can be exchanged between cells, permitting the transfer of genetic information from one microbial population to another. The fact that plasmids are self－reproducing, relatively small, and can be transferred from one cell to another makes them useful tools in genetic engineering, which has become the technology for constructing microorganisms with new capabilities.

E. coli C600 used in this exercise carries pBR322 which is antibiotic－resistant plasmid. So the bacterium is resistant to tetracycline and ampicillin and can be isolated and detected. pBR322 is a common vector in genetic engineering.

In genetic engineering, plasmids carry unrelated DNA into recipient cells, which then become

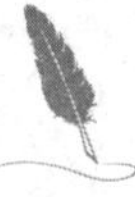

"engineered" cells. After being isolated from their host cells, the circular DNA of the plasmid is cut open (nicked) with enzymes, the restriction endonucleases, creating sites where foreign donor DNA can be inserted. Once the new DNA has been inserted into the plasmid DNA, the ligases seal the nicked ends of the DNA to recreate a circular form. In this exercise, you will follow some of the procedures used to clone genes in genetic engineering technology. First, plasmid DNA from *E. coli* cells will be isolated and purified. Second, the purified plasmids will be digested with endonucleases to produce linear fragments. These fragments and the original circular DNA will be characterized by electrophoresis on an agarose gel.

1. Isolation and Purification of Plasmid DNA There are several methods for isolation and purification of plasmid based on the difference between plasmid DNA and chromosome, including three basic steps: ①Bacteria culture and plasmid amplification. ②Harvest and lysis of bacteria. ③Purification of plasmid.

Boiling - method is used in this exercise. Bacterial cells lysed with enzymes and detergents release plasmid and chromosomal DNA into the medium as a viscous mass. Lysozyme and detergent (for example, SDS or Triton) break the peptidoglycan layer and the membrane. Boiling water bath can precipitate protein. Plasmid DNA can be separated from most of the chromosomal DNA and other cell materials (proteins, high molecular RNA) by centrifugation. Plasmid DNA remains in the supernatant solution while high molecular weight materials precipitate. The final purification step utilizes ethidium bromide - cesium chloride buoyant density centrifugation. Plasmids take up less ethidium bromide than chromosomal DNA macromolecules, which helps in the separation so that the DNA, either chromosomal or plasmid, can be recovered in essentially pure form. In this exercise, the final step in the purification procedure as outlined above will be suitable since it is not well suitable for a classroom laboratory exercise.

2. Characterization of Plasmid DNA by Electrophoretic Mobility on Agarose Gel Plasmid DNA can be detected by electrophoresis on agarose gel. DNA migrates from negative electrode to positive electrode when the pH is higher than its isoelectric point. DNA samples are mixed with a tracking dye and put into the wells on the agarose gel. Migration of DNA through the gel begins when a voltage is applied. Small fragments of DNA migrate faster than larger fragments, and covalently closed molecules migrate faster than linear and open - circular molecules. At the completion of the electrophoresis run, the gel is removed from the apparatus and stained with ethidium bromide. Ethidium bromide is an intercalating agent that is fluorescent with ultraviolet illumination, allowing visualization of DNA bands.

3. Transformation In transformation, free DNA molecules are transferred from donor to recipient bacteria. To take up DNA, a recipient cell must be competent. Natural transformation occurs in relatively few bacterial genera.

Artificial transformation is carried out in the laboratory by a variety of techniques, including treatment of the cells with calcium chloride, which renders their membranes more permeable to DNA. This approach succeeds even with species that are not naturally competent, such as *E. coli*. Relatively high concentrations of DNA, higher than would normally be present in nature, are used to increase transformation efficiency. When linear DNA fragments are to be used in transformation,

E. coli usually is rendered deficient in one or more exonuclease activities to protect the transforming fragments. It is even easier to transform bacteria with plasmid DNA since plasmid is not as easily degraded as linear fragments and can replicate within the host. This is a common method for introducing recombinant DNA into bacterial cells. DNA from any source can be introduced into bacteria by splicing it into a plasmid before transformation.

In this exercise, plasmid pBR322 is used to transform *E. coli* K12 802. The transformant acquires resistance to tetracycline and ampicillin.

Materials and Apparatus

1. **Strains** *E. coli* C600 (pBR322), *E. coli* K12 802.

2. **Media** LB broth, M9 broth, nutrient agar.

3. **Reagents** STET solution, lysozyme solution, TE solution, 1mmol/L EDTA solution, 10μg/ml ethidium bromide solution, tracking dye, electrophoresis buffer, 0.7% agarose gel, 60mmol/L $CaCl_2$ solution, 4mg/ml ampicillin solution, 5mg/ml tetracycline, 0.9% NaCl solution.

4. **Apparatus** Eppendorf (EP) tubes, microcentrifuge, UV transilluminator, horizontal slab gel electrophoresis apparatus with a power source, water bath, shaking incubator, centrifuge, pipette, petri dish, spreader.

Procedures

1. Isolation and Purification of Plasmid DNA

(1) Transfer a loopful of the culture into a sterile EP tube containing 100 μl STET solution. Add 8 μl of lysozyme solution and place at room temperature for 3min. Place into boiling water bath of 100℃ for 60s. Then quickly place into ice - water bath of 0℃ for 5min.

(2) Centrifuge at 8, 000 rpm in a microcentrifuge for 5min. Most of the chromosomal DNA and cell debris will precipitate as a white viscous clot. Pick the pellet up with a sterile tooth - stick and discard.

(3) Add 100μl of cold ethanol to the tube and mix well. Place the tube at -20℃ for 30 min. Centrifuge at 10, 000 rpm in a microcentrifuge for 5min to precipitate plasmid DNA.

(4) Decant the supernatant. Dissolve the plasmid DNA pellet in 20μl of TE solution for detection with electrophoresis.

2. Characterization of Plasmid DNA by Electrophoretic Mobility on an Agarose Gel

(1) Prepare the agarose gels for analysis: Bring 0.7g of agarose in 100ml of electrophoresis buffer to a boil to dissolve the gel.

(2) The solution is then cooled to about 50℃ and poured into a slab mold with a comb for making wells at the top of the gel.

(3) After the gel has solidified, the comb is removed and the electrophoresis chambers are filled with electrophoresis buffer.

(4) Add 10μl of tracking dye to 40μl of the plasmid DNA. Mix well. Add the mixture to the slots on the agarose gel.

(5) Set up the gel so that the tracking dye moves towards the positive electrode. Apply the voltage at 80V.

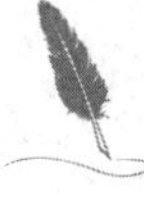

(6) Periodically observe the gel for migration of the tracking dye.

(7) After the run, turn off the power, disconnect the apparatus, and remove the gel.

(8) Stain the gel in ethidium bromide for 30min. Visualize bands under UV illumination at a wavelength of 254nm.

(9) Draw the position of wells, the bands of chromosomal DNA, plasmid DNA, RNA and the tracking dye.

3. Transformation

3.1 Preparation of competent bacteria

(1) Inoculate a loopful of agar slant culture of recipient strain into 5ml of M9 broth. Incubate with shaking at 37℃ overnight.

(2) Inoculate 0.5ml of the above culture into 250ml flask containing 5ml of M9 broth. Incubate shaking at 37℃ for 2h. Centrifuge the culture at 3500 rpm for 15min. Wash the bacteria with pre - cooled 0.9% NaCl solution and resuspend the bacteria in 0.5ml of pre - cooled $CaCl_2$ solution.

3.2 Transformation

(1) Transfer 0.1ml competent bacteria to a sterile tube and add 0.1ml DNA diluted before. Place in ice - water bath for 30min and then place in 42℃ water bath for 4min. Place in ice - water bath again for one hour.

(2) Add two fold volume of M9 broth (about 0.4ml). Incubate at 37℃ for 3h for phenotype expression.

(3) Appropriately dilute the mixture and transfer 0.1ml onto the nutrient agar plate containing ampicillin (20μg/ml) and tetracycline (25μg/ml). The same procedures are also conducted for DNA - control and recipient - control. Incubate at 37℃ overnight.

Results and Discussion

(1) The results of electrophoresis: Draw the position of the wells, the bands of chromosomal DNA, plasmid DNA, RNA and the tracking dye.

(2) The results of transformation.

Media / Test group	The growth condition on CM plate (containing Ap and Tc)
Recipient	
Plasmid DNA	
Transformation	

扫码“学一学”

(3) How to prepare competent cell of *E. coli*?

(4) Will the result be different if omitting the phenotype expression?

(5) The growth curve should be determined before transformation, why?

实验三十三　细菌转导

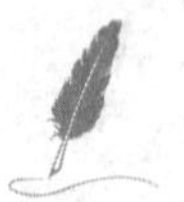

【实验目的】

熟悉局限性转导的基本原理和方法。

【实验原理】

转导是以噬菌体作为媒介，将供体菌的遗传物质传递给受体菌的过程。转导分为普遍性转导和局限性转导。本实验以局限性转导为例，用λ噬菌体专一性转导半乳糖发酵基因的现象来了解转导的基本原理，熟悉转导实验的基本方法。用大肠埃希菌 K12S（λ）gal^+ 为供体，该菌带有原噬菌体（λ），控制半乳糖发酵的基因在细菌染色体上和（λ）紧密连锁。当此溶原菌受紫外光诱导后，原噬菌体（λ）被释放出来，其中有一定比例的噬菌体携带有邻近的半乳糖发酵基因，用它感染另一不能发酵半乳糖的受体菌，就可使受体菌转变为能发酵半乳糖的菌体。过程如下：

K12S（λ）gal^+（供体）

↓UV 照射

λgal^+

↓

K12S gal^-（受体）→K12S gal^-/λgal^+ 转导子（局部杂合子）

【实验材料】

1. **菌种** 供体菌大肠埃希菌 K12S（λ）gal^+，受体菌大肠埃希菌 K12S gal^-。
2. **培养基** 肉汤培养基，加倍肉汤培养基，半乳糖 EMB 培养基。
3. **试剂** 三氯甲烷，含 Mg^{2+} 的磷酸缓冲液。
4. **器材** 离心机，离心管，吸管，毛细管，紫外灯，平皿。

【实验方法】

1. 噬菌体裂解液的制备

（1）过夜活化的供体菌斜面，取一环接种于 5ml 肉汤中，37℃摇育 6 小时。将供体菌离心集菌，3500r/min，15 分钟。

（2）沉淀物加 5ml 含 Mg^{2+} 的缓冲液，混匀。

（3）吸取 3ml 菌液置于灭菌小平皿内，打开皿盖，紫外线照射 30～50 秒（15W 距离 30cm）。

（4）照射后，加入 3ml 加倍肉汤培养基，避光培养 2～3 小时。

（5）吸取培养物 3ml 于离心管中，3500r/min，离心 15 分钟，吸出上清，加 0.1ml 三氯甲烷，剧烈振荡 30 秒，静置 5 分钟，再离心，小心把上清用无菌毛细管转移到另一试管，即得（λ）噬菌体裂解液。

2. 转导

（1）点试法（图 33－1）

①过夜活化的受体菌 K12S gal^- 斜面，取一环接种于 5ml 肉汤中，37℃摇育 6 小时。将受体菌的 6 小时培养物 5～10 倍稀释后，在含半乳糖的 EMB 平板上涂两条菌带，并把剩余菌液吸干，置孵箱中烘干（稍开盖 30 分钟）。

②滴加（λ）噬菌体裂解液 4 滴于受体菌带中，37℃培养 48 小时，观察。同时分别取一环（λ）噬菌体，供体菌，点种于半乳糖 EMB 培养基上作对照，37℃培养过夜。观察结果。

（2）涂布法

①取预先倒好的 EMB 平板 5 只，其中一只加 0.1ml 噬菌体裂解液，用于对照；两只分

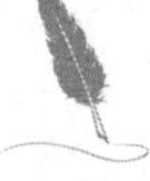

别加0.1ml经活化后的受体菌和供体菌，也用于对照；另两板加噬菌体裂解液和受体菌各0.05ml。

②用4支灭菌的涂布棒分别涂布上述各组平板，37℃培养2天，观察结果。

（3）平板注入法

①将噬菌体裂解液用肉汤稀释为10^{-1}、10^{-2}、10^{-3}、10^{-4}，从各稀释度吸取2ml裂解液于含有2ml经活化后的受体菌的离心管中，同时以只加噬菌体裂解液（2ml 10^{-1}裂解液加2ml肉汤培养液）和只加受体菌（2ml经活化后的受体菌加2ml肉汤培养液）为对照。共6支灭菌离心管，37℃保温15分钟。

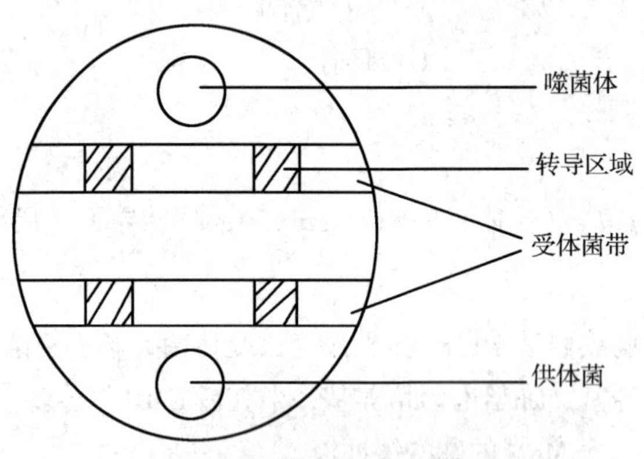

图33－1　转导点试法示意图

②取出上述6支离心管，3500r/min离心10分钟，弃上清，沉淀打匀，用生理盐水洗涤一次，3500r/min离心10分钟，弃上清，沉淀打匀，各加2ml生理盐水制成菌悬液。

③从上述菌悬液中各吸取0.1ml于预先倒好的半乳糖基本培养基平板中，转导试验每浓度各2皿，供体菌、受体菌和对照各1皿，共11皿，用7支灭菌的涂布棒分别涂布各组平板，37℃培养48小时，观察结果，计数出现的转导子数并计算转导频率。

【结果与讨论】

（1）转导点试法结果（表33－1）。

表33－1　转导点试法结果

转导实验	点试法			
	受体菌	供体菌	（λ）裂解液	受体菌＋（λ）裂解液
菌落生长情况				
菌落色泽				

（2）转导涂布法结果（表33－2）。

表33－2　转导涂布法结果

转导实验	涂布法			
	受体菌	供体菌	（λ）裂解液	受体菌＋（λ）裂解液
菌落生长情况				
菌落色泽				

（3）转导平板法结果（表 33－3）。

表 33－3　转导平板法结果

转导试验	平板注入法						
	受体菌	供体菌	（λ）裂解液	转导子数/皿			
				10^{-1}	10^{-2}	10^{-3}	10^{-4}
菌落生长情况							
转导子数（个/ml）							
转导频率 = $\frac{\text{转导子数（个/ml）}}{\text{噬菌体总数（个/ml）}} \times 100\%$							

（4）在制备噬菌体裂解液时为什么要加入三氯甲烷？

（5）怎样区分转化和转导实验？

EXPERIMENT 33　Bacterial Transduction

Purpose

To be familiar with the principle of restricted transduction and transfer method of genes from a donor bacterium to a recipient bacterium by bacteriophage λ.

Principle

In transduction, the DNA is transferred from a donor to a recipient bacterium by a bacteriophage. For transduction, a bacteriophage must acquire a portion of the genome of the host cell in which it reproduces. There are two different types of transduction, generalized and restricted, which differ in whether they can bring about the general transfer of genes or the transfer of specific genes. In each case, the bacteriophage acts as a carrier of bacterial genetic information.

Restricted transduction is made possible by an error in the lysogenic life cycle. When a prophage is induced to leave the host chromosome, excision is sometimes carried out improperly. The resulting phage genome contains portions of the bacterial chromosome next to the integration site. A transducing phage genome usually is defective and lacks some part of its attachment site.

The best－studied example of restricted transduction is lambda phage. The lambda genome inserts into the host chromosome at specific locations known as attachment or *att* sites. The *att* site for lambda is next to the *gal* and *bio* genes on the *E. coli* chromosome; consequently, restricted transducing lambda phages often carry these bacterial genes. The lysate, or product of cell lysis, resulting from the induction of lysogenized *E. coli* contains normal phage and a few defective transducing particles. These particles are called lambda *dgal* because they carry the galactose utilization genes. Because these lysates only contain a few transducing particles, they are often called low－frequency transduction lysates（LFT lysates）. Whereas the normal phage has a complete *att* site, defective transducing particles have a nonfunctional hybrid integration site that is partially bacterial and partially phage in origin. Integration of the defective phage chromosome does not readily take place. Transducing phages also may have lost some genes essential for reproduction. Stable transductants can arise from recombination between the phage and the bacterial chromosome because of

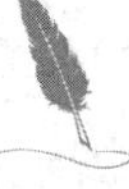

crossovers on both sides of the *gal* site.

Defective lambda phages carrying the *gal* gene can integrate if there is a normal lambda phage in the same cell. The normal phage will integrate, yielding two bacterial/phage hybrid *att* sites where the defective lambda *dgal* phage can insert. It also supplies the genes missing in the defective phage. The normal phage in this instance is termed the helper phage because it aids integration and reproduction of the defective phage. These transdutants are unstable because the prophages can be induced to excise by agents such as UV radiation. Excision, however, produces a lysate containing a fairly equal mixture of defective lambda *dgal* phage and normal helper phage. Because it is very effective in transduction, the lysate is called a high – frequency transduction lysate (HFT lysate). Reinfection of bacteria with this mixture will result in the generation of considerably more transductants. LFT lysates and those produced by generalized transduction have one transducing particle in 10^5 or 10^6 phages; HFT lysates contain transducing particles with a frequency of about 0.1 to 0.5.

Materials and Apparatus

1. **Strains** Donor: *E. coli* K12S (λ) gal^+, Recipient: *E. coli* K12Sgal^-.

2. **Media** Nutrient broth, 2 × nutrient broth, galactose EMB agar.

3. **Reagents** PBS containing Mg^{2+}, chloroform.

4. **Apparatus** Centrifuge, centrifuge tube, pipette, ultraviolet lamp, petri dish.

Procedures

1. Preparation of Transduction Lysate

(1) Transfer a loopful of overnight agar slant culture of the donor strain and inoculate into 5ml of broth. Incubate with shaking at 37℃ for 6h.

(2) Harvest the bacteria by centrifugation at 3,500rpm for 15min, resuspend them in 5ml PBS containing Mg^{2+} and mix well.

(3) Pipette 3ml the resuspended culture to a small sterile petri dish. Irradiate for 30 to 50s with the cover removed from the petri dish at a distance of 15cm from the UV lamp.

(4) After irradiation, add 3ml of broth and incubate in dark for 2 to 3h.

(5) Transfer 3ml of the culture to a centrifuge tube and centrifuge at 3, 500 rpm for 15min. Pipette the supernatant liquid and add 0.1ml of chloroform. Agitate the tube for 5min. Centrifuge again. Transfer carefully the supernatant into another tube. This is the λ lysate for transduction.

2. Bacterial Transduction

2.1 Spot method

(1) Transfer a loopful of overnight agar slant culture of the recipient strain and inoculate into 5ml broth. Incubate with shaking at 37℃ for 6h. Dilute this culture 5 to 10 fold and spread it on the surface of galactose EMB plate to form two bands and dry.

(2) Add 4 drops of λ lysate for transduction on the recipient area. Inoculate a loopful of donor culture onto the plate as donor – control. And add a drop of λ lysate for transduction onto the plate as phage – control. Incubate at 37℃ for 48h.

2.2 Spread method

(1) Prepare 5 plates of galactose EMB agar. Add 0.1ml of λ lysate for transduction onto the first plate as phage - control. Add 0.1ml donor culture onto the second plate as donor - control. Add 0.1ml recipient culture onto the third plate as recipient - control. Add 0.05ml of λ lysate for transduction and 0.05ml of recipient culture onto each of the other two plates.

(2) Spread them out with sterile glass spreader. Incubate at 37℃ for 48h.

2.3 Plate method

(1) Prepare a ten - fold serial dilution of the λ lysate for transduction. Pipette 2ml from each dilution of 10^{-1} to 10^{-4} to centrifuge tubes each containing 2ml of recipient broth culture. At the same time make the phage - control tube and the recipient - control tube.

(2) Keep these six centrifuge tubes at 37℃ for 15min. Centrifuge at 3500 rpm for 10min. Discard the supernatant and resuspend the bacteria. Wash with 0.9% NaCl. Centrifuge again and resuspend the bacteria with 2ml of 0.9% NaCl.

(3) Pipette from each suspension onto the galactose EMB plates and spread out with spreaders. Make 2 plates for each concentration of transduction. 1 plate for each control. Incubate at 37℃ for 48h. After incubation, count the colonies of transductants and calculate transduction rate.

Results and Discussion

(1) The results of spot test.

Transduction	Spot test			
	Recipient	Donor	(λ) lysate	Recipient + (λ) lysate
Growth of colonies				
Color of colonies				

(2) The results of spread test.

Transduction	Spread test			
	Recipient	Donor	(λ) lysate	Recipient + (λ) lysate
Growth of colonies				
Color of colonies				

(3) The results of plate test.

Transduction	Plate test						
Growth of colonies	Recipient	Donor	(λ) lysate	Number of transductant/plate			
				10^{-1}	10^{-2}	10^{-3}	10^{-4}
Color of colonies							
Transduction							

$$\text{Transduction ratio} = \frac{\text{Number of transductant/ml}}{\text{Number of phage/ml}} \times 100\%$$

(4) Why add chloroform in preparation of the λ lysate for transduction?

(5) How can you differentiate experimentally between transformation and transduction?

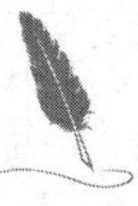

扫码“学一学”

实验三十四 枯草杆菌原生质体的制备和再生

【实验目的】

熟悉细菌原生质体制备和再生的基本原理和方法。

【实验原理】

微生物原生质体技术包括原生质体的制备、再生、融合、诱变、再生育种、转化和固定化等。

原生质体技术的关键是对细胞壁进行消化，以形成大量的原生质体，并使原生质体能高频率地再生细胞壁，回复到正常细胞状态。当细胞壁去除后，原生质体具有以下特征：一是无细胞壁障碍，可对膜和细胞器进行基础研究，同时可进行遗传操作；二是具有全能性，能在人工条件控制下，进行大量快速繁殖；三是可诱导融合，形成杂种细胞，为体细胞杂交提供实验材料。因此，原生质体技术无论在理论上或实践上都日益受到重视，在基因定位、酶的定位、细胞壁的合成和微生物遗传育种等工作中应用相当广泛。

通常用溶菌酶消除坚固的细菌细胞壁，细胞在高渗液中形成原生质体，然后在高渗的丰富的培养基保障原生质体再生细胞壁。由于缺乏细胞壁的保护，原生质体对外界的渗透压十分敏感，制备好的原生质体必须保存在高渗溶液中，而在低渗条件（如水）或 SDS 作用下，即可破裂。利用此法即可计算原生质体形成率及再生率。

【实验材料】

1. **菌种** 枯草芽孢杆菌 168。

2. **培养基** LB 培养基（液体和固体），HM 再生培养基（LB 培养基加 0.5mol/L 蔗糖和 20 mmol/L $MgCl_2 \cdot 6H_2O$），HM 半固体培养基。

3. **试剂** SMM 溶液（0.5mol/L 蔗糖，0.02mol/L 顺丁烯二酸盐，0.02mol/L $MgCl_2 \cdot 6H_2O$，用 NaOH 调 pH 为 6.5），SMMP 液（5 倍浓 LB 液体培养基 2 份，SMM 液 7.5 份，2% 牛血清白蛋白 0.5 份（用膜滤器除菌）），溶菌酶液（5mg/ml 用 SMMP 配制）。

4. **器材** 恒温水浴，离心机，吸管，平皿，试管等。

【实验方法】

1. 原生质体形成

（1）取斜面菌少量，接种至 5ml LB 液体培养基内，37℃，180r/min 摇育过夜。

（2）将菌悬液按 2% 接种量接种至装有 40ml LB 液体培养基的三角瓶中，继续摇育约 3 小时，至 $OD_{570}=0.4\sim0.6$。

（3）吸取菌悬液 10ml，3500r/min，离心 15 分钟，弃上清，沉淀用 SMM 洗一次，重新悬浮于 1ml SMMP 液。

（4）吸 0.1ml 菌悬液加入至 0.9ml 生理盐水的试管中，10 倍系列稀释至 10^{-6}，取 10^{-6} 稀释度的菌液 0.1ml，加入平皿，随即倾注融化并冷至 50℃ 的 LB 培养基约 10ml，摇匀待凝，做 2 个平板，37℃ 培养过夜，观察结果，并计数。

（5）余下 0.9ml，加溶菌酶 0.1ml，使终浓度为 0.5mg/ml，保温 45 分钟，镜检，几乎 100% 形成原生质体，由杆状变成球状。

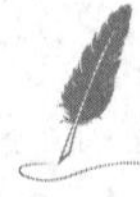

（6）随即 3500r/min 离心 10 分钟，沉淀悬浮于原体积（0.9ml 的 SMMP 液），即得原

生质体悬液。

2. **原生质体再生**

（1）吸取0.2ml原生质体悬液，加入1.8ml无菌水的试管中，作10倍稀释至10^{-2}。放置30分钟，使原生质体破裂，取适当稀释度的菌液0.1ml，加入平皿中，倾注约10ml的LB培养基，摇匀，待凝，37℃培养24小时，计数。

（2）吸取0.2ml原生质体悬液，用SMMP液10倍稀释至10^{-4}～10^{-5}。用双层平板法（先在平皿中倒入HM培养基15ml作为底层，再取适当稀释度菌液0.1ml，加入装有5ml冷至48℃的HM半固体培养基试管中，迅速摇匀，倾注底层平板上），经37℃培养48小时，计数。

【结果与讨论】

（1）将实验结果填入表34-1。

表34-1 实验结果

<table>
<tr><td colspan="2">酶作用前</td><td colspan="6">酶作用后</td><td>形成率（%）</td><td>再生率（%）</td></tr>
<tr><td colspan="2">稀释度</td><td colspan="3">水稀释</td><td colspan="3">SMMP稀释</td><td rowspan="2">$\frac{A-B}{A}\times 100\%$</td><td rowspan="2">$\frac{C-B}{A-B}\times 100\%$</td></tr>
<tr><td>10^{-6}（菌数/皿）</td><td>原液（个/ml）A</td><td>10^{-1}（菌数/皿）</td><td>10^{-2}（菌数/皿）</td><td>原液（个/ml）B</td><td>10^{-4}（菌数/皿）</td><td>10^{-5}（菌数/皿）</td><td>原液（个/ml）C</td></tr>
<tr><td></td><td></td><td></td><td></td><td></td><td></td><td></td><td></td><td></td><td></td></tr>
</table>

注：A：酶作用前的菌数/ml = 平均数/皿/加菌量×稀释倍数；

B：酶作用后的非原生质体数/ml；

C：酶作用后原生质体数/ml + 非原生质体数/ml。

（2）在制备原生质体为什么要加入蔗糖？

EXPERIMENT 34 Formation and Regeneration of *Bacillus subtilis* Protoplast

Purpose

To be familiar with the principle and methods for the formation and regeneration of bacterial protoplast.

Principle

Protoplast technology includes protoplast preparation, regeneration, fusion, mutagenesis, breeding, transformation and immobilization.

The key of protoplast technology is to digest cell wall to form a large number of protoplasts and to make protoplast regenerate cell wall with high efficiency and grow back to normal cells. When the cell wall is removed, the resulting protoplast has the following characteristics: First, cell-based research on membrane and organelle and genetic manipulation may be carried out without cell wall barriers; Second, protoplasts are totipotent and could massively reproduce in artificial conditions; Third, protoplast fusion could be induced to form a hybrid cell for somatic cell hybridization. Therefore, the protoplast technology is more and more important in theory and prac-

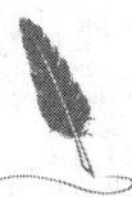

tice, such as gene mapping, enzyme targeting, cell wall synthesis and microbial genetics and breeding.

Usually lysozyme is used to eliminate the solid bacterial cell wall. Formation and regeneration of protoplasts are under hypertonic condition. Lack of cell wall protection, protoplast is very sensitive to osmotic pressure and must be well preserved in hypertonic solution. Protoplast will rupture in hypotonic conditions (such as water) or SDS. So the rate of protoplast formation and regeneration can be calculated.

Materials and Apparatus

1. Strains *Bacillus subtilis* 168.

2. Media LB broth and agar; HM regeneration medium: LB agar with 0.5mol/L sucrose and 20 mmol/L $MgCl_2 \cdot 6H_2O$; HM regeneration medium (semi – solid).

3. Reagents SMM Solution: 0.5mol/L sucrose, 0.02mol/L maleic acid, 0.02mol/L $MgCl_2$ $6H_2O$, adjusted pH with NaOH to 6.5; SMMP solution: 5 – fold concentrated LB broth : SMM solution : 2% bovine serum albumin = 2 : 7.5 : 0.5, with membrane filter sterilization; Lysozyme solution: 5 mg/ml prepared with SMMP solution.

4. Apparatus Thermostatic water bath, centrifuge, pipette, petridish, tube, *etc.*

Procedures

1. Formation of Protoplasts

(1) Inoculate a loopful of agar slant culture to 5ml LB broth and incubate at 37℃, 180rpm/min.

(2) Inoculate the above culture into a flask containing 40ml LB broth. Incubate at 37℃ for 3h with shaking (OD_{570} = 0.4 ~ 0.6).

(3) Pipette 10ml culture and centrifuge at 3,500rpm for 15min. Discard the supernatant. Wash the sediment with SMM solution and resuspend in 1ml SMMP solution.

(4) Pipette 0.1ml bacterial suspension to 0.9% NaCl solution, with 10 – fold serial dilution to 10^{-6}. Pipette 0.1 ml to petri dish and pour 10ml LB agar that is melted and cooled to about 50℃, mix. Make 2 plates. Observe and count after 37℃ overnight cultivation.

(5) Add lysozyme solution 0.1ml to the remaining 0.9ml to make a final concentration of 0.5mg/ml. Incubate for 45min and then examine under a microscope. Almost 100% bacteria form of protoplasts with change in shape from rod to ball.

(6) Centrifuge at 3,500rpm for 10min. Resuspend the sediment in 0.9ml SMMP solution to obtain the protoplasts suspension.

2. Regeneration of Protoplasts

(1) Pipette the protoplasts suspension 0.2ml to 1.8ml sterile water, 10 – fold dilute to 10^{-2}. Lay for 30min. So the protoplasts rupture. Pipette 0.1ml bacteria solution with appropriate dilution to a petri dish and pour about 10ml LB agar. Incubate at 37℃ for 24h and count.

(2) Pipette 0.2ml protoplasts suspension to 1.8ml SMMP solution, with 10 – fold dilution to 10^{-4} ~ 10^{-5}. Pour 15ml HM regeneration agar to Petri dish as bottom layer. Pipette 0.1ml bacteria solution with appropriate dilution to the tube containing 5ml HM semi – solid regeneration medium. Mix quickly and pour onto the bottom layer. Incubate at 37℃ for 48h and count.

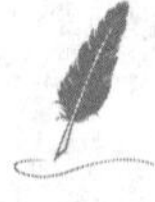

Results and Discussion

（1）The results of protoplasts formation and regeneration.

<table>
<tr><td colspan="2">Before the addition of lysozyme</td><td colspan="6">After the addition of lysozyme</td><td>Formation rate（%）</td><td>Regeneration rate（%）</td></tr>
<tr><td colspan="2">Dilution degree</td><td colspan="3">Dilute with water</td><td colspan="3">Dilute with SMMP</td><td rowspan="3">$\frac{A-B}{A}$ ×100%</td><td rowspan="3">$\frac{C-B}{A-B}$ ×100%</td></tr>
<tr><td>10^{-6}（CFU/plate）</td><td>original bacteria（CFU/ml）A</td><td>10^{-1}（CFU/plate）</td><td>10^{-2}（CFU/plate）</td><td>original bacteria（CFU/ml）B</td><td>10^{-4}（CFU/plate）</td><td>10^{-5}（CFU/plate）</td><td>original bacteria（CFU/ml）C</td></tr>
<tr><td></td><td></td><td></td><td></td><td></td><td></td><td></td><td></td></tr>
</table>

注：A：CFU/ml before the addition of lysozyme = average/plate/bacterial suspension ×dilution fold；

B：non – protoplasts after the addition of lysozyme /ml；

C：protoplasts after the addition of lysozyme /ml + non – protoplasts after the addition of lysozyme /ml。

（2）Why is sucrose added in protoplasts formation and regeneration?

实验三十五　利用 16S rRNA 基因序列进行细菌分类鉴定

扫码“学一学”

【实验目的】

（1）熟悉微生物分子鉴定的原理和意义。

（2）熟悉利用 16S rRNA 基因进行微生物分子鉴定的操作方法。

（3）了解运用软件构建系统发育树并对微生物进行系统发育关系分析。

【实验原理】

传统的微生物分类鉴定方法主要是以微生物形态结构特征和生理生化特性等表型特征为依据，烦琐费时，且有时结果不确定。近年来随着核酸技术的发展，核酸序列分析已经用于细菌鉴定、种系发生及分类。而其中 16S rRNA 基因常被用于细菌鉴定（真核微生物为 18S rRNA）。

随着分子生物学技术和方法发展，生物系统分类基础发生了重大变化，对微生物的分类鉴定已不再局限于表型特征，而是进入了表型特征和分子特征相结合的世代。从分子水平上研究生物大分子特征，为微生物分类鉴定提供了简便、准确的技术和方法，其中 16S rRNA 基因序列分析技术已广泛应用于微生物分类鉴定工作中。

16S rRNA 即 16S ribosomal RNA，是原核核糖体 30s 小亚基的组成部分，参与蛋白质的合成。16S rRNA 分子中既包含高度保守的序列区域，又有中度保守和高度变化的序列区域，16S rRNA 大小适中，约 1.5kb，既能体现不同菌种属之间的差异，又便于序列分析。

16S rRNA 中可变区序列因细菌不同而异，恒定区基本保守，所以可利用恒定区序列设计引物，将 16S rRNA 基因片段扩增出来，利用可变区序列的差异来对不同属、种的微生物进行分类鉴定。一般认为，16S rRNA 基因序列同源性小于 97%，可以认为属于不同的种，同源性小于 93% ~95%，可以认为属于不同的属。

16S rRNA 基因序列分析技术的基本原理是从待鉴定的微生物中扩增 16S rRNA 基因片段，通过克隆、测序获得 16S rRNA 基因序列信息，再与 GenBank 等数据库中的 16S rRNA 基因序列进行比对和同源性分析比较，构建系统发育树，了解该微生物与其他微生物之间

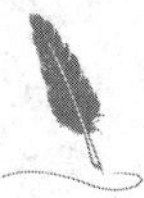

在遗传进化过程中的亲缘关系（系统发育关系），从而达到对其分类鉴定的目的。

本实验以大肠埃希菌的鉴定为例介绍利用16S rRNA基因序列分析技术进行微生物鉴定的实验方法。

【实验材料】

1. **菌株** 大肠埃希菌。

2. **培养基** 营养肉汤培养基，营养琼脂培养基。

3. **试剂** 细菌基因组DNA提取试剂盒，PCR Buffer，DNA marker，Taq酶，dNTP，Genfinder染料，PCR纯化试剂盒，琼脂糖等。

4. **器材** PCR仪、电泳仪、电泳槽、高速冷冻离心机、凝胶成像系统、超净工作台、恒温培养箱、摇床、电子天平、紫外检测灯。灭菌 ddH_2O，无菌水，灭菌的Eppendorf管，移液管，试管，离心管，天平，接种环，酒精灯等。

5. **PCR引物** 选用通用引物，fD1：5′-AGAGTTTGATCCTGGCTCAG-3′；rP2：5′-ACGGCTACCTTGTTACGACTT-3′。

【实验方法】

1. 大肠埃希菌培养

（1）接种大肠埃希菌于营养琼脂平板，37℃培养24小时。

（2）挑取营养琼脂平板上的单菌落接种于5ml营养肉汤试管中，37℃、200r/min，摇床培养15小时。

2. 16S rRNA基因序列的扩增、检测

（1）将培养15小时的大肠埃希菌在4℃、8000r/min条件下离心，收集菌体，用灭菌水洗涤两次。

（2）参照试剂盒说明提取基因组DNA，用0.7%的琼脂糖凝胶电泳检测基因组DNA。

（3）PCR反应：PCR反应体系（50μl）：10×PCR Buffer 5μl，10 mmol/μl dNTP 1μl，正向引物和反向引物各1μl，模板DNA 1μl，Taq酶（2U/μl）1μl，ddH_2O 补足至50μl。PCR反应条件：94℃ 5分钟，58℃ 1分钟，72℃ 2分钟，35个循环，最后72℃延伸10分钟。

（4）用1%琼脂糖凝胶电泳检测PCR产物。

（5）参照试剂盒说明纯化PCR产物。

3. 16S rRNA基因序列的测序 纯化后的PCR产物交测序公司完成测序工作。

4. 序列分析与系统发育树的构建

（1）将测得的序列输入GenBank用Blast软件进行相似性比较。

（2）用Clustal X软件进行多重序列比对分析。

（3）利用建树软件如Mega2.1构建系统发育树，进行系统发育关系分析。

【结果与讨论】

（1）将PCR产物的测序结果打印出来，并分析序列特征。

（2）将基于16S rRNA基因构建的系统发育树打印出来，并对系统发育关系进行分析。

（3）利用16S rRNA基因序列分析技术获得的鉴定结果与原来结果是否一致？若不一致加以分析，如何确定其准确的分类地位？

（4）利用16S rRNA基因序列分析技术进行鉴定时，一般都不直接测定16S rRNA序列，为什么？

EXPERIMENT 35　Bacterial Identification with 16S rRNA Gene

Purpose

(1) To be familiar with the principle and significance of molecular identification of microorganisms.

(2) To be familiar with the operation of molecular identification using 16S rRNA gene.

(3) To understand how to construct the phylogenetic tree and analyze the relationship of system development.

Principle

The traditional identification of microorganisms is usually performed by phenotypic methods based on colonial morphology in agar plates and biochemical tests which are time consuming, laborious and sometimes inconclusive.

In recent years, with the development of nucleic acid technique, DNA sequence analysis has been used for bacterial identification, phylogeny and classification. Polymerase chain reaction (PCR) protocols based on 16S rRNA gene sequences were developed for identification of bacteria (18S rRNA for eukaryotic microorganisms). 16S ribosomal RNA (or 16S rRNA) is a component of the 30S small subunit of prokaryotic ribosomes involved in protein synthesis. 16S rRNA gene is used as the standard for classification and identification of microbes, because it is universally distributed, highly conserved with proper changes between different species of bacteria and archaea and its moderate size (about 1,500 bp) is enough for informatics purposes and convenient for sequence analysis.

Universal primers are designed against the constant region sequence of 16S rDNA for PCR amplification. The hypervariable regions provide species - specific signature sequences for microbial identification and classification. 16S rRNA gene sequencing has become prevalent in microbiology as a rapid and cheap alternative to phenotypic methods of bacterial identification. It is also capable of reclassifying bacteria into completely new species and describing new species that have never been successfully cultured. Type strains of 16S rRNA gene sequences for most bacteria and archaea are available on public databases such as NCBI.

Generally, the sequence of 16S rRNA gene sequence data on an individual strain with a closest neighbor exhibiting a similarity score of less than 97% represents a new species while similarity of less than 93% ~ 95% means a new genus.

The basic principle of 16S rRNA gene sequence analysis technology is: the amplification of 16S rRNA gene fragments from the microbes to be identified, cloning and sequencing the 16S rRNA gene sequence information, comparison and analysis of homology with the 16S rRNA gene sequence retrieved from GenBank databases using BLAST software, classification and identification by construction the phylogenetic tree to understand the genetic evolution and relationship between microorganisms.

The identification of *Escherichia coli* is taken as an example to introduce the method of identification by 16S rRNA gene sequences in this experiment.

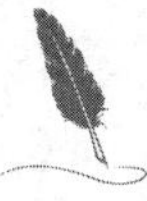

Materials andApparatus

1. Strain *Escherichia coli.*

2. Media Nutrient broth, nutrient agar.

3. Reagent bacterial genomic DNA extraction kit, PCR Buffer, DNA marker, Taq enzyme, dNTP, Genfinder dye, PCR purification kit, agarose, ddH_2O, Eppendorf tube, pipette, tube, inoculating loop, burner.

4. Apparatus PCR instrument, electrophoresis instrument, high speed refrigerated centrifuge, gel imaging system, clean bench, incubator, shaker, balance, electronic balance, UV detection lamp.

5. PCR primers selected universal primers, fD1: 5′ - AGAGTTTGATCCTGGCTCAG - 3′, rP2: 5′ - ACGGCTACCTTGTTACGACTT - 3′.

Procedures

1. *Escherichia coli* culture

(1) Inoculate *Escherichia coli* on the surface of nutrient agar plate. Incubate at 37℃ for 24h.

(2) Pick the single colony and transfer in 5 ml nutrient broth. Cultivate at 37℃ and 200r/min for 15h.

2. Amplification and detection of 16S rRNA gene sequence

(1) Centrifuge the culture at 4℃ and 8000r/min. Collect the pellet and wash twice.

(2) Extract genomic DNA according to Kit instruction. Test with 0.7% agarose gel electrophoresis.

(3) PCR reaction system (50μl): 10 × PCR Buffer 5μl, 10mmol/μl dNTP 1μl, forward primer and reverse primer, each 1μl, DNA template 1μl, Taq enzyme (2U/μl) 1μl, ddH_2O up to 50μl. Denaturation at 94℃ for 5 min, annealing at 58℃ for 1 min and extension at 72℃ for 2 min, for 35 cycles, followed by 10 min extension at 72℃.

(4) Detect the amplified products in 1% agarose gel electophoresis.

(5) Purify according to kit instruction.

3. 16S rRNA gene sequencing

Sequence analysis of the purified PCR products is carried out by sequencing company.

4. Sequence analysis and phylogenetic tree construction

(1) The DNA sequences, exclusive of primers, are compared to all bacterial sequences available in the GenBank databases by using the BLAST 2.0 program.

(2) Multiple sequence alignment is conducted by Clustal X software.

(3) Construct phylogenetic tree using software such as Mega2.1 and analyze the phylogenetic relationship.

扫码“练一练”

Results and Discussion

(1) Print the PCR product sequencing results and analyze the sequence.

(2) Print the phylogenetic tree based on 16S rRNA gene sequence and analyze the phylogenetic relationship.

(3) Is the identification using 16S rRNA gene sequence analysis consistent with the original results? If not, how to ensure the taxonomic status?

(4) Why not test 16S rRNA sequence directly when identifying with 16S rRNA gene?

第六部分　免疫学实验

免疫学广泛应用于生命科学多个领域。它不仅是一门研究机体免疫系统结构和功能的科学，同时也是一门实验科学。对免疫学实验手段的掌握，有助于药学领域的许多工作，如药物免疫功能的测定、疫苗及免疫调节药物的评价、药物的免疫安全性评估、生物制品的研发等。本部分包含了固有免疫、适应性体液免疫、适应性细胞免疫共三方面的实验内容。

实验三十六　抗原与免疫血清的制备

扫码“学一学”

将抗原注射于动物体内，使其产生相应的抗体。待动物血清中产生大量的抗体时，采集动物血液，分离析出血清，此即含抗体的抗血清或称免疫血清。特异性强、效价高的免疫血清在微生物鉴定、疾病诊断与治疗以及抗原分析等方面均有很大用途。

【实验目的】

掌握抗原与抗体的制备方法。

【实验原理】

免疫动物产生抗体的量，一方面可因动物的种属、年龄、营养状况等不同而异，另一方面还与抗原的种类、接种量、接种途径、接种次数以及接种间隔的时间有关。适宜剂量的抗原经正确的接种途径和间隔时间可使免疫动物激发有效的应答而产生大量的抗体。

本实验所用抗原是细菌（9×10^{8} CFU/ml）和血细胞（10%绵羊红细胞），其免疫原性较强，不需使用弗氏佐剂。抗原初次注射后，至少经过一周左右潜伏期，血清内即可检测到相应抗体，以后逐渐上升到达平台期，但是抗体含量不高，而且平台期不长，抗体水平逐渐下降。再次接种抗原后，抗体含量迅速上升到达平台期（远高于初次接种），而且维持时间也长。因此，制备抗体一般需要多次接种抗原，以获得高效价的抗体。

针对细菌的免疫血清称为抗菌血清，针对红细胞的免疫血清称为溶血素。

【实验材料】

1. 试剂　大肠埃希菌24小时斜面培养物，肉汤培养基，硫柳汞，0.5%石炭酸生理盐水，10%绵羊红细胞悬液（由羊颈静脉以无菌方法取血，置于灭菌的含有玻璃珠的锥形瓶中，振摇去其纤维，使其不凝固，并用生理盐水洗涤三次，配成绵羊红细胞悬液）。

2. 其他　2kg左右的健康雄家兔或未孕的健康雌家兔，McFarland比浊管，酒精棉花，碘酒棉花，消毒干棉花，灭菌吸管，毛细滴管，试管，离心管，2ml和20ml注射器针头，灭菌细口瓶，离心机等。

【实验方法】

（一）抗菌免疫血清的制备

1. 抗原的制备

（1）吸取灭菌的0.5%石炭酸生理盐水5ml，注入大肠埃希菌斜面培养物上，将菌苔洗下。

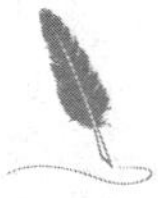

（2）用无菌毛细滴管吸取洗下的菌液，注入无菌小试管。

（3）将此含有菌液的小试管放60℃的水浴箱中1小时，并不时摇动。

（4）与比浊管对照，比浊，判定含菌液试管中细菌的含量。

（5）用0.5%石炭酸生理盐水将菌液稀释至9×10^{8} CFU/ml。

（6）无菌试验　将已稀释好的菌悬液接种少量于肉汤培养基内，37℃培养24～48小时，观察有无细菌生长，如无细菌生长，即可放冰箱4℃备用。

2. 免疫血清的制备

（1）注射动物　用消毒注射器抽取制备好的大肠埃希菌抗原（抽取前摇匀），按表36－1所列剂量与日程注射家兔耳静脉。第14日，自耳静脉采血1ml，分离血清，测其凝集效价，如合格即可大量采血。第16日采血。

表36－1　免疫家兔的抗原注射量与日程

日程	菌液注射剂量（ml）
第1日	0.2
第2日	0.4
第3日	0.6
第4日	0.8

（2）家兔心脏采血　助手的左手紧攥家兔的颈部及两只前腿，右手握家兔后肢，使家兔仰卧，胸腹部向上，固定。或将家兔仰卧手术台上，用绳缚其四肢而固定。

用左手在家兔肋骨左侧探得心脏搏动最剧烈处剪毛，然后分别用碘酒棉花与酒精棉花消毒此部位，将右手所执注射器（注射器为20ml，针头长约35～40mm，可作采家兔心血之用）从心脏搏动最剧烈的肋骨间隙刺入心脏，若针刺准确，则此时心血涌入注射器中，徐徐抽取血液，达足量（一般每兔可抽20ml而不影响存活）时迅速拔出注射器，针刺处按以清洁干棉球，并立即将所得的血液注入灭菌的大试管或平皿内。凝固后放入4℃冰箱中，使其自然析出血清。

（3）制备血清　自上述得凝固血液的容器中，用已灭菌的毛细滴管分出血清，若血清中带有红细胞，则须离心沉淀以去掉红细胞。然后将血清装入灭菌细口瓶中，并测定抗血清的效价（见凝集反应实验）。加入防腐剂，使血清含有1/10000硫柳汞。用蜡封瓶口，贴上标签，注明抗血清名称、凝集效价及日期，放冰箱备用。

（二）溶血素的制备

采用静脉注射方法，在第1、6、11、16日每日注射3ml绵羊红细胞悬液，再于第19～21日取血测定其中抗体含量，如效价在1∶16以上即达到要求，应及时采血。采血方法同上。

【结果与讨论】

（1）制备大肠埃希菌抗原时，使用石炭酸生理盐水和60℃加热1小时的目的是什么？

（2）在动物体内制备免疫血清为什么要多次注射？

PART SIX　Experiments of Immunology

Immunology is widely used in many fields of life science. It is not only a science that studies the rules of antigen recognition and response, but also an experimental science. The mastery of immunological experiments is conducive to many works in the field of pharmacy, such as the determination of drug immune function, evaluation of vaccine and immunomodulatory drugs, assessment of immunological safety of drugs, development of biological products, *etc.* This part includes three aspects of experiment: innate immunity, adaptive humoral immunity and adaptive cell immunity.

EXPERIMENT 36　Preparations of Antigen and Antiserum

Injecting antigen into animals will induce antibody. When a large quantity of antibody is produced in animal serum, collect animal blood and separate the serum. This serum is called antiserum or immunoserum and is used widely in microorganism identification, disease diagnosis and treatment, and antigen analysis.

Purpose

To be familiar with the preparation of antigens and antibodies.

Principle

The quantity of antibodies varies not only with animal species, age and nutrition, but also with the types of antigens, dose and route of injection, as well as times and interval of injection. Appropriate doses of antigen and appropriate intervals of injection can stimulate the effective response and produce large amounts of antibodies in the immunized animal.

The antigens in this experiment are bacteria (9×10^8 CFU/ml) and blood cells (10%). Because the immunogenicity is powerful, Freund adjuvant is not needed. In primary injection, after a period of inducement, the antibody in serum could be detected. The quantities of antibodies will increase gradually, but the total amount is not high, then it will decline. In secondary injection, the total amount of antibody will quickly rise to the highest point and maintain for a long time. Therefore, more injections of antigens are needed to get higher titer of immunoserum.

The immunoserum against bacteria is called anti - bacterial serum. The immunoserum against red blood cell is called haemolysin.

Materials and Apparatus

1. Reagent　the slant culture of *E. coli* (cultured for 24h), broth, thimerosal, 0.5% carbolic acid saline, 10% sheep red blood cell.

2. Others　healthy male or female rabbit, weight 2kg. McFarland turbidity compare tubes, alcohol - saturated cotton applicator, cotton applicator saturated with tincture of iodine, sterile dry cotton swab, sterile pipette, capillary tube pipette with pipettor, tubes, centrifuge tube, 2ml and 20ml syringe and needle, sterile bottle, sterile petri dish, centrifuge, 60℃ water bath.

Procedures

1. Preparation of anti - bacterial serum

1.1　Prepare antigens

(1) Add 5ml 0.5% sterile carbolic acid saline into the slant culture of *E. coli* to suspend bacteria.

(2) Transfer the suspension with sterile capillary tube pipettes to sterile tubes.

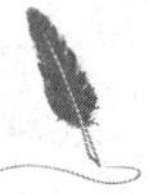

(3) Place tubes into 60℃ water bath for 1 hour. Shake frequently.

(4) Compare tubes turbidity with McFarland turbidity to measure concentrations of bacteria in tubes.

(5) Dilute bacteria with 0. 5% sterile carbolic acid saline into 900 000, 000 CFU/ml.

(6) Culture some diluted bacterial suspension into broth culture for 24 ~ 48h. If no growth was observed, store the diluted bacteria into refrigerator.

1. 2 Prepare immunoserum

(1) Inject animals

Sterilize syringes and needles. Inject the diluted bacterial suspension into the ear vein of the rabbit (Table 36 – 1) . On day 14, 1 ml blood is withdrawn from the ear vein, followed by separation of serum and determination and its agglutination titer. If the titer reaches standard, gather large quantity of serum and, gather serum on the sixteenth day.

Table 36 – 1 The injection quantities of antigen and times in immune rabbit.

Time	The injection quantity of bacterial suspension (ml)
Day 1	0. 2
Day 2	0. 4
Day 3	0. 6
Day 4	0. 8

(2) Withdraw blood from the heart of the rabbit

Let the assistant grasp rabbit neck and two forelegs with left hand, grasp rabbit hind leg with right hand to make rabbit lie supine, then fix it. Or make rabbit lie supine on operating table, fix its four limbs with ropes.

Look for a place in rabbit' s left rib where the most violent heart beat can be felt. Cut the feather and sterilize with cotton applicators saturated with tincture of iodine and alcohol – saturated cotton applicators. Stab into the heart of the rabbit through intercostal space with a 20ml syringe. If the stab is accurate, the heart blood will gush into the syringe. Draw the syringe slowly to get enough blood (a rabbit can remain alive after withdrawal of 20ml blood) . Then pull out the syringe quickly and press on the stab place with sterile dry cotton swab. Aseptically add the rabbit blood into a sterile petri dish. Make the biggest blood slope under 37℃. After stiff, put it at 4℃ ~6℃ to let the serum separate naturally.

(3) Prepare the serum

Transfer the serum with sterile capillary burette into sterile bottles. If there are red blood cells in the serum, centrifuge to get rid of it. Determine the titer of antiserum (reference the method in agglutination reaction) . Add thimerosal into the serum. The concentration of thimerosal is 1/10000. Seal the bottle with wax. Paste labels that indicate name, titer and date. Store it in refrigerator.

2. Preparation of haemolysin Intravenously inject 3ml 10 % sheep red blood cell on day 1, day 6, day 11 and day 16. At day 19 ~ 21, withdraw small volumes of rabbit blood and determine the titer. If the titer is higher than 1∶16, collect the blood as mentioned above.

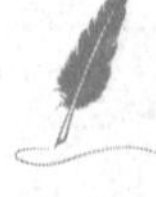

Results and Discussion

(1) For preparation of *E. coli* antigens, why carbolic acid saline and heating at 60℃ for 1h are applied?

(2) Why multiple injections are needed for in vivo preparation of immunoserum?

实验三十七　吞噬细胞功能的测定

扫码"学一学"

固有性免疫是机体针对异物的天然防御功能，主要包括吞噬作用、生理屏障、体液因子作用和自然杀伤作用等。其中吞噬细胞主要包括单核吞噬细胞系统和中性粒细胞，具有吞噬和消化病原体、细胞碎片的能力，在固有免疫中扮演重要角色。

Ⅰ　中性粒细胞的吞噬作用

【实验目的】

检测中性粒细胞的吞噬功能。

【实验原理】

在体外，将葡萄球菌与新鲜血液混合，血液中的中性粒细胞即可吞噬球菌。结果可通过染色观察到。因此可通过测定吞噬细胞的吞噬功能，来了解机体的免疫状态或判断药物对机体免疫功能的影响。

【实验材料】

1. **菌种**　葡萄球菌培养物。

2. **其他**　新鲜血液，肝素抗凝剂，无菌生理盐水，玻片，滴管，载玻片，Wright's 染液，无菌水，明视野显微镜。

扫码"看一看"

【实验方法】

(1) 将试验菌种（葡萄球菌）接种于适宜的培养基中，培养，以比浊法调整菌液浓度，约至 5×10^8CFU/ml，加热 100℃、15 分钟杀菌。灭活菌悬液 4℃保存备用。

(2) 取新鲜外周血（人指尖或耳垂）2~3 滴置凹玻片中，加一滴肝素混匀抗凝（也可用 3.8% 枸橼酸钠），然后加菌液 2~3 滴，混匀后放于潮湿的容器中，37℃ 20~30 分钟，每 10 分钟摇动一次。

(3) 悬液一滴，在玻片上推成薄膜（图 37-1），晾干，加 Wright's 染液，1 分钟后加等量的生理盐水，吹匀。5~10 分钟后弃去染液，水冲，吸水纸吸干，油镜镜检。

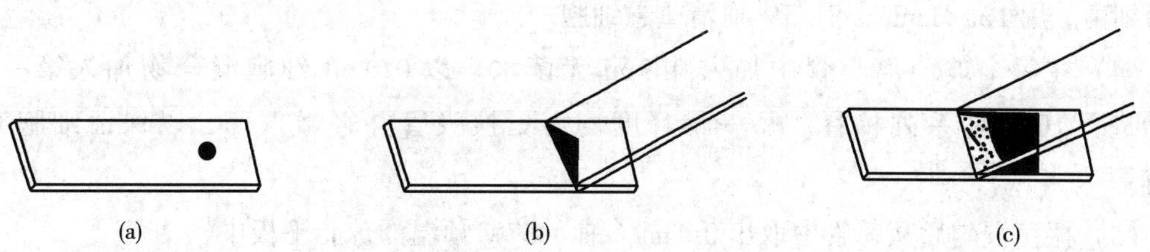

图 37-1　推片制作示意图

(4) 镜检视野中有大量红细胞存在，被染成深蓝色的、颗粒极小的葡萄球菌散在于细胞间。寻找不同视野，可发现蓝色无细胞浆的小淋巴细胞和紫红色的中性粒细胞（细胞核为分叶状），中性粒细胞中可找到许多深蓝色葡萄球菌。

（5）如欲了解机体免疫功能的强弱，可以观察100个吞噬细胞，计算吞噬百分数（吞噬率）或吞噬指数：

吞噬率 = 吞噬了细菌的吞噬细胞数/观察到的吞噬细胞总数

吞噬指数 = 被吞噬的细菌总数/观察到的吞噬细胞总数

正常参考值，吞噬率在61.39% ~64.11%，吞噬指数在1.009 ~1.107。

【结果与讨论】

（1）记录实验结果，作图描述嗜中性粒细胞的吞噬作用，计算吞噬指数和吞噬率。

（2）为什么吞噬细胞在机体免疫应答过程中起重要作用?

Ⅱ 巨噬细胞杀菌功能的检测

【实验目的】

检测巨噬细胞的杀菌作用。

【实验原理】

巨噬细胞具有吞噬和杀伤细菌的作用。这一作用可通过巨噬细胞吞噬细菌的数量与孵育较长时间后细菌数量的比较来确定。

【实验材料】

1. 菌种 大肠埃希菌培养物。

2. 试剂 Hank's液，血清（临用前融化冰浴），Hank's液/5%血清（冰浴），营养琼脂培养基，无菌水。

3. 其他 外周血分离的单核细胞（细胞密度2.5×10^{3}CFU/ml），1.5ml Eppendorf管，振荡器，10ml无菌玻璃离心管（配螺口塞），比浊管，滴管。

【实验方法】

（1）混悬振摇过夜培养的大肠埃希菌培养物，使细菌成为单细胞悬液。以Hank's液制备成2.5×10^{7}CFU/ml的稀释液，取0.1ml加入1.5ml Eppendorf管中。

（2）在Eppendorf管中，依次加入：0.1ml单核巨噬细胞、50μl冰预冷的血清，加Hank's液至总体积1ml，混匀。

（3）将小管在37℃振荡15 ~20分钟，4℃，1000r/min离心8分钟，去上清，去除胞外多余细菌。用1ml Hank's液/5%血清重悬细胞。

（4）在每个玻璃离心管中加入0.9ml无菌水。以0.1ml细胞混合物加入第一管，开始进行10倍的系列稀释。每一稀释度均需更换吸管并轻微振荡，以保证细胞充分裂解。

（5）振荡混匀后从每管中取出0.1ml，铺入37℃预温的琼脂平板中。

（6）同时，盖紧Eppendorf管，置于37℃，孵育90 ~120分钟。

（7）试管置冰上以使细菌生长停止。按照（4）~（5）步的方法制备系列稀释液，并铺入平板。

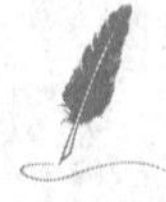

（8）37℃培养24 ~48小时。计数并比较菌落数。

【结果与讨论】

记录巨噬细胞杀伤细菌的实验结果，并分析两次琼脂平板中菌落数差异的原因。

EXPERIMENT 37 Assay of the Function of Phagocytes

Innate immunity refers to the inborn ability that can resist a foreign matter. It mainly includes phagocytosis, physiologic barriers, humoral proteins effect and natural killing, *etc.* Phagocytes mainly include mononuclear – phagocyte system and neutrophils, which can engulf and digest pathogen, cellular debris, *etc.* They play an important role in innate immunity.

Ⅰ Phagocytosis of neutrophils

Purpose

To understand the function of neutrophils.

Principle

When fresh blood is mixed with *staphylococcus in vitro*, neutrophils in blood will engulf the coccus. The results can be observed by staining. Through these results, we can determine the immunity state of a body or the effect of medicines on body' s immunity.

Materials and Apparatus

1. Culture culture of *Staphylococcus.*

2. Apparatus fresh blood, heparin, sterile physiological water, slide, Wright' s stain, bright – field microscope, pipette, sterile water.

Procedures

(1) Prepare the cultures of *Staphylococcus* with 5×10^8 CFU/ml. Store at 4℃ after treatment at 100℃ for 15min.

(2) Drip 2 ~ 3 drops of fresh blood on the slide, mix it with a drop of heparin. Then add 2 ~ 3 drops of coccus into the blood, mix and then put into a wet box for 20 ~ 30min at 37℃, wave the slide every 10min.

(3) Drag a drop of sample over a surface of a slide to form a continuous smear (Fig. 37 – 1). Stain it with Wright' s stain for 1min, then add an equal quantity of water, discard the fluid on the slide after 5 ~ 10min, gently wash and air dry the slide. Observe the slide under an oil – immersion len.

(4) In fields of vision, there are mass of red blood cell and small dark blue particles (cocci). After searching in different fields, you will find lymphocytes, which are blue and have no cytoplasm, and neutrophils, which are purplish red and have a multilobed nucleus. There are many cocci in neutrophils.

(5) The percentage of phagocytosis and the index of it are related to thepotency of body' s immunity. You may observe 100 phagocytes, and calculate as follows:

Percentage of phagocytosis = the number of phagocytes that engulf bacteria/the total number of phagocytes.

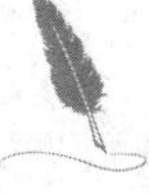

Index of phagocytosis = the number of engulfed bacteria / the total number of phagocytes.

The normal reference of percentage of phagocytosis is between 61.39% ~ 64.11%, The normal reference of index of phagocytosis is between 1.009 ~ 1.107.

Results and Discussion

(1) Drawa diagram of phagocytosis and calculate the percentage and index of phagocytosis.

(2) Why are phagocytes so important in immune response ?

Ⅱ Assay of Bactericidal Activity of Macrophage

Purpose

To understand the bactericidal activity of macrophages.

Principle

Macrophages can engulf bacteria and kill them. This ability is measured by quantitating cell - associated bacteria after a brief phagocytosis period, then determining how many organisms remain after a longer incubation.

Materials and Apparatus

1. Culture culture of *E. coli*.

2. Reagent Hanks' Balanced Salt Solution, normal serum, freshly thawed and kept on ice, Hanks' solution /5 % normal serum, ice - cold, broth agar medium, sterile water.

3. Others Monocytes from human PBMC (2.5×10^7 CFU/ml), 1.5ml Eppendorf tube, Labquake shaker, 10ml sterile glass tube with screw cap, McFarland turbidity compare tubes, pipettes.

Procedures

(1) Vortex overnight culture of *E. coli* and prepare a dilution of 2.5×10^7 CFU/ml with Hanks' solution. Before removing it, vortex the cultures to ensure that bacteria are added as single cells. Add 0.1ml dilution into an Eppendorf tube.

(2) In the Eppendorf tube, mix the following: 0.1ml monocytes, 50μl ice - cold normal serum. Add Hanks' solution to 1 ml and seal caps tightly.

(3) Place tubes in Labquake shaker and rotate 15 to 20min at 37℃. Centrifuge tubes at 1000rpm, 4℃ for 8min. Remove supernatant and resuspend cells in 1ml Hanks' solution/5% serum.

(4) Set up four screw - cap glass tubes containing 0.9ml sterile water each. Starting with 0.1ml of cell mixture, make four 1/10 serial dilutions into these tubes, using a new pipet for each dilution and vortexing briefly (to ensure adequate cell lysis) between dilutions.

(5) Briefly vortex each tube and plate 0.1ml, in duplicate, on broth plates prewarmed to 37℃.

(6) Cap and tightly seal undiluted sample tubes. Incubate samples at 37℃ for 90 to 120min.

(7) Place tubes on ice to stop bacterial growth. Prepare serial dilutions and plate samples as described in step 4 ~ 5.

(8) Incubate at 37℃ for 24 to 48h. Count the colonies and compare the number of colonies at step 5 to the number of colonies at step 7.

Results and Discussion

Record the results of the macrophage killing. And analyze the reasons for the difference in colony number between different times.

扫码“学一学”

实验三十八 体液因子的免疫功能测定

体液中有着多种免疫因子，如补体、溶菌酶、干扰素等。它们具有调理吞噬、介导对靶细胞的杀伤、裂解细菌以及启动炎症反应等多种作用。

Ⅰ 补体溶血反应

【实验目的】

熟悉补体的溶血作用。

【实验原理】

扫码“看一看”

补体的活性可通过绵羊红细胞、溶血素以及豚鼠来源补体间相互作用导致的溶血现象来测定。绵羊红细胞和溶血素的混合，可导致凝集现象出现。如果向系统中添加补体，溶血作用发生。溶血作用常用于测定总补体活性或溶血素的效价。

【实验材料】

绵羊红细胞悬液，溶血素（经56℃加热30分钟处理），补体（来自豚鼠血清）；10ml玻璃试管，无菌生理盐水，无菌吸管，移液管，37℃水浴箱等。

【实验方法】

（1）取小试管三支，按表38－1所示加入各组分。

表38－1 补体溶血反应检测

管号	2%羊红细胞（ml）	溶血素（2单位）	补体（2单位）	生理盐水（ml）	结果
1	0.5	0.5	0.5	0.5	
2	0.5	0.5	－	1.0	
3	0.5	－	0.5	1.0	

（2）操作完毕后，将上述试管放37℃水浴15～30分钟，观察有无溶血现象（如细胞溶解，混浊液变为红色透明的液体）。

【结果和讨论】

根据实验结果，完成表38－1。

Ⅱ 溶菌酶的溶菌作用

【实验目的】

熟悉溶菌酶活性的检测方法。

【实验原理】

溶菌酶广泛存在于机体的泪液、唾液、痰、乳汁、血清等处，是一种重要的体液免疫因子。它能特异性地裂解革兰阳性菌细胞壁肽聚糖分子间的β－1，4－糖苷键，而对革兰阴性细菌细胞壁作用微弱。溶菌酶活性可通过检查其对指定敏感菌株裂解作用来进行测定。

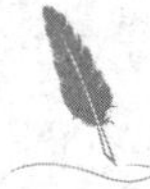

【实验材料】

1. **菌种** 溶壁微球菌（*Micrococcus lysodeikiticus*）菌液，大肠埃希菌菌液。

2. **其他** 1%高层琼脂（以1g优质琼脂溶解于100ml、15mol/L、pH6.4磷酸缓冲液制成），无菌生理盐水，无菌平皿，无菌小滤纸片，无菌吸管，镊子。

【实验方法】

（1）取1%高层琼脂一支加热融化，待冷至50℃左右时，加入溶壁微球菌菌液1ml，倾注成含菌平板。

（2）用镊子夹取滤纸片，沾以唾液（滤纸片应完全湿润），放置于含菌平板的适当区域内。

（3）同时用滤纸片沾取生理盐水，放置于同一平板另一区内，作为对照。

（4）置37℃培养18～24小时，观察结果。如为定量测定，需与溶菌酶标准品对比进行实验。

（5）用大肠埃希菌菌液重复上述步骤。

【结果与讨论】

（1）记录实验结果，并将溶菌酶的溶菌作用实验结果作图。

（2）为什么溶菌酶对溶壁微球菌的效果与对大肠埃希菌的效果不同？

EXPERIMENT 38 Assay of Immune Functions of Humoral Factors

There are many immune factors in humor, such as complement, lysozyme, interferon, *etc.* Their activities fall into a number of broad categories including production and regulation of inflammation, opsonization of foreign materials for phagocytosis, mediation of direct cytotoxicity against cells and lysing the bacteria cell wall.

Ⅰ The hemolytic assay of complment

Purpose

To be familiar with the hemolytic activity of complement.

Principle

Complement activity can be measured and quantitated using hemolytic assays with sheep erythrocytes, and a complement source, usually guinea pig serum. When mixing the sheep erythrocytes with hemolysin, the agglutination will been found. And if complement is added, hemolysis will occur. The hemolytic assay is used in measuring activities of complement or potency of hemolysin, *etc.*

Material

The suspended sheep erythrocytes; hemolysin (56℃ water bath 30min); complement (from guinea pig serum); 10ml glass tube; sterile physiological saline, sterile pipette, 37℃ water bath.

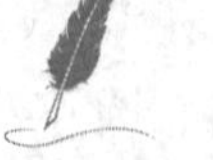

Procedure

(1) Add the materials into three glass tubes according to table 38 – 1:

Table 38 – 1 The hemolytic assay of complement

Tube number	2% sheep erythrocytes (ml)	hemolysin (2 unit)	complement (2 unit)	saline (ml)	phenomenon
1	0.5	0.5	0.5	0.5	
2	0.5	0.5	–	1.0	
3	0.5	–	0.5	1.0	

(2) Place in 37℃ water bath for 15 ~ 30 minutes. Observe the phenomenon (if hemolysis occurs, the solution will appear transparent and red).

Results and discussion

Finish table 38 – 1.

Ⅱ Lysozyme

Purpose

To be familiar with detection of the potency of lysozyme in saliva.

Principle

Lysozyme is an important kind of humoral protein, which has innate immunity effect. It is a natural component of tears, saliva, phlegm, milk, serum *etc.* Lysozyme specifically degrade the β – 1, 4 – glycosidic bond in peptidoglycan, the main component of the gram – negative bacteria. Its effect to lyse the gram – negative bacteria cell wall is weak.

The potency of lysozyme can be tested through determining the lysozyme's lyse effect to sensitive bacteria.

Materials and Apparatus

1. Culture culture of *Micrococcus lysodeikiticus*, culture of *E. coli.*

2. Apparatus saliva, 1% high – layer agar (1 g agar dissolved in 100ml, 15 mol/L, pH 6.4 phosphate buffer), sterile petri dish, small sterile filter paper, sterile physiological saline, sterile pipette, sterile tweezer.

Procedures

(1) Prepare 1% high – layer agar plate with *Micrococcus lysodeikiticus.*

(2) Place a slice of filter paper, dampen with saliva thoroughly, on the dish, by using twee zers.

(3) Place a slice of filter paper, dampen with sterile physiological saline thoroughly, on the same dish, by using tweezers.

(4) Incubate the dish for 18 ~ 24h at 37℃. Observe the result. If you want to test quantity, you should set up a positive control with standard sample.

(5) Repeat the same procedures with cultures of *E. coli.*

Results and Discussion

(1) Draw the diagram of lyse.

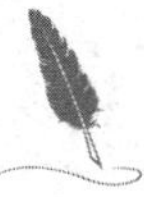

(2) Why the lysozyme effect to *Micrococcus lysodeikiticus* and to culture of *E. coli* is difference?

实验三十九　体液免疫功能检测（1）

抗原抗体反应又称血清学技术包括凝集反应、沉淀反应、中和反应、补体参与的反应和免疫标记技术。颗粒状抗原（如细菌、红细胞）与相应抗体在电解质（生理盐水）参与下产生大小不等的凝块，称为凝集反应。可溶性抗原（如多糖、蛋白质、类脂等）与相应的抗体混合，在适量电解质的存在下，二者比例适合即有沉淀物出现，称为沉淀反应。凝集反应、沉淀反应、中和反应、补体参与的反应是经典的血清学反应，在实验室研究和临床诊断工作中应用广泛。

Ⅰ　凝集反应

【实验目的】

（1）了解凝集反应类别。

（2）掌握玻片凝集与试管凝集的操作与结果观察方法。

【基本原理】

凝集反应可分为直接凝集反应、间接凝集反应和协同凝集反应等。直接凝集反应为最简便、常用的一种实验方法，在操作上可分为玻片法与试管法两种。前者多用已知免疫血清来诊断抗原（如未知的细菌），为诊断肠道传染病时鉴定病人标准中肠道细菌的重要手段，也用于人类血型的测定， 其突出优点是极为快速。试管法多用已知抗原来检测抗体。例如诊断伤寒、副伤寒的肥达反应便是试管凝集反应。试管法可定量。试验时将待检血清用生理盐水作稀释，然后加入等量的标准抗原混合，在一定温度下经一定时间后观察结果。血清发生明显凝集反应的最大稀释度即为血清中抗体的效价。

【实验材料】

1. 菌种　伤寒杆菌（*Salmonella typhi*）培养物。

2. 试剂　伤寒杆菌“H”诊断血清，生理盐水。

3. 其他　洁净玻片，接种环，酒精灯，蜡笔，洁净用小试管（测血清），大试管，1ml吸管，10ml 吸管、试管架等。

【实验方法】

1. 玻片凝集反应

（1）取玻片一张用蜡笔划分为两区，一端标记“S”，即伤寒杆菌。两边各放盐水一小滴。

（2）于“S”端加一接种环伤寒杆菌“H”诊断血清，另一端加生理盐水对照。

（3）用接种环取伤寒杆菌分别于“S”端及盐水端研磨均匀。

（4）轻轻摇动玻片，数分钟后，肉眼观察结果（观察后玻片应做消毒处理）。

（5）如菌体凝集成肉眼可见的颗粒团块或絮状，其周围液体澄清，则为阳性反应。生理盐水对照不应发生凝集，为阴性反应。

2. 试管凝集反应

（1）取洁净小试管 8 支，列于试管架上，依次注明号码，用 1ml 吸管吸取 0. 5ml 生理盐水加于每支试管。用 10ml 吸管吸取 9ml 生理盐水，加入 1 支大试管中。

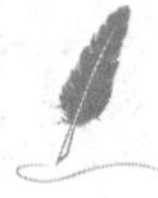

（2）用1ml吸管吸取伤寒杆菌“H”诊断血清1ml加入大试管中，用吸管反复吹吸三次，使血清与盐水充分混合，然后吸出0.5ml加入第1管，同样予以充分混合后吸出0.5ml加入第2管。依此类推，稀释到第7管。自第7管中吸出0.5ml弃去，第8管不加血清作对照，此时第1管到第7管的血清稀释倍数为1∶20，1∶40……1∶1280，每支容量为0.5ml。

（3）用吸管吸取伤寒杆菌菌液，加入各管中，每管0.5ml（由第8管对照管开始向前加），晃动试管架混匀。此时血清稀释倍数又增加一倍，为1∶40，1∶80……1∶2560。

（4）将试管置于37℃水浴箱水浴2～4小时，取出后观察试管底部结果，勿振摇。如所有的菌细胞都凝集成团沉于试管底部，可判断结果为4+。对照管应混浊，如雾状。

（5）血清抗体效价为出现明显凝集现象（++）的血清最高稀释度。

【结果与讨论】

（1）记录实验结果，图示玻片凝集反应。

（2）列表表示试管凝集反应的结果，并作出结论。

（3）如何利用凝集反应测定血型?

Ⅱ　沉淀反应

【实验目的】

（1）了解常见的沉淀反应类别。

（2）掌握环状沉淀反应、单向和双向琼脂扩散实验的应用、操作与观察结果的方法。

【实验原理】

环状沉淀反应是在溶液中进行的简单的沉淀实验。将免疫血清加到试管底部，将稀释的含有可溶性抗原的材料小心重叠其上，让抗原与抗体在两液体的界面相遇，形成白色沉淀环。如抗原系列稀释后进行试验，可对抗原半定量测定。环状沉淀反应广泛用于法医学血迹鉴定和食品真伪鉴别等。

琼脂扩散法分单向和双向两种。单向琼脂扩散是指抗原或抗体这两种成分中只有一种成分扩散的方法。将一定量的抗体混合于加热的琼脂中，倾注于玻板上。凝固后，在琼脂板上适当位置打孔。将抗原材料加入琼脂板的小孔内，孔中抗原向四周扩散，与琼脂板中的抗体相遇，在比例合适处呈现白色沉淀环，沉淀环的直径与抗原的浓度成正比。可先用不同浓度的标准抗原绘制标准曲线，未知标本的抗原含量就可从标准曲线中求出。可用于血清中免疫球蛋白（IgG、IgA、IgM）、AFP或其他可溶性抗原的定量测定。

双向琼脂扩散指抗原和抗体在同一凝胶内扩散，彼此相遇后，在比例合适处出现特异性的沉淀线。双向琼脂扩散实验不但可对抗原或抗体进行定性鉴定和效价测定，还可对抗原或抗体进行纯度分析、相对分子质量估计和同时对两种不同来源的抗原或抗体进行比较，分析其所含成分的异同等。

【实验材料】

1. 试剂　羊血清，抗羊血清，生理盐水，标准羊血清（已知浓度），3%琼脂糖（以pH9.6，0.1mol/L巴比妥-巴比妥钠缓冲液配），牛血清，马血清。

2. 其他　毛细吸管，沉淀反应用小试管，试管架，玻片，凝胶打孔器（直径3mm），载玻片，水平台，水浴箱，37℃恒温箱，10ml吸管，5μl加样器。

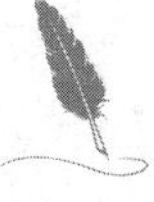

【实验方法】

1. 环状沉淀实验

（1）用细长的毛细滴管吸取抗体（抗羊血清），插入沉淀管管底，徐徐滴入，每管约0.2ml。

（2）取等量羊血清，轻轻加于抗羊血清上方。注意务必使抗原和抗体间能显示出清楚的两层，不可产生气泡，以免抗原和抗体二者接触不均匀而影响结果。

（3）对照管以生理盐水（或人血清）代替羊血清。

（4）静置5分钟后，观察抗原和抗体的接触面，如有白色细微的环状沉淀，即为阳性。半小时后再观察一次。

2. 单向琼脂扩散实验

（1）取干净干燥载玻片，置水平台上备用。

（2）将3%琼脂糖融化，56℃水浴中保温。

（3）取1.5ml琼脂糖加到56℃预热玻璃管中，加入等量抗羊血清，充分混匀后铺于玻片上。

（4）待凝胶凝固后打孔（图39－1），孔距1.2～1.5cm，用记号笔在琼脂板的底面将孔编号。

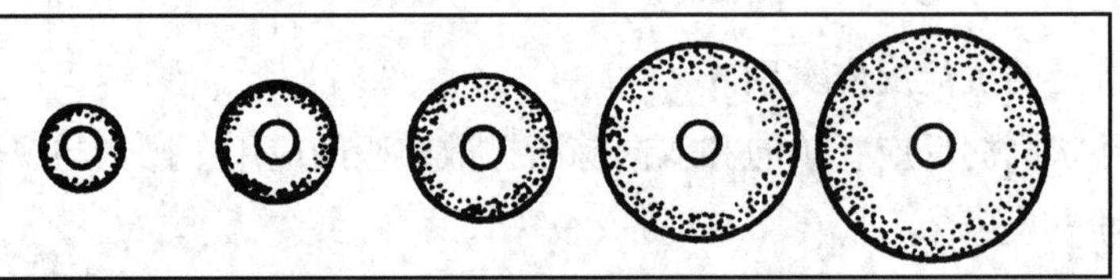

图39－1　单向琼脂扩散结果示意图

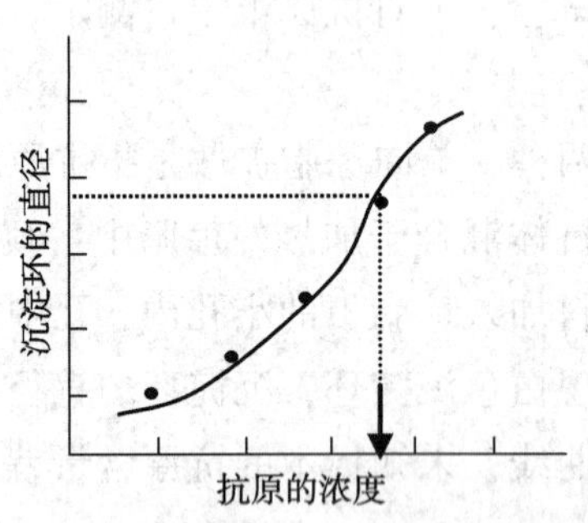

图39－2　单向琼脂扩散标准曲线图

（5）将系列稀释的标准羊血清和待检羊血清分别加到凝胶孔中，每孔5μl。

（6）将凝胶板置于湿盒内，37℃ 24小时后，观察结果，测量沉淀环直径。

（7）绘制标准曲线（图39－2），并求出待测羊血清浓度。

3. 双向琼脂扩散实验

（1）取干净干燥平皿，置水平台上备用。

（2）将琼脂糖融化，取15ml琼脂糖铺于平皿上。

（3）凝胶凝固后打孔（图39－3），孔距1.0cm，用记号笔在琼脂板的底面将孔编号。

（4）中心孔中加5μl抗羊血清，周围分别加羊血清、牛血清、马血清和缓冲液各5μl

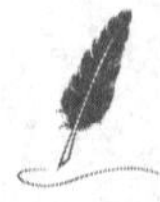

（实验前可先将抗原、抗体做系列稀释，以获得适宜的抗原抗体比例）。

（5）将凝胶板置于湿盒内，37℃ 24 小时后，观察结果。

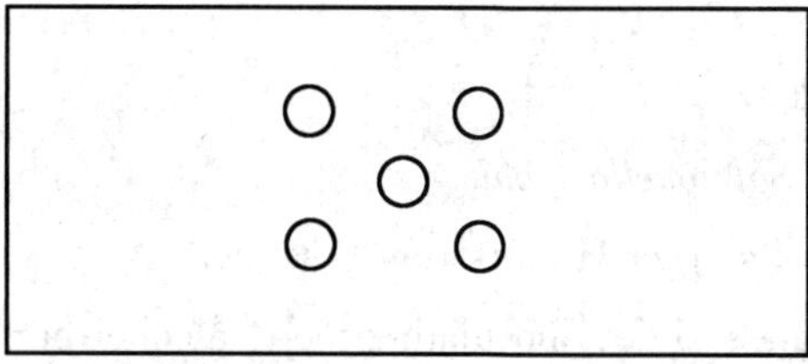

图 39－3　双向琼脂扩散打孔图

【结果与讨论】

（1）详细记录三个实验的结果。

（2）根据双向琼脂扩散实验的结果，分析羊血清与牛血清、马血清之间有无共同成分。抗羊血清的纯度如何？

EXPERIMENT 39　Immune Functions by Antibody（1）

Antigen－antibody reactions are called serological techniques. They include agglutination, precipitation reaction neutralization reaotion, complement hemolysis and immunolabelling technique. Agglutination is the formation of a clumping of particles after the combination of a particle antigen such as bacteria and red blood cell with specific antibodies in the presence of electrolytes. Precipitation is formation of insoluble precipitate after combination of a soluble antigen such as polysaccharide, protein and lipoid with specific antibodies in the presence of electrolytes. Precipitation reaction is one of the basic methods in clinical tests. Agglutination reaction, nevtralization reaction and complement hemolysis precipitation reaction are classical serological reactions and are very useful in the research work and the diagnosis of certain diseases.

Ⅰ　Agglutination Reactions

Purpose

（1）To be familiar with the types of the agglutination reactions.

（2）To grasp slide agglutination test and tube agglutination test.

Principle

Agglutination reactions can be divided into direct agglutination, indirect passive agglutination and co－agglutination The direct agglutination reaction is the simplest agglutination and used widely, including the slide agglutination test and the tube agglutination test. The slide test is often used to diagnose antigens, such as unknown bacteria, with the known antiserum. It is an important method for detecting bacteria that live in intestines and also can be used in determining human blood types. The most outstanding advantage of the slide test is rapidity. The tube test is often employed to diagnose antibody with known antigen. For example, the Widal tube agglutination test can

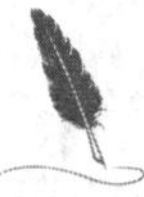

identify *Salmonella*, and it is qualitative. In the tube test, a specific amount of antigen is added to a series of tubes, and serial dilutions of serum are then added to each tube and mixed. The greatest dilution of serum showing an agglutination reaction is determined, and the dilution is the titer of the antibody in the serum.

Materials and Apparatus

1. **Culture** culture of *Salmonella typhi.*

2. **Reagents** *Salmonella typhi* H antiserum , saline.

3. **Apparatus** clean glass slide, inoculating loop, alcohol burner, wax pencil, clean serological test tube, a large test tube, 1 - ml pipette, 10ml pipette and test tube rack.

Procedures

1. The slide agglutination reaction

(1) Mark a line in the middle of the slide to divide it into two sections, mark one end of the slide S (*Salmonella*) . Place a drop of the saline to each half of the slide.

(2) Place one loopful of *Salmonella typhi* H antiserum on the S end, saline is added to other end as control.

(3) Suspend a loopful of *Salmonella typhi* culture at the control end. Then suspend another loop of *Salmonella typhi* H antiserum in the S end. Mix each of the drops thoroughly.

(4) Pick up the slide and rock them back and forth gently. After a few minutes, observe the result with the unaided eye. (After observing, the slide should been sterilized.)

(5) If large clumps are formed and the medium is clear, agglutination occurs. The result is positive. The control result should be negative.

2. The tube agglutination reaction

(1) Using the wax pencil, label eight clean serology test tubes with the number 1 ~8. Pipette 0. 5ml of saline to each tube.

(2) Add 1ml of *Salmonella typhi* H antiserum to the large test tube. Mix by drawing the solution into the serological pipette and slowly blow it out for three times. Then transfer 0. 5ml with the same pipette to the first serological test tube. Mix and then transfer 0. 5ml aliquot to tube 2. Continue this procedure to tube 7, and discard 0. 5ml from tube 7 after mixing. The tube 8 is the antigen control tube without antiserum. Tubes 1 ~7 constitute a dilution series from 1/20, to 1/40 and finally to1/1280. Each tube contains 0. 5ml liquid.

(3) Add 0. 5ml of *Salmonella typhi* culture to each tube (from tube 8 to tube 1) . Mix by gently shaking the test tube rack to agitate all tubes. Tubes 1 ~7 constitute a dilution series from 1/40 to 1/80 and finally to 1/2560.

(4) Incubate the tubes in a 37℃ water bath for 2 ~4h. Then observe the result. Observe the bottom of each tube without shaking. A tube would be given a 4 + ranking if all cells had clumped and settled to the bottom of the tube. The control is seen as a compact bottom with a cloudy supernatant.

(5) The titer of the antiserum is the highest dilution showing agglutination (+ +) .

Results and Discussion

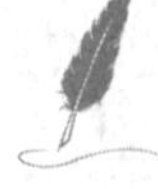

(1) Draw the result of the slide agglutination reaction.

(2) Tabulate the tube agglutination reaction result.

(3) How to identify blood type by agglutination reactions ?

Ⅱ Precipitation Reactions

Purpose

(1) To be familiar with the precipitation reactions.

(2) To grasp the ring test, the simple diffusion test and the double diffusion test.

Principles

The ring test is a simple precipitation reaction that occurs in solution. Antiserum is introduced into a small - diameter test tube, and the antigen is then carefully added to form a distinct layer at the interface between the two reagents. The antigen can be determined semi - quantitatively if a series of dilutions of the antigen is used. This method is extensively used in the bloodstain identification in forensic medicine and foodstuff.

Immunodiffusion includes simple diffusion test and double diffusion test. In the simple diffusion test, either antigen or antibody mixed through the support of diffusion. It can be used for quantitative analysis of antigen or antibody. Mix some antibody with thawed agar and pour them in slides. After solidify, make wells on agar and add antigen into the wells. The antigen in wells can diffuse. The precipitation ring will be formed. The direct proportion can be found between the diameter of precipitation rings and the antigen. Draw a standard curve with an antigen with known concentration and the diameter of precipitation rings and then the unknown concentration of antigen can be obtained from the curve. It can be used for the detection of immunoglobulin (IgG, IgA and IgM), AFP or other soluble antigens in serum.

In the double diffusion, antigen and antibody are placed and diffused in the same agar. As they meet, the precipitation lines will be formed in the area with suitable concentrations. The double diffusion can be used to qualitatively analyze the antigen or antibody, determine the titers, analyze purity, estimate molecular weight and compare antigens or antibodies of different origins.

Materials and Apparatus

1. Reagent goat serum, anti - goat whole serum, 0.85% saline, standard goat serum (with known concentration), 3% agarose (make up with pH 8.6, 0.1mol/L barbital - barbital sodium buffer), bovine serum, horse's serum.

2. Apparatus capillary, test tube, test tube rack, slide, cork borer (with the diameter of 3mm), horizontal table, water bath, 37℃ incubator, 10ml pipette, 5ml pipette.

Procedures

1. The ring test

(1) Pipette 0.2ml anti - goat serum using a capillary pipette and add it into a test tube.

(2) Carefully add goat serum using another capillary pipette to form a layer over the antiserum. Avoid bubbles.

(3) In the control tube, goat serum is replaced by saline or human serum.

(4) After 5min, observe the interface between the serum and antiserum. White precipitation ring indicates a positive result. After 30min, observe again.

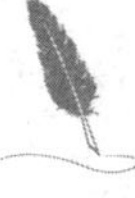

2. The simple diffusion

(1) Put clear and dry slide on a horizontal table.

(2) Thaw 3% agarose and keep it warm in 56℃ water bath.

(3) Add 1.5ml agarose to tubes preheated at 56℃, then add 1.5ml antiserum. Mix it and pour a slide.

(4) After the agar has hardened, cut holes with a cork borer (Fig. 39-1) with the centers of two neighboring holes about 1.2~1.5cm apart, label the slides.

(5) Add serially diluted standard goat serum and the goat serum (with known concentration) into the holes, each for 5μl.

(6) Incubate the slide at 37℃ for 24h in a damp petri dish. Then observe the results, measure the diameter of precipitation rings and calculate the concentration of the antibody in the goat serum (Fig. 39-2).

3. The double immunodiffusion

(1) Put clear and dry slide on a horizontal table.

(2) Thaw 1% agarose and pour 15ml agarose to a petri dish.

(3) After the agar has hardened, cut holes with a cork borer (Fig. 39-3) with the center of two neighboring holes about 1.0 cm apart, label the holes.

(4) Add 5μl antigoat serum into the central hole. Add 5μl goat serum, bovine serum, horse serum and buffer in the surrounding holes.

(5) Incubate the dishes at 37℃ for 24h in a damp box. Then observe the results.

Results and Discussion

(1) Record results of these three experiments.

(2) According to the results of the double diffusion, is there any common ingredients among goat serum, bovine serum and horse serum, and what is the purity of the antigoat serum?

实验四十 体液免疫功能检测（2）

扫码“学一学”

Ⅰ 间接 ELISA 法检测 AFP

【实验目的】

掌握 ELISA 的原理和实验方法。

【实验原理】

酶联免疫吸附试验是以酶标记的抗原或抗体去检测液体中的未知抗体或抗原，随后加入酶的底物，使产生有色产物，颜色的深浅与抗原或抗体的量成正比，可直接目测结果，也可通过酶标仪进行测定。此法可定性，也可定量，在实验室研究和临床诊断中应用非常广泛。标记酶的抗体及底物一般可直接购买。酶联免疫法有直接法、间接法等。本试验利用间接 ELISA 法检测样品中的 AFP（甲胎蛋白）。

【实验材料】

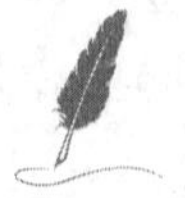

1. 试剂　鼠抗 AFP 单抗，羊抗鼠 HRP 酶标 IgG，酶作用底物（A 液：联苯二胺；B

液：过氧化氢），洗涤液（pH7.4，0.01mol/L Tris－HCl 缓冲液），终止液（2mol/L H_2SO_4），AFP 标准品，阳性对照血清（来自孕妇），阴性对照血清（来自健康人群），血清样品。

2. 其他　已包被抗 AFP 抗体的聚苯乙烯酶联免疫反应用小皿，移液管。

【实验方法】

（1）向反应用小皿中加入血清或 AFP 标准品 2 滴，室温下 3 分钟后弃去，洗涤液洗三次，弃去。

（2）加入 1 滴酶标抗 AFP，室温下 5 分钟后弃去，水洗三遍，弃去。

（3）加入 1 滴 A 液和 1 滴 B 液，5 分钟后加入终止液 1 滴，观察结果。黄色者为阳性。

【结果与讨论】

（1）记录本次实验结果。

（2）为什么可在妊娠女性血液中检测到 AFP？AFP 检测的意义何在？

Ⅱ　胶体金技术检测 HCG

【实验目的】

掌握胶体金技术快速检测抗原的方法。

【实验原理】

人类绒毛膜性腺激素（HCG）是胎盘发育过程中分泌的一类糖蛋白激素。由于 HCG 在怀孕后立刻出现且浓度在孕早期快速升高，使得它成为孕早期检测的极佳标记。胶体金技术是一个简便快速的抗原检测方式，可用于检测尿液样本中的 HCG 含量。妊娠检测试纸条是胶体金技术应用于早早孕检测的商品化试剂盒。

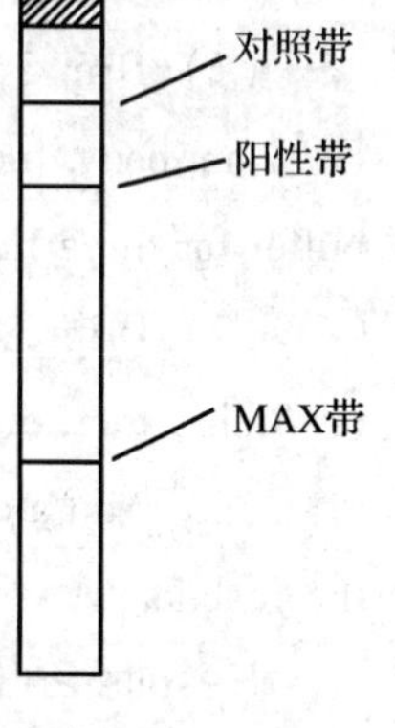

图 40－1　胶体金试纸条的结果示意图

【实验材料】

尿液收集杯，早早孕试纸条。

【实验方法】

（1）以小杯收集尿液样本。

（2）将试纸条垂直小心地插入样本液中。将标有箭头的一端对准尿液。注意不要将 MAX 线（标记线）位置浸没。

（3）约 3 分钟后取出试纸条，平摊于洁净、干燥、不吸水的表面。

（4）待反应完全结束，着色带显现。读取结果（图 40－1）。

不同样品的检测可能导致 3 种不同的结果产生。如试纸条上出现对照带和阳性带，表明样品为 HCG 阳性。如试纸条上仅出现对照带，表明样品为 HCG 阴性。如两条带均不显现，表明试纸条失效。

【结果与讨论】

1. 记录本次实验结果。

2. 为什么 HCG 可用于妊娠期的检测？

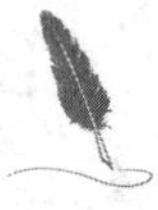

EXPERIMENT 40 Immune Functions of Antibodies (2)

Ⅰ Detection of AFP by Indirect ELISA

Purpose

To grasp a method for the identification of antigens or antibodies by using ELISA.

Principle

The procedures of ELISA include reaction between enzyme – linked specific antigen or antibody and unknown antibody or antigen, subsequent addition of the substrate of the linked enzyme and development of colored products. The depth of the color is proportional to the quantity of the antigen or antibody. The results can be observed by eyes or determined spectrophotometrically. This method is a widely accepted for the detection of specific antigens or antibodies. And it can be used for qualitative or quantitative analysis. The antibody labelled with enzyme and the substrate, are easily available. This test can be performed as an indirect immunoabsorbent assay, a direct immunoabsorbent assay, *etc.* In this exercise, it will be used to detect AFP in samples.

Materials and Apparatus

1. **Reagent** Mouse anti – AFP McAb, goat anti – mouse IgG/HRP, substrate (A: OPD and B: H_2O_2), washing buffer (pH7.4, 0.01mol/L Tris – HCl), stop buffer (2mol/L H_2SO_4), standard AFP, the positive serum (from pregnant woman), the negative control serum (from healthy man), serum samples.

2. **Apparatus** microtiter plates (binding anti – AFP antibody), clear pipette.

Procedures

(1) Drip 2 drops of serum or standard AFP into microtiter plates preincubated with anti – HCG antibody. Incubate in room temperature for 3min, then discard supernatant. Wash with washing buffer for three times.

(2) Drip a drop of mouse anti – AFP McAb labeled with HPR. Incubate at room temperature for 5min, then discard it. Wash for three times.

(3) Add a drop of OPD and a drop of H_2O_2. After 5min, add a drop of 2 mol/L H_2SO_4 to stop the reaction. A yellow color indicates the positive result.

Results and Discussion

(1) Record the results of this exercise.

(2) Why AFP can be detected in pregnant woman? What is the significance of AFP detection?

Ⅱ Detection of HCG by Colloidal Gold Technique

Purpose

To grasp a method for the identification of antigens by using colloidal gold technique.

Principle

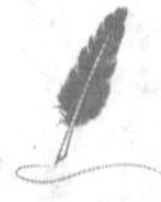

Human chorionic gonadotropin (HCG) is a glycoprotein hormone secreted by the developing placenta shortly after fertilization. It has become an excellent indicator of early pregnancy detection because it usually occurs immediately after pregnancy and its concentration rises rapidly in early pregnancy.

Colloidal gold technique is a simple and rapid method for the detection of antigen. It can be used to test the HCG in urine specimen. Pregnancy Test Strip is a test kit for the determination of HCG to diagnose early pregnancy.

Materials and Apparatus

Sample collection cup, HCG Strip.

Procedures

(1) Collect the urine sample in a sample collection cup.

(2) Holding the strip vertically, carefully dip it into the sample. Insert the strip into the urine sample with the arrow pointing towards the urine. Do not immerse the MAX Line (Marker Line).

(3) Take the strip out after 3 minutes and lay the strip flat on a clean, dry, non-absorbent surface.

(4) Colored band appears immediately after the reaction is completed. Then read the results (see Fig. 40-1).

对照带

阳性带

MAX带

There are three possible results when different samples are tested. If the control line and positive line appear on the strip, the sample is HCG positive. If only the control line appears on the strip, the sample is HCG negative. If none of these two lines appear, the test strip fails.

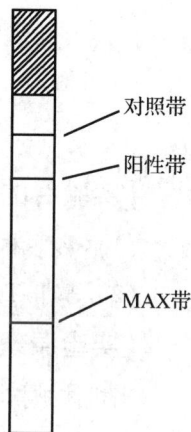

Results and Discussion

(1) Record the results of this experiment.

(2) Why HCG test can be used to diagnose pregnancy?

扫码“学一学”

实验四十一　细胞免疫功能检测（1）——体外试验

Ⅰ　E 玫瑰花环试验

【实验目的】

熟悉鉴别 T 淋巴细胞的 E 玫瑰花环试验。

【基本原理】

T 淋巴细胞鉴定有多种方法。人的 T 细胞可以结合绵羊红细胞，形成玫瑰花环。利用该原理设计的 E 玫瑰花环试验不但可用来检测人 T 细胞的免疫功能，还是一种重要的 T 细胞计数方法。此外，B 淋巴细胞可通过补体参与的 EAC 玫瑰花环试验进行鉴定。

【实验材料】

1. **细胞**　外周血单个核细胞（PBMC，以 RPMI 1640 悬浮）。

2. **试剂**　绵羊红细胞（SRBC，用阿氏液保存），Hank's 液，RPMI 1640 培养液，胎牛血清（FCS，56℃灭活 1 小时），无菌双蒸水，吉姆萨－瑞氏染液。

3. **其他**　离心机，洁净载玻片，吸管，圆底离心管，显微镜。

【实验方法】

(1) 取 10ml SRBC，置于 20ml 离心管中。用 Hank's 液装满离心管，1000×g 离心 10 分钟。

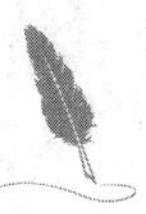

去上清，加 Hank's 液，以吸管悬浮细胞。1000 × *g* 离心 10 分钟。重复上述洗涤过程 1 次。

（2）以 RPMI1640 悬浮 SRBC 至终浓度 2% V/V，4℃保存（可保存 5 ~ 7 日）。

（3）将≤2×10^7 PBMC 置圆底离心管中，400 × g 离心 10 分钟。去上清，以 RPMI 1640 悬浮细胞至终浓度 1×10^7 cells/ml。

（4）将 2ml FCS，2ml SRBC，1×10^7 PBMC 混匀。混合物在 37℃水浴孵育 10 分钟。200 × g 4℃离心 5 分钟。在冰上孵育 1 小时。

（5）悬浮沉淀，加 0.8% 戊二醛 0.1ml，混匀，4℃固定 15 分钟。

（6）在洁净载玻片上滴一小滴细胞悬液。空气干燥后，以吉姆萨 – 瑞氏染液染色。冲洗并干燥后，显微镜观察 PBMC 中的 T 淋巴细胞。

【结果与讨论】

图示 E 玫瑰花环。

Ⅱ 淋巴细胞体外转化试验

【实验目的】

（1）熟悉淋巴细胞转化试验的原理。

（2）掌握 T 淋巴细胞体外转化实验的方法。

【实验原理】

当机体被抗原或有丝分裂原（如结核菌素、PHA 等）刺激后，淋巴细胞能够转化为淋巴母细胞，并进一步发育成致敏淋巴细胞。在一定程度上，这种转化现象代表着机体的细胞免疫状态。在体外试验中，通过加入合适的刺激物，T 细胞也可发生转化并显示出形态上的改变。目前，常用的体外检测细胞免疫功能的方法是 PHA 诱导的 T 淋巴细胞转化试验。可通过三种不同的方法检测细胞转化率：形态学观察法、MTT 法和同位素标记法。本实验采用的是形态观察法。

【实验材料】

1. **细胞** 外周血单个核细胞（PBMC，以 RPMI 1640 悬浮）。

2. **试剂** 吉姆萨 – 瑞氏染液，RPMI 1640 培养液，肝素（400U/ml），PHA（1mg/ml），2.5% 碘酒，75% 乙醇。

3. **其他** 玻片，无菌棉签，无菌注射器，毛细吸管，96 孔培养板，CO_2 恒温培养箱，移液管。

【实验方法】

（1）以 RPMI 1640 悬浮 PBMC 至终浓度 1×10^6 cells/ml。在 96 孔板的每孔中加入 100μl。

（2）在孔中加入 PHA 至终浓度 10μg/ml。每个样品制 3 个平行孔。

（3）37℃孵育 72 小时。

（4）离心 3000r/min，10 分钟，去上清。

（5）以残余液体悬浮细胞，取少量滴于玻片上，涂片，干燥。

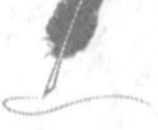

（6）吉姆萨 – 瑞氏染液染色。

（7）显微镜观察淋巴细胞的转化情况，一般计数 100 ~ 200 个淋巴细胞，然后计算转化率。正常情况下，PHA 刺激淋巴细胞的转化率在 60% ~80% 。

（转化的淋巴细胞形态特点：体积增大，比原来的成熟淋巴细胞大 2 ~3 倍；核膜清晰，染色体疏散呈网络状结构；胞浆丰富，染色为嗜碱性。）

【结果与讨论】

（1）计算淋巴细胞的转化率。

（2）在何种条件下，T、B 淋巴细胞会发生转化？

EXPERIMENT 41 Immune Function by Cellular Immunity（1）——*in Vitro*

Ⅰ Erythrocyte rosette test

Purpose

To be familiar with the methods for identification of T cell ——the erythrocyte rosette formation test.

Principle

There are many methods for identification of human T cells. The erythrocyte rosette formation test can be used to detect the cellular immune function in human and animal cells. And it's also an important method for counting T cells. An EAC rosette formation test is used to identify B cell.

Materials and Apparatus

1. Culture Peripheral blood mononuclear cells（PBMC）suspended in complete RPMI 1640 medium）.

2. Reagents SRBC in Alsevers solution, Hanks'（balanced salt solution）, complete RPMI1640 medium, fetal calf serum（FCS, heat - inactivated 1 hr at 56℃）, sterile distilled water, Giemsa - Wright dye.

3. Apparatus centrifuge, clean glass slide, clean glass slide, pipette, round - bottom centrifuge tube, microscope.

Procedures

（1）Place 10ml SRBC in Alsevers solution in a 20ml centrifuge tube. Fill tube with Hanks' and centrifuge 10 min at 1000 × g. Remove supernatant, and use pipet to resuspend cells in Hanks' solution. Centrifuge 10min at 1000 × g. Repeat this washing process once.

（2）Add complete RPMI 1640 to the pelleted SRBC（final concentration 2% v/v）. Store at 4℃ for further use（can be stored for 5 to 7 days）.

（3）Transfer ≤ 2×10^7 PBMC to a round - bottom centrifuge tube. Centrifuge for 10min at 400 × g. Remove supernatant and resuspend cells in complete RPMI 1640 at a final concentration of 1×10^7 cells/ml.

（4）Add 2ml heat - inactivated FCS and 2ml of SRBC for each 1×10^7 PBMC. Incubate the mixture 10min in a 37℃ water bath. Centrifuge for 5min at 200 × g, 4℃. Incubate for 1 hr on ice.

（5）Resuspend the precipitate and add 0. 1ml 0. 8% glutaraldehyde, mix and fix at 4℃ for 15min.

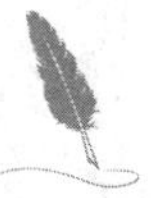

(6) Drip a small drop of suspension on a clean slide. After air dry, stain it with Giemsa – Wright dye. Wash, dry and then observe with microscope.

Results and Discussion

Draw the erythrocyte rosettes.

Ⅱ Lymphocyte transformation test *in vitro*

Purpose

(1) To be familiar with the priciple of lymphocyte transformation test.

(2) To grasp the lymphocyte transformation test *in vitro*.

Principles

When the body is stimulated by antigen or mitogen (such as the tuberculin or PHA, *etc.*), lymphocytes can be transformed into lymphoblastoid cells, and further into sensitized lymphocytes. To a certain extent, this transformation represents the state of the body's cellular immunity. By adding appropriate stimulus, T cells can be also transformed *in vitro* and undergo morphological changes. At present, the regular method for examining the cellular immunity is PHA – induced T lymphocyte transformation test. Cell transfomation rates can be measured by 3 different methods: morphological examination, MTT assay and isotopic tracer method. In this experiment, the morphological changes can be observed.

Materials and Apparatus

1. Culture Peripheral blood mononuclear cells (PBMC) in complete RPMI 1640 medium.

2. Reagent Giemsa – Wright dye, RPMI1640, heparin (400 unit/ml), PHA (1mg/ml), 2.5% tincture of iodine, 75% alcohol.

3. Apparatus slide, sterile cotton, sterile syringe, capillary, 96 – well plate, CO_2 incubator, pipette.

Procedures

(1) Resuspend PBMC in complete RPMI 1640 to a final concentration of 1×10^6 cells/ml. Add 100μl to each well of a 96 – well plate.

(2) Add PHA to each well to a final concentration of 10μg/ml. Three parallel wells are used for each sample.

(3) Incubate at 37℃ for 72h.

(4) Centrifuge at 3000r/min for 10min, remove supernatant.

(5) Resuspend cells with remnant liquid. Drip a drop on a slide, smear and dry.

(6) Stain with Giemsa – Wright dye.

(7) Observe with a microscope, count at least 100 ~ 200 lymphocytes, then calculate the conversion rate. Normal conversion rate is 60% ~ 80%.

(Morphological characteristics of transformated lymphocytes: 2 ~ 3 fold increase in volume compared with the original maturity lymphocytes; clearly visible nuclear membrane, loose and network – like nuclear chromatin; abundant cytoplasm and basophilic staining.)

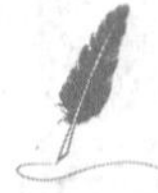

Results and Discussion

（1）Calculate the lymphocyte conversion rate.

（2）Under what conditions will T and B lymphocytes undergo transformation?

实验四十二　细胞免疫功能检测（2）——细胞因子检测

扫码“学一学”

【实验目的】

（1）熟悉生物活性法检测 IL－2 的原理。

（2）掌握生物活性法 IL－2 检测的技术及计算方法。

【基本原理】

白细胞介素 2（IL－2）是一种 T 细胞源性的细胞因子，对多种免疫细胞都有促进生长和促进分化的作用。一些肿瘤细胞株必须依赖于 IL－2 才能生长，如 CTLL、CTB6、F12、CTLL－2 等。因此本实验以 CTLL－2 的增殖情况来检验IL－2 的生物活性。

MTT（四甲基偶氮唑蓝）法是实验室常用的检测手段，通过标准比色可以测量琥珀酸脱氢酶活性（该酶可将 MTT 降解为紫蓝色的结晶）。琥珀酸脱氢酶的活性不但与细胞生长和活力成正比，而且可用于检测潜在药物和其他有毒物质对细胞的毒性。

【实验材料】

1. **细胞**　CTLL－2 细胞。

2. **试剂**　IL－2 样品，IL－2 标准品，5mg/ml MTT 溶液，10% 牛血清 RPMI1640 培养液，DMSO。

3. **其他**　离心机，离心管，洁净载玻片，移液管，显微镜，毛细吸管，96 孔板，细胞计数板，CO_2 培养箱，酶标仪（570nm 和 630nm 滤光片）。

【实验方法】

（1）用 10% 牛血清 RPMI－1640 培养液洗涤 CTLL－2 细胞 2 次，1000r/min，离心 10 分钟，移去含 IL－2 的原始培养基质。

（2）以含 10% 牛血清的 RPMI1640 调整细胞浓度至 1×10^5/ml。

（3）将 IL－2 样品和标准品不同稀释度加入 96 孔板中。每孔 50μl，设置 3 个复孔。同时设培养基质对照。

（4）加 CTLL－2 细胞悬浮液 50μl/孔。37℃ 5% CO_2 培养 24 小时。

（5）加 10μl MTT 溶液至每孔，继续孵育 4h。

（6）移去 50μl 上清，然后添加 50μl DMSO，置室温 10～20 分钟。混匀使产物完全溶解。

（7）1 小时后，以酶标仪测 OD 值。取 3 个复孔的均值为每种样品的 OD 值。

最终 OD 值为 $OD_{570nm}-OD_{630nm}$ 再减去培养液对照孔 OD 值。

$$\text{IL}-2\text{样品活性单位（U/ml）}=\frac{\text{样品最大 OD 值 50\% 的样品稀释度}}{\text{标准品最大 OD 值 50\% 的标准品稀释度}}\times\text{IL}-2\text{标准品活性}$$

【结果与讨论】

（1）计算 IL－2 样品的活性单位。

（2）常用检测细胞因子活性的不同方法有哪些？

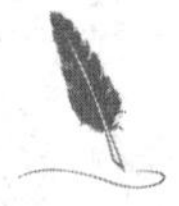

EXPERIMENT 42 Immune Function by Cellular Immunity (2) ——Detection of Cytokines Levels

Purpose

1. To be familiar with the principle of bioactivity detection of IL－2.

2. To grasp the bioactivity detection and calculation of IL－2.

Principle

Interleukin－2 (IL－2) is a T cell－derived cytokine known to promote growth and differentiation of many immune cells. The growth of some tumor cell lines are depended on IL－2, such as CTLL, CTB6, F12 and CTLL－2. So the biological activities of IL－2 can been tested by CTLL proliferation.

The MTT assay is a laboratory test and a standard colorimetric assay for measuring the activity of succinate dehydrogenase that reduce MTT to formazan. The activity of succinate dehydrogenase is directly proportional to cell proliferation. It can be used to determine cytotoxicity of potential medicinal agents and other toxic materials.

Materials and Apparatus

1. Culture　CTLL－2 cells.

2. Reagents　IL－2 sample, IL－2 standards, 5mg/ml MTT solution, complete 10% FCS－RPMI 1640 medium, DMSO.

3. Apparatus　centrifuge, centrifuge tube, clean glass slide, pipette, capillary, 96－well plate, microscope, cell counting chamber, CO_2 incubator, microtiter plate reader (570nm filter or 630nm filter).

Procedures

(1) Wash CTLL－2 cells with 10% FCS－RPMI 1640 culture medium twice. Centrifuge at 1000r/min for 5min to remove the original growth medium, which contains IL－2.

(2) Adjust cell concentration to 1×10^5/ml with 10% FCS－RPMI 1640 culture medium.

(3) Add the dilutions of the IL－2 sample and the standard respectively in 96－well plate, 50μl per well in triplicate. At the same time, set the culture medium control.

(4) Add 50μl/well with CTLL－2 cell suspension, cultivate at 37℃ and 5% CO_2 for 24h.

(5) Add 10μl MTT solution to each well and continue to incubate for 4 hours.

(6) Discard 50μl supernatant, then add 50μl DMSO and place at room temperature for 10～20min. Mix to make the product fully dissolved.

(7) After 1 hour, measure OD values with a microtiter plate reader. OD value of each sample shall be taken as the average of 3 parallel wells.

The final OD value = OD_{570nm} － OD_{630nm} － the control OD.

The activity units of IL－2 samples (U / ml) =

$$\frac{\text{Dilution factor of the sample with 50\% maximum OD value of standard}}{\text{Dilution factor of the standard with 50\% maximum OD value of standard}}\times\text{the activity of IL}-2$$

standard

Results and Discussion

(1) Calculate the activity units of IL－2 samples.

(2) What are the available methods for determination of cytokine activity?

扫码“学一学”

实验四十三　细胞免疫功能检测（3）——体内试验

Ⅰ　豚鼠结核菌素试验

【实验目的】

掌握结核菌素试验的方法。

【基本原理】

豚鼠对结核杆菌具有高度敏感性，其感染后的病理变化与人类疾病相似。豚鼠结核菌素试验是分离、鉴定和诊断结核杆菌，筛选抗结核杆菌药物的最佳动物模型。

结核菌素是结核杆菌的组成成分。人体感染结核杆菌或接种卡介苗后，将产生致敏T细胞。致敏T细胞再次接触结核菌素或结核杆菌后，能够释放大量淋巴因子，并形成单个核细胞浸润的炎症反应。因此，结核菌素试验也对测定细胞免疫功能有参考意义。

【实验材料】

豚鼠两只，1∶1000稀释的旧结核菌素（OT），卡介苗注射器及针头，剪刀，碘酒棉球，酒精棉球。

【实验方法】

(1) 试验正式进行前两个月，准备两只豚鼠。其中一只皮内注射卡介苗致敏。

(2) 实验当天，以卡介苗注射器对两只豚鼠分别注射0.1ml 1∶1000的旧结核菌素。

(3) 注射后48～72小时，观察注射位置的皮肤红肿、肿块大小等反应现象。

【结果与讨论】

(1) 记录结核菌素试验的结果。

(2) 简述结核菌素试验的技术和临床意义。

Ⅱ　体内淋巴细胞转化试验

【实验目的】

掌握体内淋巴细胞转化实验的方法。

【基本原理】

人外周血T淋巴细胞在体内遇到PHA或ConA，将转化为淋巴母细胞。通过外周血涂片染色，可进行淋巴细胞计数和转化率计算。转化率将反映机体细胞免疫水平，可作为机体免疫功能检测的指标。

【实验材料】

1. 试剂　吉姆萨－瑞氏染液，ConA（0.5mg/ml），heparin（400unit/ml）。

2. 其他　玻片，棉球，离心机，显微镜，细胞计数板。

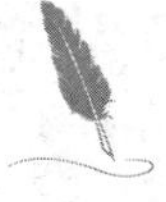

【实验方法】

(1) 试验正式进行前3天，对实验组小鼠腹腔注射ConA 0.3～0.5mg。

(2) 摘取小鼠眼球，取外周血，滴加入预先加入肝素的试管。

(3) 涂片　取一滴外周血滴入玻片中央。推片，干燥。

(4) 固定　滴加1～2滴甲醇，干燥。

(5) 染色　滴加2滴吉姆萨－瑞氏染液，同时滴加两滴水。染色5～10分钟。

(6) 洗涤　然后用吸水纸轻轻吸干玻片上的水分。

(7) 显微镜观察，计数转化的细胞，然后计算转化率。

$$转化率=\frac{转化的淋巴细胞数量}{转化的淋巴细胞数量+未转化的淋巴细胞数量}\times 100\%$$

【结果与讨论】

计算并比较试验组和对照组的淋巴细胞转化率。

EXPERIMENT 43　Immune Function by Cellular Immunity (3) ——*in Vivo*

Ⅰ　Tuberculin test in guinea pigs

Purpose

To grasp Tuberculin test method.

Principle

Guinea pigs have a high degree of sensitivity to *Mycobacterium tuberculosis*. And its pathological changes after infection are similar to human disease. *Mycobacterium tuberculosis* in guinea pigs is the best animal model for separation, identification, diagnosis of tubercle bacillus and for screening of anti－TB drugs.

Tuberculin is a component of *Mycobacterium tuberculosis*. During TB infection or BCG vaccination, T cells are sensitized. After re－exposure to TB or tuberculin, the Tuberculin sensitized T cells can release a variety of lymphokines and will form mononuclear cell－based inflammatory cell infiltration. Therefore, the tuberculin test has reference value for the determination of cellular immune function.

Materials and Apparatus

Two guinea pigs, 1:1000 dilution of old tuberculin (Old tuberculin, OT), BCG syringe and needle, scissor, iodine swab, alcohol swab

Procedures

(1) Keep two guinea pigs two months before this experiment. One of them is sensitized by an intradermal injection of BCG.

(2) Use BCG syringe to inject both guinea pigs with 0.1ml 1:1000 diluted old tuberculin.

(3) 48～72h after injection, observe skin reactions at the injection site to see whether swelling occurs and how large is the swelling area.

Results and Discussion

(1) Record the result of tuberculin test.

(2) Briefly describe the technique and clinical significance of tuberculin test.

Ⅱ Lymphocyte transformation test *in vivo*

Purpose

To grasp lymphocyte transformation test *in vivo*.

Principles

When incubated with PHA or ConA, peripheral blood T lymphocytes *in vivo* will transform to lymphoblastoid cell. Through the peripheral blood smear staining, lymphocyte count and the conversion rate can be calculated. Conversion rate can reflect the level of cellular immunity, and often seen as an indicator of cellular immunity.

Materials and Apparatus

1. **Reagent**: Giemsa - Wright dye, ConA (0.5mg/ml), heparin (400unit/ml).

2. **Apparatus**: slide, straw, centrifuge, microscope, cell count board.

Procedures

(1) Three days before the experiment, the mouse of experimental group was intraperitoneal injected with ConA 0.3 ~ 0.5mg.

(2) During the experiment, collect peripheral blood of mice by removing the eyeball, and then add to heparin tube.

(3) Smear: Take a small drop of blood in the center of a slide. Smear the blood and air dry.

(4) Fix: drip 1 ~ 2 drops of methanol on the smear, air dry.

(5) Stain: add 2 drops of Giemsa - Wright dye on the smear, plus 2 drops of water at the same time. Dye for 5 ~ 10 minutes.

(6) Wash and then gently dry the slide with absorbent paper.

(7) Observe transformed lymphoid cell with a microscope. Count the transformed cell and then calculate the conversion rate.

$$\text{Conversion rate} = \frac{\text{Number of transformed lymphocytes}}{\text{Number of transformed lymphocytes} + \text{Number of non-transformed lymphocytes}} \times 100\%$$

扫码“学一学”

Results and Discussion

Calculate and compare lymphocyte conversion rate of the experimental group and the control group.

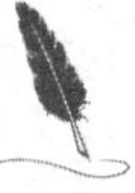

第七部分 药学微生物学实验

微生物在自然界中分布极为广泛，无论是在土壤、水体、空气等环境都存在，大多数微生物对人类、动物和植物有益，如，微生物能产生抗生素、蛋白酶、淀粉酶等酶制剂，被广泛应用于工业生产；通过基因工程菌的构建可以高产干扰素、胰岛素等生物制品。少数微生物对人类有害，如病原微生物、抗药菌及发酵工业中噬菌体的污染。

本部分包括两部分：①药物的体外抗菌活性测定，常用的方法有连续稀释法和琼脂扩散法；②《中华人民共和国药典》2020 年版对药品的卫生学标准做了明确规定，这里主要介绍无菌的药品的无菌检查，非无菌产品的微生物限度检查。

扫码“学一学”

实验四十四 药物的体外抗菌试验

【实验目的】

（1）掌握琼脂扩散渗透法测定药物体外抗菌活性的原理。

（2）熟悉常用体外抗菌活性的测定方法。

（3）熟悉液体二倍稀释法测定抗生素的最低抑菌浓度（MIC）。

【实验原理】

药物的体外抗菌实验（antimicrobial test *in vitro*）是在体外测定微生物对药物敏感程度的实验。药物的体外抗菌实验不仅有助于临床选择用药，而且还可用于新药研发、抗菌谱测定、药物含量测定、血药浓度测定等方面。

药物体外抗菌活性的测定方法很多，一般有两大类：琼脂扩散渗透法和系列浓度稀释法。

琼脂扩散渗透法是利用药物能够渗透到琼脂培养基的性质，将试验菌混入琼脂培养基后倾注倒平板，或将试验菌涂布于琼脂平板的表面，然后用不同的方法将药物置于含有试验菌的琼脂平板上。根据加药的操作方法不同分为滤纸片法、打洞法、挖沟法、管碟法和移块法等，经适宜温度培养后观察药物的抑菌能力。本实验主要介绍其中的滤纸片法和挖沟法。

系列浓度稀释法常用于测定药物的最低抑菌浓度（minimum inhibitory concentration，MIC）或最低杀菌浓度（minimum bactericidal concentration，MBC）。药物的最低抑菌浓度是指药物能够抑制微生物生长的最低浓度；可杀灭细菌的最低药物浓度为最低杀菌浓度。MIC（MBC）可以评价药物抑菌作用的程度，常以μg/ml 或 U/ml 表示。其值越小，则抑菌作用越强。常见的测定方法有：试管稀释法、平板稀释法、斜面混入法和微孔板法等。本试验主要介绍试管稀释法和微孔板法。

【实验材料】

1. 菌种 金黄色葡萄球菌、表皮葡萄球菌和大肠埃希菌临床菌株的 8 小时牛肉膏蛋白胨肉汤培养物，金黄色葡萄球菌（ATCC 25925）、大肠埃希菌（ATCC 25922）、表皮葡萄球

菌（ATCC 49134）标准菌株的8小时肉汤培养物。

2. 培养基及试剂 肉汤琼脂培养基等，待测药物青霉素G（β-内酰胺类）、链霉素（氨基糖苷类）、阿奇霉素（大环内酯类）和左旋氧氟沙星（喹诺酮类）、0.1%苯扎溴铵（新洁尔灭）、0.1%龙胆紫、2.5%碘液、0.85%生理盐水、板蓝根浸煮剂等）。

3. 仪器 恒温培养箱，超净工作台，酶标仪，微量移液器，游标卡尺等。

4. 其他 无菌平皿，无菌吸管，无菌试管，无菌接种铲，无菌滤纸片、接种环、镊子等。

【实验方法】

1. 滤纸片法 滤纸片法是琼脂扩散法中最常用的方法，适用于初步判断药物是否有抗菌作用的初筛试验及临床药敏试验。可进行多种药物或一种药物的不同浓度对同一种试验菌的抗菌试验。

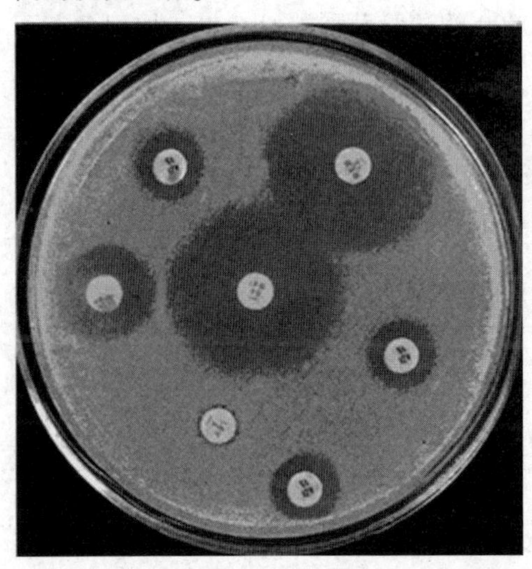

图44-1 滤纸片法

(1) 用滴管分别取金黄色葡萄球菌和大肠埃希菌（临床菌株）肉汤培养物4~5滴，加到两个灭菌的空平皿中，每皿加入15~20ml已溶化并冷却至50℃左右的培养基，制成含菌平板，冷凝备用。

(2) 用无菌镊子夹取滤纸片，分别浸入0.1%新洁尔灭、0.1%龙胆紫、2.5%碘液、0.85%生理盐水中，在盛药平皿内壁上除去多余药液后，分别贴在含菌平板表面，并作好标记，见图44-1，37℃培养20小时。

(3) 观察滤纸片周围的抑菌圈。滤纸片边缘到抑菌圈边缘的距离在1mm以上者为阳性（+），即微生物对药物敏感；反之为阴性（-），即微生物对药物不敏感。

扫码“看一看”

2. 挖沟法 本法适用于半流动性药物或中药浸煮剂的抗菌试验。可在同一平板上试验一种药物对几种试验菌的抗菌作用。本实验建议选用板蓝根浸煮剂。

(1) 在琼脂平板中央，用无菌接种铲挖一条长沟，将沟内琼脂全部挖出。

(2) 将待测药物加入此沟内。

(3) 在沟两侧垂直划线接种各种试验菌，见图44-2。

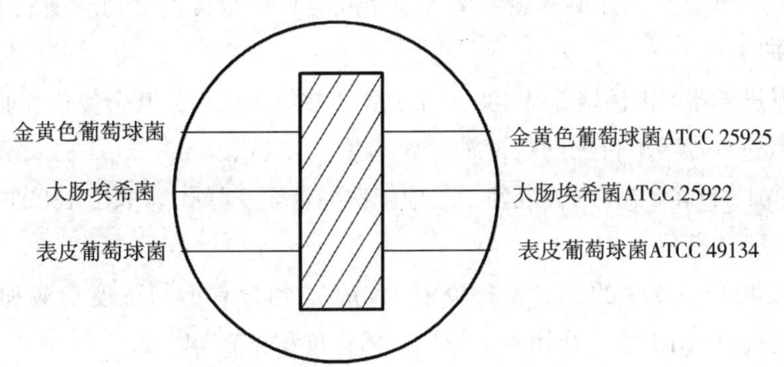

图44-2 挖沟法

(4) 若为细菌则37℃培养24~48小时；若为放线菌或真菌则28℃培养48~72小时。

（5）观察沟两边所生长的试验菌距离沟的抑菌距离，从而判断待测药物对这些菌的抗菌能力。

3. 试管稀释法 该方法是在一系列试管中，采用二倍稀释法，用液体培养基连续稀释药物，然后在每一试管中加入一定量的试验菌，经培养后，肉眼观察能抑制试验菌生长的最低浓度即为该药物的MIC。本法所用药物可选链霉素，试验菌可选用大肠埃希菌。

（1）取10支小试管，编号1~10。

（2）用5ml移液管取肉汤培养基1.8ml加到第1管中，其余各管各加1ml。

（3）用1ml无菌移液管吸取待测药物溶液（1280 μg/ml）0.2ml加入第1管内混匀，从第1管取出1ml加到第2管内，混匀，其他依次稀释至9号管（取出1ml扔掉），10号管为空白对照，不加药物。

（4）用另一支1ml无菌移液管，分别吸取1∶10000的试验菌稀释液0.1ml加到含有不同浓度药液和对照小试管中，加入顺序为从对照管（10号）开始到1号管，稀释过程见表44－1。

（5）37℃培养20小时，对照管中微生物应正常生长，液体变混浊。观察其他管中药物对测试菌生长的抑制作用，以抑制细菌生长的最低药物浓度为MIC值。

表44－1 试管稀释法系列稀释过程

管号	1	2	3	4	5	6	7	8	9	10
肉汤培养基（ml）	1.8	1.0	1.0	1.0	1.0	1.0	1.0	1.0	1.0	1.0
药液（ml）	0.2 →	1.0→	1.0→	1.0→	1.0→	1.0→	1.0→	1.0→	1.0→ 弃掉	
大肠埃希菌（ml）	0.1	0.1	0.1	0.1	0.1	0.1	0.1	0.1	0.1	0.1
药物终浓度（μg/ml）	128	64	32	16	8	4	2	1	0.5	0
每管总体积（ml）	1.1	1.1	1.1	1.1	1.1	1.1	1.1	1.1	1.1	1.1

4. 微孔板法 微孔板是一种聚氯乙烯塑料板，通常使用96孔板，可用于同时测定多种药物的最低抑菌浓度。微孔板法综合了常规测定法的优势，测试速度快、结果准确、重现性好，具有良好的实用性。本法可用于同时测定多种药物的MIC值，是一种高通量测定法。

本次实验我们采用微孔板法测定青霉素G（β－内酰胺类）、链霉素（氨基糖苷类）、阿奇霉素（大环内酯类）和左旋氧氟沙星（喹诺酮类）对金黄色葡萄球菌的MIC值；这里以链霉素为例讲解。

（1）用微量进样器取肉汤培养基180 μl加到第1排第1孔中，其余各孔各加100μl。

（2）用微量进样器吸取待测药物溶液（链霉素：1280μg/ml）20μl加入第一孔内混匀，从孔中取出100μl加到第二孔内，混匀，其他依次稀释至9号孔（取出100μl扔掉），10号孔为空白对照，不加药物。

（3）分别吸取1∶10000的试验菌稀释液100μl加到含有不同浓度药液和对照小孔中，加入顺序为从对照孔（10号）开始到1号孔。稀释过程见表44－2。

（4）37℃培养20小时，对照孔的微生物应正常生长，液体变为混浊。观察其他孔中药物对测试菌生长的抑制作用，以抑制细菌生长的最低药物浓度为MIC值。

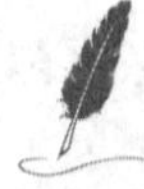

表 44－2　微孔板法系列稀释过程

孔号	1	2	3	4	5	6	7	8	9	10
肉汤培养基（μl）	180	100	100	100	100	100	100	100	100	100
药液（μl）	20 →	100→	100→	100→	100→	100→	100→	100→	100→ 弃掉	
试验菌（μl）	100	100	100	100	100	100	100	100	100	100
药物终浓度（μg/ml）	128	64	32	16	8	4	2	1	0.5	0
每管总体积（μl）	200	200	200	200	200	200	200	200	200	200

【结果与讨论】

（1）各种化学药品对金黄色葡萄球菌的抑菌作用（表 44－3）。

表 44－3　各种化学药品时金黄色葡萄球菌的抑菌作用

化学药品	抑菌圈直径（mm）
0.1% 新洁尔灭	
0.1% 龙胆紫	
2.5% 碘液	
0.85% 生理盐水	

（2）观察挖沟法实验中沟两边所生长的试验菌离沟的抑菌距离，判断板蓝根浸煮剂对这些试验菌的抑菌能力大小。

（3）观察试管稀释法实验中各试管菌液的生长状况，计算测试药物链霉素的最低抑菌浓度。

（4）在本实验中，如果抑菌圈内无菌生长，是否说明微生物已经被杀死？如何通过实验加以确定，请自行设计实验。

（5）如何判断试验中导致细菌不生长的药物浓度是抑菌还是杀菌？MIC 大，还是 MBC 大？

PART SEVEN　General Microbial Experiments in Pharmaceutics

Microbes can be found in soil, water and air. Most are beneficial to human, for instant, they can provide antibiotics, enzymes and genetic engineered biopharmaceuticals. However, few microorganisms are harmful like pathogens, and contaminations.

This part includes two sections which are: ①determination of antibacterial activity of drugs *in vitro* (serial dilution and agar diffusion methods); ②sterility test and microbial limit test of drugs in Pharmacopoeia of the People's Republic of China (2020 edition).

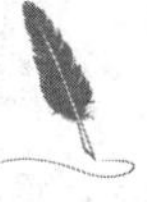

EXPERIMENT 44 Determination of Antimicrobial Activity *in Vitro* of Pharmaceutical Preparations

Purposes

(1) To understand the principles of determination of antimicrobial activity by disk diffusion method.

(2) To be familiar with the common methods for determination of antimicrobial activity *in vitro*.

(3) To be familiar with the tube double dilution method for the determination of minimum inhibitory concentration (MIC).

Principles

In vitro antimicrobial tests evaluate the effectiveness of selected antibacterial agents against bacteria. Antimicrobial sensitivity tests are widely used in new drug development and provide guidance for clinical application, such as screening of antibacterial agents, determination of antibacterial spectrum, susceptibility test and plasma concentration determination.

Many methods are available to determine antimicrobial activity *in vitro*, which are mainly classified into tube dilution tests and disk diffusion test (Bauer – Kirby test).

The principle of the disk diffusion test is as follows: when the antibiotic is placed on agar containg the test bacteria, the antibiotic diffuses radially outward through the agar, producing an antibiotic concentration gradient. A clear zone or ring is present around the antibiotic after incubation if the agent inhibits bacterial growth. The wider the zone surrounding the antibiotic, the more susceptible the bacterium is. It is divided into the paper – disk diffusion test, agar plate dig groove method, cylinder plate method and moving – agar block test. Here, the paper – disk diffusion test and agar plate dig groove method will be introduced.

The serial dilution tests are usually used to determine minimum inhibitory concentration (MIC) and minimum bactericidal concentration (MBC). MIC is the lowest concentration of the antibiotic capable of preventing growth of the test organism. MBC is the lowest concentration of the antibiotic that results in no growth (turbidity) of the subcultures. We can assess the extent of bacterial inhibition by MIC (MBC), usually in μg/ml or U/ml. The smaller the MIC and MBC, the higher the antimicrobial activities.

The commonly used methods are disk dilution test, broth dilution test, infiltrating – agar slant test, microtiter plate method and so on. Disk dilution test and microtiter plate method are introduced here.

Materials and Apparatus

1. Strains 8h nutrient broth cultures of clinical strains of *Staphylococcus aureus*, *Staphylococcus epidermidis*, *Escherichia coli*, and standard strains of *Staphylococcus aureus* (ATCC 25925), *Escherichia coli* (ATCC 25922) and *Staphylococcus epidermidis* (ATCC 49134).

2. Media and Reagents Nutrient agar media; test drugs: Penicillin G (β – lactam), streptomycin (aminoglycosides), azithromycin (macrolides) and levofloxacin (quinolones), 0.1%

Benzalkonium Bromide, 0.1% Gentian Violet, 2.5% Iodine solution, 0.85% normal saline, Isatis root.

3. Apparatus Incubator, clean bench, microplate reader, micropipettor, vernier caliper, *etc.*

4. Others Sterile petri dish, sterile pipette, sterile test tube, sterile glass spade, sterile paper slip, inoculating loop, tweezer, *etc.*

Procedures

1. The paper – disk diffusion test Paper – disk diffusion test is the most commonly used method in dish diffusion test and is applicable to preliminarily screen for new drugs for their antimicrobial effectivness and clinical drug susceptibility. It can also be used to carry out antimicrobial test for different drugs or different concentrations of the same drug against the same microorganism.

(1) Transfer 4 ~ 5 drops of *S. aureus* and *E. coli* broth culture respectively to two sterile empty dishes, pour 15 ~ 20 ml nutrient agar medium (50℃) onto each plate and mix gently

(2) Steep paper disks in 0.1% Benzalkonium Bromide, 0.1% Gentian Violet, 2.5% Iodine solution, or 0.85% normal saline, place on the plates and then label them. Incubate at 37℃ for 20h (Figure 44 – 1).

(3) Observe the zones of inhibition surrounding the paper discs. If the distance between the rim of the paper disc and the rim of inhibitory zone are larger than 1 mm, it is a positive result indicating the sensitivity of the microorganism is to the drug. Otherwise it will be negative.

2. Agar plate digs groove method This method is applicable to the antimicrobial test of semi – fluid or the soak of Chinese medicinal materials. It can examine the effects of one drug on several different tested bacteria on the same agar plate.

(1) Dig out the agar in the center of the agar plate with a sterile spade to produce a ditch.

(2) Add the tested drug to the ditch to its full capacity. Note: do not spill over the ditch.

(3) Inoculate a variety of tested bacteria on both side of the ditch (See Figure 44 – 2).

(4) Incubate for 24 ~ 48 h at 37℃ in case of bacteria, incubate for 48 ~ 72h at 28℃ in case of actinomycetes or fungi.

(5) Observe the inhibitory distance between the ditch and the tested bacteria on both sides of the ditch, and then assess antimicrobial ability of tested drugs.

3. The broth dilution test In a series of test tubes, the testing drugs are double diluted with broth culture medium. Add a certain amount of tested bacteria to each test tube and incubate. The minimum concentration of the drug that can inhibit the growth of bacteria observed by naked eyes is MIC. We select *Escherichia coli* as tested microbe and streptomycin as tested drug.

(1) Take 10 test tubes, label them with 1 ~ 10.

(2) Add 1.8ml broth culture medium to No. 1 tube and add 1ml broth culture medium respectively to other tubes.

(3) Add 0.2ml tested drug solution (1280μg/ml) to No. 1 tube, mix evenly, transfer 1ml from No. 1 tube to the second tube, and mix well. Continue until the ninth tube (with 1ml removed). The No. 10 tube is the blank control without any drug.

(4) Add 0.1ml diluted solution of the test bacteria (1: 10000) to 10 tubes respectively,

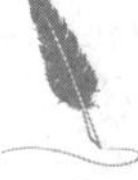

start from tube 10 to 1 (Table 44 – 1).

(5) Incubate at 37℃ for 20h. The bacteria in the blank control should grow well and the liquid becomes opaque. Observe the antimicrobial activity of tested drug in other tubes and record MIC.

Table 44 – 1 the broth dilution test

TubeNo.	1	2	3	4	5	6	7	8	9	10
broth culture (ml)	1.8	1.0	1.0	1.0	1.0	1.0	1.0	1.0	1.0	1.0
drug sample (ml)	0.2									
diluting	→	1.0→	1.0→	1.0→	1.0→	1.0→	1.0→	1.0→	1.0→ throw away	
Escherichia coli (ml)	0.1	0.1	0.1	0.1	0.1	0.1	0.1	0.1	0.1	0.1
concentration of drug (μg/ml)	128	64	32	16	8	4	2	1	0.5	0
total volume (ml)	1.1	1.1	1.1	1.1	1.1	1.1	1.1	1.1	1.1	1.1

4. Microtiter Plate Method Microtiters plates, a kind of polyvinyl chloride plastic plates (PVC) such as 96 – well plates, are widely used to determine the MIC of many drugs at the same time. Microtiter plate method combines the advantages of conventional methods together and characterized by fast testing speed, high measuring accuracy, good reproducibility and better practicability. This method could significantly improve the efficiency of screening multiple drugs.

In this experiment, we will determine the MIC of penicillin G, streptomycin, azithromycin and levofloxacin against tested microbes by microtiter plate method. Take the streptomycin as an example.

(1) Add 180μl broth culture to well 1 on the first row, and add 100μl broth culture medium respectively to the other wells on the same row.

(2) Add 20μl tested drug solution (streptomycin : 1280μg/ml) to well 1, mix evenly, transfer 100μl from well 1 to the second well, and mix well. Continue until the ninth well (with 100μl removed). The No. 10 well is the blank control without any drug.

(3) Add 100 μl diluted solution of test bacteria (1∶10000) to 10 wells respectively, start from well 10 to 1 (Table 44 – 2).

Table 44 – 2 microtiter plate method

Well No.	1	2	3	4	5	6	7	8	9	10
broth culture (μL)	180	100	100	100	100	100	100	100	100	100
drug sample (μL)	20									
diluting	→	100→	100→	100→	100→	100→	100→	100→	100→ throw away	
E. coli (μL)	100	100	100	100	100	100	100	100	100	100
drugconcentration (μg/ml)	128	64	32	16	8	4	2	1	0.5	0
total volume (μL)	200	200	200	200	200	200	200	200	200	200

(4) Incubate at 37℃ for 20h. The bacteria in the blank control should grow well and the liquid becomes opaque. Observe the antimicrobial activity of the tested drugs in other wells and record their MIC.

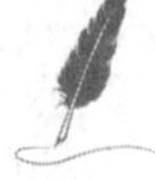

Results and Discussion

(1) The antimicrobial effects of chemical drugs on *S. aureus*

Chemical drugs	Diameter of inhibition zone (mm)
0.1% Benzalkonium Bromide	
0.1% Gentian Violet	
2.5% Iodine solution	
0.85% normal saline	

(2) Observe the distance between the ditch and the bacteria grown on both sides of the ditch, asses the inhibitory ability of the tested drug against different bacteria.

(3) Observe the growth of bacteria in each tube, record MIC for streptomycin.

(4) In this experiment, if there is no growth of bacteria within the inhibition zone, can you get the conclusion that those bacteria are killed ? How to prove it ?

(5) Please design another experiment to prove whether the drug exhibit a bacteriostatic or bactericidal effect? Which value is larger, MIC or MBC?

实验四十五　抗生素效价的测定

扫码"学一学"

【实验目的】

(1) 掌握管碟法测定抗生素效价的原理。

(2) 熟悉微生物法测定抗生素效价的方法。

【实验原理】

抗生素效价测定法是在特定条件下，根据量反应平行线原理设计，通过检测抗生素对微生物的抑制作用，计算抗生素的效价。

抗生素的微生物检定包括两种方法：管碟法和浊度法。

1. 管碟法　管碟法系利用抗生素在琼脂培养基中的扩散作用，比较标准品与供试品两者对接种的试验菌产生抑菌圈的大小，以测定供试品效价的一种方法。

在含有高度敏感性试验菌的琼脂平板上放置小钢管（也称牛津杯）（内径6.0mm ± 0.1mm，外径7.8 ± 0.1mm，高10mm ± 0.1mm），管内放入标准品和被检品溶液，经16～18小时恒温培养，抗生素扩散的有效范围内则产生透明的无菌生长的抑菌圈。抑菌圈的直径大小与抗生素的浓度相关，也与抗生素的扩散系数、扩散时间、培养基的厚度及抗生素的最低抑菌浓度等因素有关，比较抗生素标准品与检品的抑菌圈大小，可计算出抗生素的效价。

管碟法的特点是灵敏度高，能直接测定抗生素的抗菌活性，因此作为国际通用的方法被列入各国药典中。

管碟法测定抗生素的效价又分为一剂量法、二剂量法和三剂量法。其中二剂量法最为常用，又称四点法。将抗生素标准品和被检品各稀释成一定浓度比例（2:1或4:1）的两种溶液，在同一平板上比较其抗菌活性，再根据抗生素浓度对数和抑菌圈直径成直线关系的原理来计算检品效价。

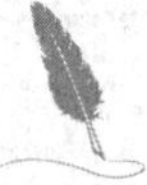

取含菌的双层平板培养基，每个平板表面放置4个小钢管，管内分别放入检品高、低

剂量和标准品高、低剂量溶液。

先测量出四点的抑菌圈直径，按下列公式计算出检品的效价。

（1）求出 W 和 V

$$W=(SH+UH)-(SL+UL)$$
$$V=(UH+UL)-(SH+SL)$$

其中，UH 为检品高剂量之抑菌圈直径，UL 为检品低剂量之抑菌圈直径，SH 为标准品高剂量之抑菌圈直径，SL 为标准品低剂量之抑菌圈直径。

（2）求出 θ

$$\theta=D\cdot \text{antilog}\ (IV/W)$$

其中，θ 为检品和标准品的效价比，D 为标准品高剂量与检品高剂量之比，一般为 1，I 为高低剂量之比的对数，即 log2 或 log4。

（3）求出 Pr

$$Pr=Ar\times\theta$$

其中，Pr 为检品实际单位数，Ar 为检品标示量或估计单位。

2. 浊度法 本法系利用抗生素在液体培养基中对试验菌生长的抑制作用，通过测定培养后细菌浊度值的大小，比较标准品与供试品对试验菌生长抑制的程度，以测定供试品效价的一种方法。

药典中规定在测定抗生素效价时，对所用的标准品、试验菌、培养基、培养条件及药物的浓度范围都有相应的要求。本试验主要参照 2020 年版药典，采用管蝶法测定四环素检品的效价。

【实验材料】

1. 菌种 藤黄微球菌（*Micrococcus luteus*）［CMCC（B）28 001］肉汤琼脂斜面。

2. 培养基及试剂

（1）试剂 四环素检品及标准品（高剂量、低剂量，高剂量与低剂量之比为 2∶1，浓度范围为 10.0～40.0 Unit/mg），无菌生理盐水（0.85%）。

（2）培养基

蛋白胨	6g
牛肉浸膏	1.5g
酵母抽提物	3g
葡萄糖	1g
琼脂	15～16g
水	1000ml

除琼脂外，混合上述各成分，调节 pH 为 6.7～7.0。加入琼脂，加热溶化，调节 pH，使灭菌后 pH 为 6.5～6.6，在 115℃灭菌 30 分钟。

3. 仪器 恒温培养箱，超净工作台，游标卡尺等。

4. 其他 无菌平皿，牛津杯（小钢管），无菌陶土盖，无菌吸管，镊子，滴管等。

【实验方法】

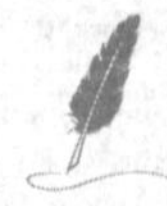

采用管碟法的二剂量法测定四环素的效价。

1. 制备菌悬液 取藤黄微球菌［CMCC（B）28001］的营养琼脂斜面培养物，接种于营养琼脂斜面上，26℃～27℃培养24小时，临用时，用0.85%灭菌氯化钠溶液将菌苔洗下，备用。

2. 标准品溶液的制备　四环素标准品的使用参照标准品说明书的规定。临用时，按照药典的规定用指定的缓冲液（pH6.0）稀释。

3. 供试品溶液的制备　精密称取供试品适量，用规定的溶剂（pH6.0）溶解后，再按估计效价或标示量的规定稀释至与标准品相当的浓度（10.0～40.0Unit/ml）。

4. 制备双层平板　取无菌平皿（直径90mm、高16～17mm）4个，分别加入20ml加热溶化的培养基，放置水平台上凝固后作为底层。另取检定用培养基适量，加热溶化后，冷却至50℃左右，加入上述制备好的试验菌悬液适量（二剂量法标准品的高剂量所致抑菌圈直径在18～22mm为宜），摇匀，在底层平板上加5ml并使之均匀摊平，作为菌层。放置水平台上凝固待凝。采用无菌操作技术，在每一双碟中以等距离均匀安置4个不锈钢小管（内径为6.0mm±0.1mm，高为10.0mm±0.1mm，外径为7.8mm±0.1mm）［图45－1(a)］，用陶土盖覆盖备用。

5. 检定　在每1双碟中的对角的2个不锈钢小管中分别滴加高浓度与低浓度的标准品溶液，其余的2个小管中分别滴加相应的高低两种浓度的供试品溶液；高、低浓度的剂距为2∶1或4∶1。在35℃～37℃下培养14～16小时后，测量各个抑菌圈直径［图45－1(b)］，照生物鉴定统计法进行可靠性测验及效价计算。

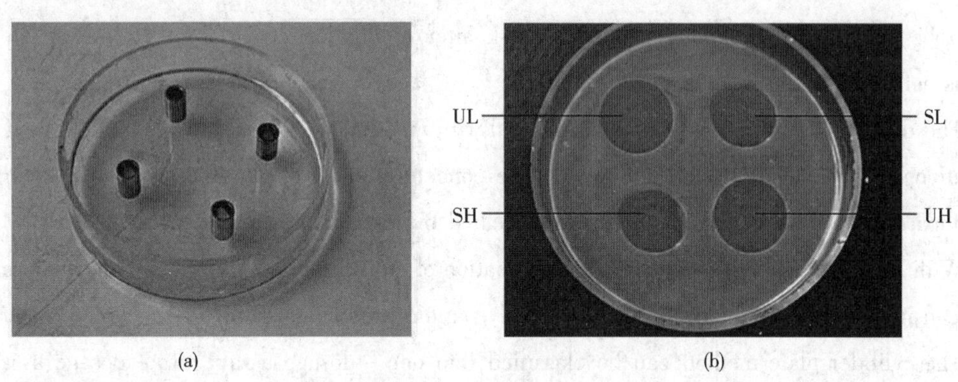

图45－1　管碟法

【结果与讨论】

（1）将抑菌圈直径记录于表45－1。

表45－1　抑菌圈直径

碟号	UH（mm）	UL（mm）	SH（mm）	SL（mm）
1				
2				
3				
4				
Σ				

（2）根据实验原理中的公式计算四环素的效价（已知四环素标准品1000Unit/mg）。

（3）在实际操作中，哪些因素对生物效价测定有影响？

（4）抗生素的效价测定，除了微生物法外还有哪些方法？

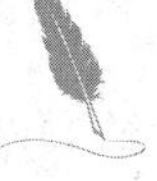

Experiment 45 Assay of Antibiotic Potency

Purposes

(1) To grasp the principles of antibiotic potency assay by cylinder plate method.

(2) To be familiar with the method of microbiological assay of antibiotics.

Principles

The potency of antibiotics may be demonstrated under suitable conditions by their inhibitory effect on microorganisms. The assay is designed on the basis of the principle of parallel line model. Two kinds of methods are often employed, the agar diffusion method (the cylinder plate method) and the turbidimetric method.

1. Cylinder Plate Method The agar diffusion method is a methodused to determine the potency of an antibiotic and is based on the comparison of the size of inhibitions zone created by the test drug and the standard antibiotic against the susceptible microorganism.

Cylinder plate method is based on the agar diffusion method. Four stainless tubes (inner diameter 6.0 ± 0.1 mm, outer diameter 7.8 ± 0.1 mm, height 10.0 ± 0.1 mm) are placed on the agar plate previously inoculated with the sensitive bacteria. Then solutions of tested antibiotics and standard antibiotics are added into the tubes. The antibiotics in the tubes will diffuse radically and a clear zone will present around an antibiotic disk after incubation at 37℃ for 16 ~ 18h. The clear zone is called inhibition zone.

The diameter of inhibition zone is associated with medium thickness, diffusion coefficient, concentration and MIC of the tested antibiotics. The concentration of the antibiotics can be determined by comparing the diameter of inhibition zone created by test samples and standards

With its high sensitivity and direct determination of antibacterial activity, cylinder plate method has been included in the pharmacopoeia of many nations as an internationally accepted method.

The cylinder plate method can be classified into one – dosage assay, two – dosage assay and three – dosage assay. Two – dosage assay is the most commonly used one, and is also called four dots method. Standard antibiotics and test samples are diluted to the concentration ratio of 2:1 or 4:1 and compare their antimicrobial activity with antibiotics sample on the same plate. The concentration of the antibiotic is calculated according to the linear relationship between logarithm of antibiotic concentration and diameter of the inhibition zone.

In this experiment, four stainless tubes are placed on double layer agar plate containingsensitive bacteria in upper layer, two tubes for high concentration and the other two for low concentration.

After determining the diameter of the inhibition zone, we can calculate the antibiotics concentration as follows:

(1) Calculate W and V:

$$W = (SH + UH) - (SL + UL)$$

$$V = (UH + UL) - (SH + SL)$$

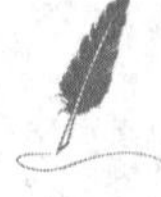

Where UH and UL are the inhibitory diameters of high and low concentration of antibiotics sample, SH and SL are the inhibitory diameters of high and low concentration of standard antibiotics.

(2) Calculate θ:

$$\theta = D \times \text{antilog}\ (IV / W)$$

Where θ is the potency ratio of antibiotics sample to standard antibiotics, D is ratio of the high dose of antibiotics sample to the high hose of standard antibiotics, which usually equals one, I is the logarithm of the ratio of high dose to low dose, which is usually log2 or log4.

(3) Calculate Pr:

$$Pr = Ar \times \theta$$

Where Pr is the actual unit of antibiotics sample and Ar is the labelled amount.

2. Turbidimetric Method The turbidimetric method is a method to determine the potency of an antibiotic, depends upon the preparation being examined that inhibits the growth of a microbial culture in a fluid medium and that of the standard preparation of that antibiotic which are in the same degree of inhibition expressed by the turbidity of the microbial culture which can be measured photometrically. The turbidimetric method is proved to be convenient, accurate and rapid.

The reference, tested microorganisms, culture medium, incubation condition and concentration of antibiotics are strictly required in the pharmacopoeia 2020 when determining antibiotics potency. This experiment mainly introduces the determination of tetracyclines potency by cylinder plate method.

Materials and Apparatus

1. Strains Broth slant cultures of *Micrococcus luteus* [CMCC (B) 28001].

2. Media and Reagents

(1) Reagents tetracycline sample and Reference (the ratio of high dosage to low dosage is 2:1, concentration range of tetracycline is 10.0 ~ 40.0 u/mg), 0.85% sterile normal saline.

(2) Medium

Peptone	6g
Beef extract	1.5g
Yeast extract	3g
Glucose	1g
Agar	15 ~ 16g
Water	1000ml

Mix the above ingredients with the exception of agar; Adjust the pH value to 6.7 ~ 7.0. Add agar, heat to dissolve, then mix thoroughly and adjust the pH of the solution in order that it is 6.5 ~ 6.6 after sterilization. Sterilize the medium at 115℃ for 30min.

3. Apparatus Incubator, clean bench, vernier caliper, *etc.*

4. Others Sterile plate, Oxford cup, sterile clay lid, sterile pipette, tweezer, dropper, *etc.*

Procedures

2 - dose assay

Determination of the potency of tetracycline sample by 2 - dose assay.

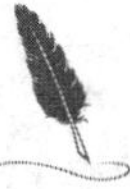

1. Inoculum Preparation of *Micrococcus luteus* suspension Transfer *Micrococcus luteus* [CMCC (B) 28001] from the nutrient agar slant onto a fresh slant surface, incubate at 26℃ ~ 27℃ for 24h. Wash off the growth with sterile water or 0. 85% sterile normal saline immediately before use.

2. Reference preparation The reference substances (tetracycline) should be handled as directed in the package inserts. Solutions of the reference substance are prepared using sterile buffers described (pH 6. 0) above and diluted immediately before use.

3. Test preparation Dissolve anaccurately weighed quantity of tetracycline in the sterile buffers (pH 6. 0) and dilute to approximately the same concentration as that of the reference preparation (Concentration: 10. 0 ~ 40. 0Unit/ml).

4. Preparation of inoculated plates Fill 4petri dishes (with flat bottom, 90mm diameter, 16 ~ 17mm high) with 20ml of melted medium listed in Materials and Apparatus. Place the dishes on a horizontal platform. Then add to each plate 5ml of the same medium which has previously been inoculated at 48℃ ~ 50℃ with an inoculum of the test organism. The concentration of the inoculum should be so selected that the sharpest zones of inhibition are obtained. The diameters of the inhibition zones produced by the high dose of the reference preparation are 18 ~ 22mm in 2 – dose assay, Spread the medium evenly over the entire surface and allow to cool on a horizontal platform. Place 4 stainless steel cylinders (6. 0mm ± 0. 1mm in internal diameter, 7. 8mm ± 0. 1mm in external diameter and 10. 0mm ±0. 1mm in height) on the surface of each plate at equal distance (Figure 45 – 1a) then cover them with clay lids.

5. Measure Take no less than 4 inoculated plates prepared as above, fill two of the diagonal cylinders on each plate with the high or low dose of the reference preparation, fill the remaining cylinders with the high or low dose of the test preparation. The dose levels should be in the ratio of 2 : 1 or 4 : 1. Incubate the plate at 35℃ ~ 37℃ for 14 ~ 16h. Measure the diameter of the inhibition zones (Figure 45 – 1b). Carry out the statistical analysis of variance and calculate the potency of tetracycline.

Results and Discussion

(1) Record diameter of inhibition zone

NO.	UH (mm)	UL (mm)	SH (mm)	SL (mm)
1				
2				
3				
4				
Σ				

(2) Calculate the potency of tetracycline (standard tetracycline: 1000Unit /mg).

(3) What are the factors affecting biological activity in practical operation?

(4) Apart from microbiological methods, are there any other methods for the detection of antibiotic potency?

扫码"学一学"

实验四十六　药物无菌检查法

【实验目的】

(1) 掌握药物制剂的无菌检查方法。

(2) 熟悉药典要求的需无菌检查的范围。

【实验原理】

无菌检查法是用于检查药典要求无菌的药品、生物制品、医疗器械、原料、辅料及其他品种是否无菌的一种方法。各种注射剂（如针剂、输液等）、手术、眼科制剂等都必须保证无菌，符合药典相关规定。

无菌检查应在无菌条件下进行，试验环境必须达到无菌检查的要求，检验全过程应严格遵守无菌操作，防止微生物污染，防止污染的措施不得影响供试品中微生物的检出。单向流空气区、工作台面及受控环境应定期按医药工业洁净室（区）悬浮粒子、浮游菌和沉降菌的测试方法的现行国家标准进行洁净度确认。隔离系统应定期按相关的要求进行验证，其内部环境的洁净度须符合无菌检查的要求。日常检验还需对试验环境进行监控测。

无菌检查是用部分样品的测定结果推断整体的含菌情况，适当的试验操作技术能确保结果的科学、准确。

1. 培养基及培养条件　见《中华人民共和国药典》2020 年版（以下简称 2020 年版药典）四部通则 1101。

2. 培养基的制备　培养基配制应按照药典处方制备，也可使用按该处方生产的符合规定的脱水培养基或成品培养基。配制后，应采用验证合格的灭菌程序灭菌。

若不及时使用，应置于无菌密闭容器中，在 2℃ ~25℃且避光的环境下保存，并在经验证的保存期内使用。

3. 培养基的适用性检查　无菌检查用的硫乙醇酸盐流体培养基及胰酪大豆胨液体培养基等应符合培养基的无菌性检查及灵敏度检查的要求。

(1) 无菌性检查　无菌性检查即每批培养基随机取不少于 5 支（瓶），置各培养基于规定的温度培养 14 天，应无菌生长。

(2) 培养基灵敏度检查　菌种培养基所用的菌株传代次数不得超过 5 代，并采用适宜的菌种保藏技术进行保存和确认，以保证菌株的生物学特性。

4. 方法适用性试验　当进行产品的无菌检查法时，应进行方法适用性试验，以确认所采用的方法适合于该产品的无菌检查。若检验程序或产品发生变化可能影响检验结果时，应重新进行方法适用性试验。

5. 供试品的无菌检查

(1) 无菌检查法包括薄膜过滤法和直接接种法。只要供试品性质允许，应采用薄膜过滤法。

(2) 供试品无菌检查所采用的检查方法和检查条件应与方法适用性试验确证的方法相同。

(3) 在 2020 年版药典中，对无菌检查所用供试品的检验数量和检验量也有严格规定，且针对不同性质的供试品要求作适当的处理。

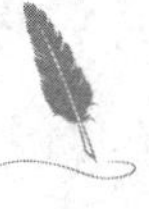

(4) 阳性对照与阴性对照　选用合适的阳性对照菌进行验证，以证明所采用的培养基

和检验方法适合于该药品的无菌检查。

阳性对照：根据供试品特性选择阳性对照菌。无抑菌作用及抗革兰阳性菌为主的供试品，以金黄色葡萄球菌为对照菌；抗革兰阴性菌为主的供试品，以大肠埃希菌为对照菌；抗厌氧菌的供试品，以生孢梭菌为对照菌；抗真菌的供试品，以白色念珠菌为对照菌。阳性对照试验的加菌量不大于100cfu。阳性对照管培养不超过5天，应生长良好。

阴性对照 供试品无菌检查时，应取相应溶剂和稀释剂、冲洗液同法操作，阴性对照不得有菌生长。

【实验材料】

1. 菌种 金黄色葡萄球菌（*Staphylococcus aureus*）［CMCC（B）26 003］、铜绿假单胞菌（*Pseudomonas aeruginosa*）［CMCC（B）10 104］，枯草芽孢杆菌（*Bacillus subtilis*）［CM-CC（B）63 501］，生孢梭菌（*Clostridium sporogenes*）［CMCC（B）64 941］，白色念珠菌（*Candida albicans*）［CMCC（F）98 001］，黑曲霉（*Aspergillus niger*）［CMCC（F）98 003］。

2. 培养基及试剂 硫乙醇酸盐流体培养基，胰酪大豆胨液体或琼脂培养基，沙氏葡萄糖液体或琼脂培养基。冲洗液：组氨酸－卵磷脂－聚山梨酯80混合溶液，0.05%（V：V）聚山梨酯80的0.9%（W：V）的氯化钠溶液，利福霉素钠注射液，0.9%（W：V）氯化钠注射液。

3. 仪器 恒温培养箱，集菌仪，封闭式薄膜过滤器等。

4. 其他 试管，灭菌吸管等。

【实验方法】

1. 菌液制备 接种金黄色葡萄球菌、铜绿假单胞菌、枯草芽孢杆菌的新鲜斜面培养物至或胰酪大豆胨液体培养基或胰酪大豆琼脂培养基中，30℃～35℃培养18～24小时。接种生孢梭菌的新鲜斜面培养物至硫乙醇酸盐流体培养基内，30℃～35℃培养18～24小时。接种白色念珠菌的新鲜斜面培养物至沙氏葡萄糖液体培养基或沙氏葡萄糖琼脂斜面培养基上，20℃～25℃培养2～3天。上述培养物用0.9%无菌氯化钠溶液制成适宜浓度的菌悬液。接种黑曲霉的新鲜斜面培养物至沙氏葡萄糖琼脂斜面培养基或马铃薯葡萄糖琼脂培养基上，20℃～25℃培养5～7天，或直到获得丰富的孢子，加入适量含0.05%（ml/ml）聚山梨酯80的0.9%（W/V）的氯化钠溶液，将孢子洗脱。然后采用适宜的方法吸出孢子悬液到无菌试管中。用含0.05%）（ml/ml）聚山梨酯80的0.9%（W/V）无菌氯化钠溶液制成适宜浓度的孢子悬液。

2. 验证方法

（1）培养基的适用性检查

①无菌性检查：每批培养基随机取不少于5支（瓶），置各培养基规定的温度培养14天，应无菌生长。

②灵敏度检查：取适宜装量的硫乙醇酸盐流体培养基7支，分别接种不大于100cfu的金黄色葡萄球菌、铜绿假单胞菌、生孢梭菌各2支，另1支不接种作为空白对照，培养不超过3天；取适宜装量的胰酪大豆胨液体培养基7支，分别接种不大于100cfu的枯草芽孢杆菌、白色念珠菌、黑曲霉各2支，另1支不接种作为空白对照，培养不超过5天。

结果判定：空白对照管应无菌生长，若加菌的培养基管均生长良好，判该培养基的灵

敏度检查符合规定。

（2）方法适用性试验　按“供试品的无菌检查”的规定及下列要求进行操作。对每一试验菌应逐一进行方法确认。

薄膜过滤法：取每种培养基规定接种的供试品总量按薄膜过滤法过滤，冲洗，在最后一次的冲洗液中加入不大于100cfu的各试验菌，过滤。加培养基至滤筒内，接种金黄色葡萄球菌、大肠埃希菌、生孢梭菌的滤筒内加硫乙 醇酸盐流体培养基；接种枯草芽孢杆菌、白色念珠菌、黑曲霉的滤筒内加胰酪大豆胨液体培养基。另取一装有同体积培养基的容器，加入等量试验菌，作为对照。置规定温度培养不超过5天。

直接接种法：取符合直接接种法培养基用量要求的硫乙醇酸盐流体培养基6管，分别接入不大于100cfu的金黄色葡萄球菌、大肠埃希菌、生孢梭菌各2管，取符合直接接种法培养基用量要求的胰酪大豆胨液体培养基6管，分别接入不大于100cfu的枯草芽孢杆菌、白色念珠菌、黑曲霉各2管。其中1管按供试品的无菌检查技术接入每支培养基规定的供试品接种量，另1管作为对照，置规定的温度培养3~5天。

结果判断：与对照管比较，如含供试品各容器中的试验菌均生长良好，则说明供试品的该检验量在该检验条件下无抑菌作用或其抑菌作用可以忽略不计，照此检查方法和检查条件进行供试品的无菌检查。

（3）供试品的无菌检查

①利福霉素钠注射液作无菌检查（薄膜过滤法）：本实验采用薄膜过滤法对利福霉素钠注射液作无菌检查。参照2020年版药典选用金黄色葡萄球菌为阳性对照菌。且无菌检查所用培养基及稀释剂均符合2020年版药典规定要求。

薄膜过滤法应优先采用封闭式薄膜过滤器（图46-1）。无菌检查用的滤膜孔径应不大于0.45μm，直径约为50mm。若使用其他尺寸的滤膜，应对稀释液和冲洗液体积进行调整，并重新验证。滤器及滤膜使用前应采用适宜方法灭菌。

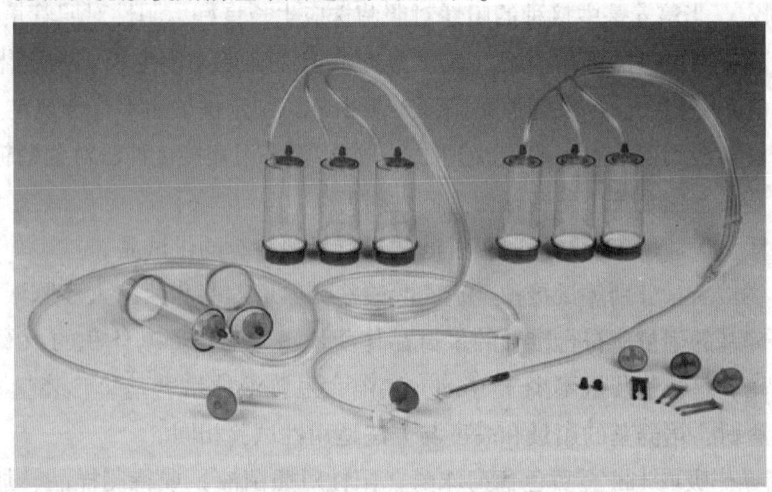

图46-1　全封闭集菌培养器

a. 供试品处理及接种培养基

a）用适宜的方法对供试品容器表面进行彻底消毒；

b）取供试品（利福霉素钠）适量，用灭菌0.9%氯化钠稀释制成每1ml中约含利福霉素5mg的溶液；

c）先用少量稀释剂润湿滤膜；以无菌操作将供试液300ml加入薄膜过滤器内，立刻

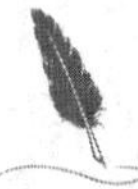

抽滤；

d）同法用100ml 组氨酸 - 卵磷脂 - 聚山梨酯 80 混合溶液冲洗滤膜，重复 3 次以上，冲洗清除残留在滤筒、滤膜上的抗生素；

e）冲洗后，2 份滤器各加入 100ml 硫乙醇酸盐流体培养基，1 份滤器加入 100ml 胰酪大豆胨液体培养基，同时以金黄色葡萄球菌为阳性对照菌。

f）另取盛有 100ml 硫乙醇酸盐流体培养基，100ml 胰酪大豆胨液体培养基的两个滤器作为阴性对照。

结果见表 46 - 1。

表 46 - 1　样品无菌检查结果

培养基	培养温度（℃）	管号	培养时间（d）													
			1	2	3	4	5	6	7	8	9	10	11	12	13	14
硫乙醇酸盐流体培养基	30 ~ 35	阳性														
		样品														
		阴性														
胰酪大豆胨液体培养基	30 ~ 35	样品														
		阴性														

b. 培养及观察：上述含培养基的容器 30℃ ~ 35℃ 培养不少于 14 天，培养期间应逐日观察并定期记录是否有菌生长。

c. 结果判定：当培养基中接种的阳性对照菌株应生长良好，阴性对照管培养基 14 天后应澄清无菌生长；而供试品管均澄清，或虽显浑浊但经确证无菌生长，判定供试品符合规定；若供试品管中任何一管呈现浑浊并确证有菌生长，判定供试品不符合规定。

②葡萄糖注射液无菌检查（直接接种法）：本实验采用直接接种法对葡萄糖注射液作无菌检查。参照药典选用金黄色葡萄球菌为阳性对照菌。

直接接种法一般适用于无法用薄膜过滤法进行无菌检查的供试品。

取规定量供试品，分别等量接种至硫乙醇酸盐流体培养基和胰酪大豆胨液体培养基中。每个容器中培养基的用量应符合接种的供试品体积不得大于培养基体积的 10%，同时，硫乙醇酸盐流体培养基每管装量不少于 15ml，胰酪大豆胨液体培养基每管装量不少于 10ml。在对供试品检查时，培养基的用量和高度与方法适用性试验相同。

a. 以无菌操作吸取 1ml 金黄色葡萄球菌（阳性对照菌液）或待测样品，加入硫乙醇酸盐流体培养基和胰酪大豆胨液体培养基中，摇匀。

b. 于 30℃ ~35℃ 培养 14 天，阳性菌对照管培养 1 天，记录实验结果。

c. 培养期间应逐日检查是否有菌生长，阳性对照管 24 小时内应有菌生长。

d. 结果判断：当阳性对照管显浑浊并确有菌生长，阴性对照管无菌生长，药物试验的各培养基管均为澄清或显浑浊，但经显微镜检查证明无菌生长，则判定被检测样品无菌试验合格。

【结果与讨论】

（1）记录利福霉素钠注射液的无菌检验结果。

（2）记录葡萄糖注射液的无菌检验结果。

（3）哪些药物需无菌检查？

（4）抗生素药物如何进行无菌检查？

EXPERIMENT 46　Sterility Test of Pharmaceutical Preparations

Purposes

（1）To grasp the methods for sterility tests of pharmaceutical preparations.

（2）To be familiar with the detecting range required in pharmacopoeia.

Principles

Sterility test is a method to detect whether pharmaceutical preparations, biological products, medical apparatus, raw materials or other articles, which are required to be sterile according to the Pharmacopoeia, are aseptic. All injections and ophthalmic and surgical preparations should be produced sterile.

Test for sterility should be carried out under strictly aseptic conditions including sterile environment and operation techniques to avoid any microbial contamination. without any effects on the detection of microbes in the testing sample Laminar air flow cabinet, working bench and background room should be monitored regularly according to current national standard such as airborne particles, airborne microbe and settling microbe in the cleaning area of the pharmaceutical industry. The isolation system should be periodically verified in accordance with relevant requirements, and the cleanliness of its internal environment should meet the requirements of sterility inspection. Daily inspection also requires monitoring and measurement of the testing environment.

Sterility test is used to guestimate the contamination of a whole product by testing a sample part. The testing results are ensured by suitable experimental techniques. In the Pharmacopoeia of the People's Republic of China (2020) (referred to as "Pharmacopoeia" in the following) Volume IV. The followings could be found:

1. Culture media and incubation conditions　Reference to the Pharmacopoeia (2020) Volume IV, general principle 1101.

2. Media for the test　Media for the test may be prepared as described in pharmacopoeia, dehydrated media or ready-to-use media may be used provided that they have the same ingredients and comply with the requirements. Media should be sterilized using a validated process. and stored in sterile sealed container, at 2℃ ~25℃ protected from light if not in use immediatelly.

3. Suitability tests of medium　The media (Fluid Thioglycollate medium and Trypone Soya-Tryptose Broth) used in the test for sterility should comply with the following sterility and sensitivity tests.

（1）Sterility test: For sterility test, no less than 5 vessels of each batch of sterilized media should be incubated for 14 days. No microbial growth should occur.

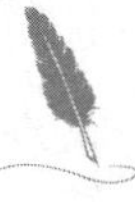

（2）Media sensitivity test: For media sensitivity test, strains with no more than 5 passages from the parent organism can be applied. Validated preservation techniques are also requsted.

4. Suitability tests of sterility testing method In the course of establishing sterility testing method for product to be examined, the method must be verified to ensure that the adopted method is suitable for sterility test of the product. Whenever there is a change of drug composition or test procedures of the test, the testing method must be revalidated.

5. Test for sterility of the product being examined

(1) The test for sterility is carried out by membrane filtration or direct inoculation methods. The membrane filtration should be applied whenever the nature of the product permits.

(2) The same method and experimental conditions used in suitability tests of sterility testing method should be also adopted in sterility test.

(3) In Pharmacopoeia (2020), number of products and/or quantity of products to be tested is strictly defined. Proper treatment of products with different natures needs to be performed.

(4) Positive control and negative control

When establishing sterility test method for product to be examined, the method must be verified with appropriate positive strain to ensure that the adopted method is suitable for sterility test of the product.

Positive control: The microorganisms for positive control should be selected according to the nature of the product being examined. *Staphylococcus aureus* is used for the product possessing no antimicrobial activity or mainly anti – gram – positive bacteria activity. *Escherichia coli* are used for the product mainly possessing anti – gram – negative bacteria activity. *Clostridium sporogenes* is used for the product possessing anti – anaerobic bacteria activity. *Candida albicans* is used for the product possessing fungistatic activity. The number of tested microorganism added should be less than 100 cfu. Incubate the positive control container for no more than 5 days, the test microorganisms should be well grown.

Negative control: A negative control should be performed with the same solvent and diluents as the test product. There should be no growth of microorganisms.

Materials and Apparatus

1. Strains *Staphylococcus aureus* [CMCC (B) 26 003], *Pseudomonas aeruginosa* [CMCC (B) 10 104], *Bacillus subtilis* [CMCC (B) 63 501], [CMCC (B) 44 102], *Clostridium sporogenes* [CMCC (B) 64 941], *Candida albicans* [CMCC (F) 98 001], *Aspergillus niger* [CMCC (F) 98 003]

2. Media and Reagents Fluid thioglycollate medium, tryptic soy broth, Sabouraud's glucose broth medium or Sabouraud's glucose agar medium; Flushing fluid: the mixed solution of histidine – lecithin – polysorbate 80; rifamycin sodium preparations, sterile 0.9% (W : V) sodium chloride solution containing 0.05% (v : v) of polysorbate 80, 0.9% (W : V) glucose injection.

3. Apparatus Incubator, sealed sterility testing system.

4. Others Test tube, sterile sucker.

Procedures

1. Preparation of inoculum Inoculate freshly cultured *Staphylococcus aureus or Pseudomonas*

or *Psendomonas aeruginosa* or *Bacillus subtilis* into tryptic soy broth medium or tryptic soy agar medium and freshly cultured *Clostridium sporogenes* into fluid thioglycollate medium and incubate at 30℃ ~ 35℃ for 18 ~ 24h. Inoculate freshly cultured *Candida albicans* into Sabouraud' s glucose broth medium or Sabouraud' s glucose agar medium and incubate at 20℃ ~ 25℃ for 2 ~ 3 days. Prepare sulitable suspension, With of the above cultures with sterile 0. 9 % (W : V) sodium chloride solution. Inoculate freshly cultured *Aspergillus niger* into Sabouraud' s glucose agar medium or potato glucose agar media, incubate at 23℃ ~ 28℃ for 5 ~ 7days until good sporulation is obtained. Wash the *Aspergillus niger* spore culture and transfer it to sterile tube, prepare spore suspension with suitable concentration with sterile 0. 9% (W: V) sodium chloride solution containing 0. 05% (v : v) of polysorbate 80.

2. Validation test

2. 1 Suitability Tests of Medium

2. 1. 1 Sterility

Incubate no less than 5 vessels of each batch of sterilized medium at the specified incubation temperature for14 days. Growth of microorganisms should not occur.

2. 1. 2 Test for sensitivity of medium

Take 7 containers of fluid thioglycollate medium, inoculate 2 containers of the medium with no more than 100cfu test microorganisms of *Staphylococcus aureus*, *Pseudomonas aeruginosa* and *Clostridium sporogenes* respectively and the remaining uninoculated culture medium (one container) is used as blank control, then incubate for not more than 3 days.

Take 7 containers of tryptic soy broth medium, inoculate 2 containers of the medium with no more than 100cfu test microorganisms of *Bacillus subtilis*, *Candida albicans* and *Aspergillus niger* respectively, and use the remaining uninoculated culture medium (one container) as blank control, incubate for not more than 5 days. Observe the test containers for growth of the microorganisms every day during the incubation.

Evaluation of results

The blank control should be free of bacterial growth. If a clearly visible growth of the microorganisms occurs in an inoculated culture medium, the medium meets the requirement of the test for sensitivity of the medium.

2. 2 Suitability tests of sterility testing method

Suitability test is conducted as described below under test for sterility of the product being examined using exactly the same methods and the following instructions. The tests should be performed separately for each of the microorganism tested.

(1) Membrane filtration

Filter a specified quantity of the test specimen with membrane filtration apparatus, rinse the membrane, add test microorganism of less than 100 cfu to the final portion of rinsing fluids, filter again. Add fluid thioglycollate medium into the filtration apparatus which inoculate with *Staphylococcus aureus*, *Escherichia coli* and *Clostridium sporogenes*. Add tryptic soy broth medium into the filtration apparatus which inoculate with *Bacillus subtilis*, *Candida albicans* and *Aspergillus Niger*. Use another container containing the same volume of the medium, and then add the same amount

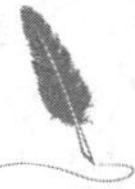

of test microorganisms as control. Incubate the containers at specified temperature for no more than 5 days.

(2) Direct Inoculation

Take 6 containers containing certain required volume of fluid thioglycollate medium for direct inoculation; inoculate 2 containers of medium with no more than 100cfu test microorganisms of *Staphylococcus aureus*, *Escherichia coli* and *Clostridium sporogenes* rseparately. Take 6 containers containing tryptic soy broth complying with the required volume for direct inoculation, inoculate 2 containers of medium with ho more than 100cfu test microorganisms of *Bacillus subtilis* , *Candida albicans* and *Aspergillus niger* separately. Add specified quantity of the product being tested to one of the inoculated containers of each test microorganism according to sterility test request of testing sample, the other inoculated container is used as control. Incubate the containers at specified temperature for 3 ~ 5 days.

(3) Evaluation of the results

Compare with the control container, if clearly visible growth of each test microorganisms is obtained in the test containers containing the product to be tested, visually either the product posseses no antimicrobial activity under the conditions of the test or such activity has been satisfactorily eliminated. The sterility test of the product being examined may then be carried out using the same method and conditions of the test.

2.3 Sterility test for of the product to be examined

2.3.1 Sterility test for rifamycin sodium preparations (membrane filtration method)

To establish a sterility test method for rifamycin sodium preparations by using a membrane filtration technique. According to the Pharmacopoeia, *Staphylococcus aureus* is used as positive control in this experiment. All the media and diluents for sterility tests comply with the stipulations in the Pharmacopoeia.

Sealed sterility testing system (Fig. 46 – 1) is preferentially used in the method of membrane filtration. The membrane used has a minimal pore size which is not greater than 0.45μm and a diameter about 50mm. When filtration membrane with other sizes is applied, validation of volume of diluents and rinses is required. The membrane and apparatus should be sterilized by appropriate ways before use.

(1) Sample preparation and medium inoculation

1) Before opening the container of the product to be tested, the exterior surfaces of containers must be thoroughly cleansed with a suitable method.

2) Take a specified quantity of samples tested (rifamycin sodium) and mix the samples into an aseptic vessels containing suitable quantity of the sterile 0.9% (w/v) NaCl (the final concentration is 5mg/ml).

3) Pre – wet the membrane with a small quantity of rinsing fluid. Aseptically transfer the mixture (300ml) to the membrane and filter immediately.

4) Wash the membrane with 100ml sterile histidine – lecithin – polysorbate 80 solution for 3 times to remove the antibiotics residual on the filter.

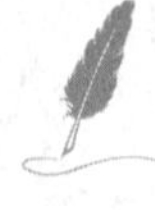

5) Transfer two of 100ml of fluid thioglycollate medium and one tryptic soy broth into the cor-

responding filter apparatus respectively after washing, set one of the containers as a positive control (*Staphylococcus aureus*).

6) Take another container with fluid thioglycollate medium and one with tryptic soy broth only as negative controls.

See Table 46 - 1.

Table 46 - 1 Sterility Test of the test product

Medium	Tm (℃)	container	Incubation time (d)													
			1	2	3	4	5	6	7	8	9	10	11	12	13	14
Fluid thioglycollate medium	30 ~ 35	positive														
		sample														
		negative														
tryptic soy broth	30 ~ 35	sample														
		negative														

(2) Incubation and observation

Incubate the above containers for at least 14 days at 30℃ ~35℃.

Observe and record each medium container for evidence of microbial growth every day or al regular intervals during the incubation period.

(3) Evaluation of the results

Except the positive control container, if no evidence of microbial growth is found in all of the test containers, the test product complies with the sterility test. If evidence of microbial growth is found in any one of the test containers, the test product does not comply with the sterility test.

2.3.2 Sterility test for glucose injection (direct inoculation method)

This experiment will carry out the sterility tests of glucose injection. *S. aureus* is used as positive test microorganism according to the Pharmacopoeia.

Direct inoculation method is usually suitable for the products which cannot be examined by membrane filtration.

Direct Inoculation method is to directly transfer the specified quantity of product tested into fluid thioglycollate medium and tryptic soy broth respectively. In each incubated container, the volume of samples tested is not more than 10% of the volume of the medium, and the volume of fluid thioglycollate medium should not be less than 15ml, the volume of tryptic soy broth should be no less than 10ml, unless otherwise specified. Use the same medium volume and height in the container as in validation test.

(1) Aseptically transfer 1ml of inoculum of *S. aureus* (positive test strain) or testing sample into the containers containing 15ml of fluid thioglycollate medium and tryptic soy broth for sterility tests.

(2) Incubate at 30℃ ~35℃ for 14d. Incubate the container of positive control for 1d, and then record the results.

(3) Observe and record each medium container for evidence of microbial growth every day during the incubation period. Microbial growth of the positive control should be obviously observed.

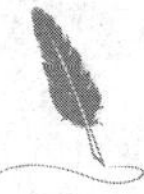

(4) Evaluation of results: Except the positive control container, if no evidence of microbial growth is found in all of the test containers, the test product complies with the test for sterility. If evidence of microbial growth is found in any one of the test containers, the test product does not comply with the test for sterility.

Results and Discussion

(1) Record the results of sterility tests on rifamycin sodium preparations.

(2) Record the results of sterility tests on glucose injection.

(3) List the range of pharmaceuticals for sterility tests in Pharmacopoeia.

(4) How to conduct sterility tests for antibiotics ?

实验四十七　药物的微生物限度检查法

扫码"学一学"

【实验目的】

(1) 掌握药物中大肠埃希菌的检验方法。

(2) 熟悉口服药物微生物限度检查中平板菌落计数法。

(3) 了解药物中控制菌的检查方法。

【实验原理】

控制菌检查法系用于在规定的试验条件下，检查供试品中是否存在特定的微生物。

口服药及外用药等均属于非规定灭菌制剂，在生产和临床使用过程中，不要求达到完全无菌，但是为了保证药品的质量，防止药品的污染，需要限制性控制微生物的数量和种类。我国2020版药典规定的检查项目包括需氧菌总数、霉菌数和酵母菌数及控制菌检查。控制菌的检验包括大肠埃希菌、沙门菌、金黄色葡萄球菌、铜绿假单胞菌、破伤风梭菌等病原菌检查等。

需氧菌总数、酵母菌和霉菌总数的测定采用平皿法或膜过滤法；根据细菌的形态结构和生理生化特性来检查控制菌的存在；《中国药典》(2020版，第四卷，通则1105、1106)中对微生物限度检查法有详细规定，包括检验量及样品的抽取、供试液的制备、培养基的适用性检查、检验方法的适用性试验等。

1. 需氧菌总数、霉菌和酵母数的检查　需氧菌总数的测定是检查每克或每毫升被检药品内所含有的活的需氧菌数，以判断供试药物被需氧菌污染的程度；霉菌和酵母菌总数的测定是考察供试药物中每克或每毫升所含的活的霉菌和酵母菌的总数，以判明供试药物被真菌污染的程度。

计数方法包括平皿法、薄膜过滤法和最可能数法（Most - Probable - Number Method，简称MPN法)。检查时，按已验证的计数方法进行供试品的需氧菌数、霉菌及酵母菌菌数的测定，且应按规定报告结果。

菌数报告规则（平皿法）需氧菌总数宜选取平均菌落数小于300cfu、酵母菌和霉菌总数宜选取平均菌落数小于100cfu的稀释级，作为菌数报告（取两位有效数字）的依据。以最高的平均菌落数乘以稀释倍数的值报告1g、1ml或10cm^{2}供试品中所含的菌数。如各稀释级的平板均无菌落生长，或仅最低稀释级的平板有菌落生长，但平均菌落数小于1时，以<1乘以最低稀释倍数的值报告菌数。

菌数报告规则（薄膜过滤法）以相当于1g、1ml或10cm^{2}供试品的菌落数报告菌数。

若滤膜上无菌落生长，以 <1 报告菌数（每张滤膜过滤 1g、1ml 或 10cm^{2}供试品），或 <1 乘以最低稀释倍数的值报告菌数。

2. 控制菌的检查　可根据细菌的形态结构和生理生化特性来检查，一般的检验程序如下：

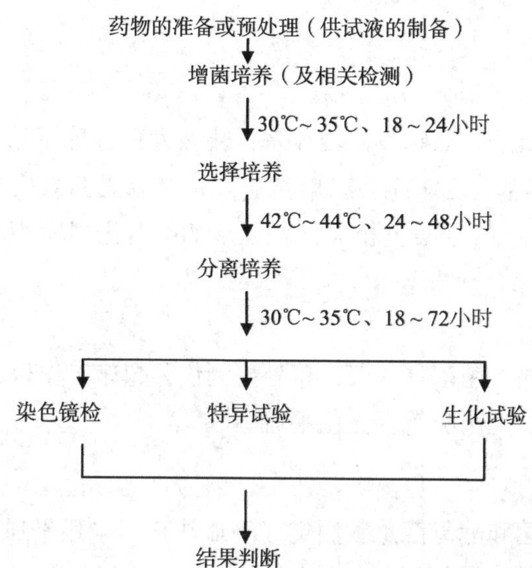

本实验只选作其中之一大肠埃希菌的检查。大肠埃希菌是口服药品的常规必检项目之一。大肠埃希菌是人和温血动物肠道内寄生的正常菌群，药品中的大肠埃希菌来源于人和温血动物的粪便。凡由供试品中检出大肠埃希菌时，表明该药品可能已被粪便污染，也就可能被存在于粪便的其他肠道致病菌所污染。患者服用这种药物后，就可能出现这些病原体感染的危险。因此，口服药品中不得检出大肠埃希菌。大肠埃希菌的检验程序如下：

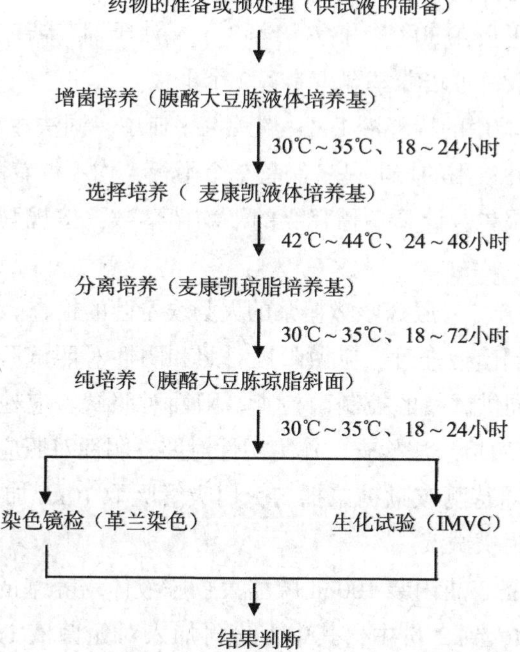

3. 培养条件　药典规定本检查法中细菌及控制菌培养温度为30℃ ~35℃；霉菌、酵母菌培养温度为23℃ ~28℃。检验结果以1g、1ml、10g、10ml、10cm^{2}为单位报告，特殊品种可以最小包装单位报告。

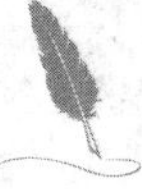

4. 药物的微生物限度标准及控制菌限度标准　控制菌的限度标准：口服药品中不得检

出大肠埃希菌；凡外用药和眼科制剂不得检出金黄色葡萄球菌和铜绿假单胞菌；含动物组织来源的制剂不得检出沙门菌。抗细菌的口服抗生素制剂应检查霉菌，每克中不得超过100个；抗真菌的口服抗生素制剂应检查细菌，每克不得超过100个；霉变、长螨者均为不合格药品。

【实验材料】

1. **菌种** 大肠埃希菌（*Escherichia coli*）[CMCC（B）44 102] 液体培养物。

2. **培养基及试剂** 胰酪大豆胨液体培养基，胰酪大豆胨琼脂培养基，沙氏葡萄糖琼脂培养基，麦康凯液体培养基，麦康凯琼脂培养基，pH 7.0 无菌氯化钠－蛋白胨缓冲液，IMViC 生化试验各培养基等；革兰染色相关试剂，IMViC 生化试验用相关试剂，灭菌生理盐水等。

3. **药物** 咳嗽糖浆。

4. **仪器** 恒温培养箱，菌落计数仪，紫外检测仪，超净工作台，显微镜等。

5. **其他** 无菌试管，无菌吸管，无菌平皿等。

【实验方法】

1. **需氧菌总数、霉菌和酵母菌总数测定（平皿法）** 采用平皿法检查口服药咳嗽糖浆的需氧氧总数、霉菌和酵母菌总数。

（1）供试液制备：将待测咳嗽糖浆摇匀，用吸管吸取10ml 加 pH7.0 无菌氯化钠－蛋白胨缓冲液至100ml，混匀，作为1∶10 的供试液。用稀释液稀释成 $1:10^2$、$1:10^3$ 等稀释级的供试液。

（2）接种：① 分别吸取上述稀释的供试品溶液各1ml 于无菌平皿中，再加入15～20ml 温度不超过45℃熔化的胰酪大豆胨琼脂或沙氏葡萄糖琼脂培养基，混匀，凝固倒置培养，胰酪大豆胨琼脂培养基平板在30℃～35℃培养3天，沙氏葡萄糖琼脂培养基平板在20℃～25℃培养5天，每稀释级每种培养基至少制备2个平板。

② 阴性对照：取试验用的稀释液1ml，置无菌平皿中，同法注入培养基作为阴性对照，凝固，倒置培养。每种计数用的培养基各制备2个平板，均不得有菌生长。

（3）计数菌落，写报告：计算各稀释级的平均菌落数，按规则报告需氧菌总数、霉菌和酵母数。

2. **大肠埃希菌的检查** 口服药咳嗽糖浆的大肠埃希菌的检查。

在对供试品进行控制菌检查时，应做阳性对照和阴性对照试验。阳性对照试验的加菌量为10～100cfu，方法同供试品的控制菌检查。阳性对照试验应检出相应的控制菌。取稀释液10ml 按照相应控制菌检查法检查，作为阴性对照。阴性对照应无菌生长。

（1）制备供试液：将待测咳嗽糖浆摇匀，用吸管吸取10ml 加 pH7.0 无菌氯化钠－蛋白胨缓冲液至100ml 作为供试液。

（2）增菌培养：准备3瓶内装100ml 胰酪大豆胨液体培养基的三角瓶。将待测咳嗽糖浆摇匀，分别取10ml 加入到2份中，其中1份再加入对照菌液1ml 做阳性对照，第3份100ml 胰酪大豆胨液体培养基中加入与供试液等量的稀释剂作阴性对照。于30℃～35℃恒温培养18～24小时（必要可延至48小时）。阴性对照瓶应无菌生长。其他2瓶培养液变浑浊表明有细菌生长。

（3）选择和分离培养：取上述预培养物1ml 接种至100ml 麦康凯液体培养基中，

42℃～44℃培养24～48 小时。取麦康凯液体培养物划线接种于麦康凯琼脂培养基平板上，30℃～35℃培养 18～72 小时。

（4）结果判定：当阳性对照的平板呈现阳性菌落时，供试品的平板无菌落生长，或有菌落但不同于表 47－1 所示的特征，可判为未检出大肠埃希菌。

表 47－1 大肠埃希菌菌落形态特征

培养基	菌落形态
麦康凯琼脂	鲜桃红色或微红色，菌落中心深桃红色，圆形，扁平，边缘整齐，表面光滑，湿润

如生长菌落与表 47－1 所列特征相符或疑似者，应挑选 2～3 个菌落分别接种于胰酪大豆胨琼脂斜面培养基，培养 18 小时，作以下检查。

（5）显微镜检：取上述斜面培养物，革兰染色后显微镜检，大肠埃希菌为革兰阴性无芽孢的短杆菌。

（6）生理生化反应：取上述斜面培养物，分别接种于乳糖发酵管，IMViC 各试验管，培养 24～48 小时观察。

大肠埃希菌可发酵乳糖产酸产气。

大肠埃希菌的 IMViC 试验结果为“＋ ＋ － －”（IMViC 分别代表：吲哚试验、甲基红试验、乙酰甲基甲醇生成试验及柠檬酸盐利用试验）。

当空白对照试验呈阴性，供试品检查为革兰阴性无芽胞杆菌；乳糖发酵产酸产气或产酸不产气；IMViC 试验为阳性、阳性、阴性、阴性或阴性、阳性、阴性、阴性，判为检出大肠埃希菌。

（7）给出检查报告：咳嗽糖浆是否检出大肠埃希菌？

【结果与讨论】

（1）计算各稀释级的平均菌落数，按规则报告需氧菌总数、霉菌和酵母菌总数；判断咳嗽糖浆的需氧菌总数、霉菌和酵母菌总数是否符合药物的微生物限度标准。

（2）记录大肠埃希菌各步检查结果，给出检验报告。

（3）如何判断某一药物中控制菌符合微生物限度标准？举例说明。

EXPERIMENT 47 Microbial Quality and Microbial limit Tests of Pharmaceutical Preparations

Purposes

1. To grasp how to examine the existence of *E. coli* in pharmaceuticals.

2. To be familiar with the plate method used for microbial limit tests of oral drugs.

3. To understand the inspection methods of specified microorganisms in pharmaceuticals.

Principles

Microbial limit tests provide tests for the existence of specified microorganisms present in non－sterile pharmaceutical products.

Oral drugs and drugs for external use are non－sterile pharmaceuticals which mean because asepsis is not necessary during manufacture process and clinical use. But specified microorganisms are not permitted or number－limited to ensure the quality of medicines. In Chinese Pharmacopoeia

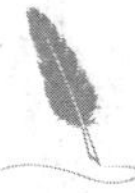

(edition 2020 Volume IV, general principle 1105, 1106), the total numbers of aerobes, molds or yeasts count, as well as the specified bacteria, are tested. Specified microorganisms include *Escherichia coli*, *Salmonella species*, *Staphylococcus aureus*, *Pseudomonas aeruginosa*, *Clostridia*. .

Plate method and membrane filtration method are used to count the total numbers of aerobes, yeasts and molds. Morphology and biochemical characteristics are applied to examine the existence of specified microbes. Mite can be identified by using a microscope. In Pharmacopoeia, quantity of products, preparation of the sample, suitability examination for count media and method validation, *etc.* are all explicitly stipulated.

1. The examination for total numbers of aerobes, molds or yeasts count The total numbers of aerobes is the number of viable aerobic microorganisms in every gram (or ml) of tested product. This will help to determine the bacterial contamination of a product. Total fungi count is the number of viable molds and yeasts in every gram (or ml) of tested product which indicates the degree of fungal contamination.

Examination method includes plate count method, membrane filtration method and Most - Probable - Number Method (MPN method) . Use validated methods to carry out total numbers of aerobes, molds and yeasts count of the test product.

(1) Microbial number report rule (plate method): Select the dilution in which the average number of colonies of aerobes is no more than 300 cfu and the yeasts and molds is no more than 100 cfu. Calculate the number of cfu per gram, per ml or per 10 cm^2 test product by multiplying the highest average number of cfu by the dilution folds. When no microbial growth occurs in any of the dilutions, or it only occurs at the lowest dilution where the average microbial number of the cfu is less than 1, report the result with 1 multiplying with the lowest dilution folds.

(2) Microbial number report rule (membrane filtration): Multiply the average microbial number by dilution folds as the number of cfu per g or per ml (10 $cm^{2)}$ test product. If no microbial growth occurs, report the result with less than 1 or 1 multiplying with the lowest dilution folds.

2. Tests for specified microorganisms According to bacterial morphological structure, testing methods is as follows:

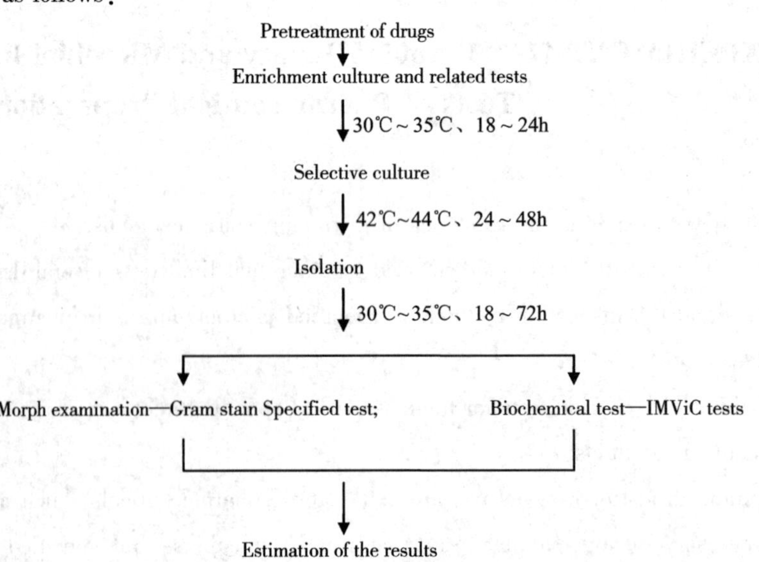

This experiment focuses on the examination of *E. coli* which is one of the specified microorgan-

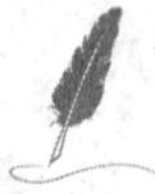

isms in microbial limit tests. *E. coli* is a normal flora in the intestinal tract of human and warm - blooded animals and commonly found in feces. Once *E. coli* is detected in pharmaceuticals, the drugs may have been contaminated by feces and the possibility of contamination by other pathogens in the intestinal tract increases drastically. The risk of pathogenic infection may occur as well. Therefore, no *E. coli* is permitted to be detected in oral drugs. The examination procedure is as follows:

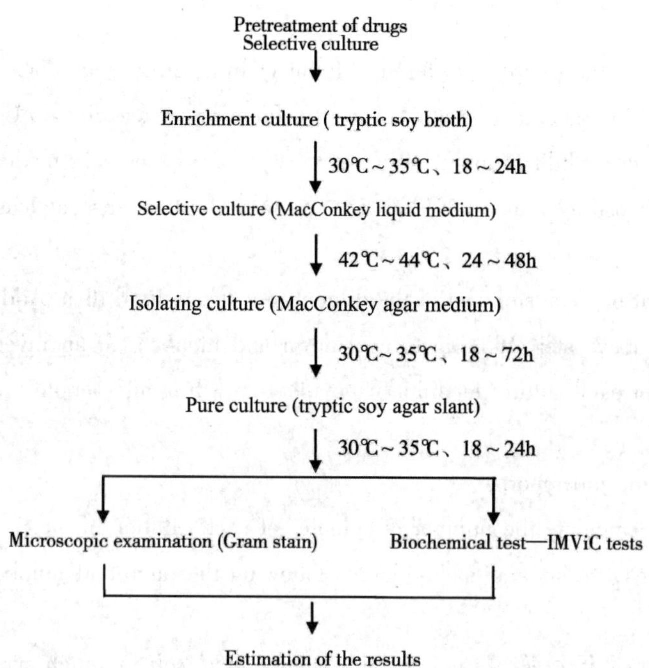

3. Incubation conditions Incubate bacteria at 30℃ ~35℃, at 23℃ ~28℃ for molds and yeasts. The test result is reported in the unit of 1g, 1ml, 10g, 10ml or $10cm^2$.

4. Microbial contamination limits of pharmaceutical preparations For the preparations for oral administration, no *E. coli* should be present, as well as *Staphylococcus aureus* and *Pseudomonas aeruginosa* for the preparation for eye administration and external use, *Salmonella species* for preparations containing animal tissues. No more than 100cfu per g of molds in anti - bacterial oral antibiotics is permitted. No more than 100cfu per g of bacteria in anti - fungal oral antibiotics is permitted. Mite should be absent in pharmaceuticals.

Materials and Apparatus

1. Strains Broth culture of *Escherichia coli* [CMCC (B) 44 102].

2. Media and Reagents Tryptic soy broth, tryptic soy agar, Sabouraud's glucose broth medium, MacConkey liquid medium, MacConkey agar medium, pH 7.0 sterile sodium chloride - peptone buffer, media for IMViC tests, reagents for Gram stain, reagents for IMViC tests, sterile normal saline.

3. Testing sample Cough syrup.

4. Apparatus Incubator, colony counter, UV lamp, clean bench, bright - field microscope.

5. Others Sterile tube, dropper, plate.

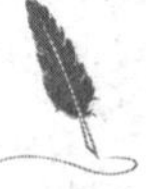

Procedures

1. The total numbers of aerobes, molds and yeasts count (plate method)

Examine the total numbers of aerobes, molds or yeasts count incough syrup by plate method.

(1) Sample preparation

Mix the testing cough syrup and transfer 10 ml of the product to 100 ml of sterile sodium chloride – peptone buffer solution (pH 7.0). Then mix well. Use this 1: 10 solution as the testing sample. Further dilution of 1: 10^2, 1: 10^3 is then performed.

(2) Inoculation

① Transfer 1ml of the sample (different dilutions) to a sterile Petri dish, then add 15 ~ 20ml melted tryptic soy agar or Sabouraud's glucose agar medium (not exceeding 45℃). Mix well and incubate upside down after solidification at 30 ℃ ~ 35 ℃ (tryptic soy agar medium) or 23 ℃ ~ 28 ℃ (Sabouraud's glucose agar medium) for 5d. For each dilution, use at least 2 Petri dishes for each culture medium.

2) Negative control: Transfer 1ml of the diluent to a sterile Petri dish. Add the culture medium and mix well as the above step. Waiting to cool down and incubate in an inverted position. Use at least 2 Petri dishes for each culture medium. No evident growth of microorganisms occurs in either of the Petri dish.

(3) Colony count and report

After counting, calculate the number of colonies of each dilution of the product, report the total numbers of aerobes, yeasts and molds counts following the microbial number report rule in the principle part.

2. Examination of *E. coli* Examine the existence of *E. coli* in cough syrup.

Positive control: Add 10 ~ 100cfu of the tested microorganisms of the positive control, and then carry out the test in the same way for specified microorganism. The tested microorganism should be detected in the positive control.

Negative control: Transfer 10 ml of diluting solution to a prescribed amount of culture media as negative control. Examine it in the same way for specified microorganism. No microbial growth occurs in the negative control.

(1) Sample preparation

Mix the test cough syrup and transfer 10ml of the product to 100ml of sterile sodium chloride – peptone buffer solution (pH 7.0). Then mix well. Use this 1:10 solution as the test sample.

(2) Enrichment culture

Prepare 3 flasks of tryptic soy broth (100ml in every flask). Mix the test sample and transfer 10 ml to the test sample and positive control flasks respectively. Add 1ml of *E. coli* inoculum to the positive control flask. Add 10 ml of diluents to the negative control. Incubate the 3 flasks at 30℃ ~ 35℃ for 18 ~ 24h (48h if necessary). No microbial growth should occur in negative control. If the other 2 flasks become turbid, microbial growth occurs.

(3) Selective and isolation culture

Transfer 1ml of the enrichment culture to 100ml of MacConkey liquid medium, and incubate at 42℃ ~ 44℃ for 24 ~ 48h. Take the inoculum mentioned above and streak on MacConkey agar medi-

um plate, incubate them at 30℃ ~35℃ for 18 ~72h.

(4) Evaluation of results

When colonies of positive control show the same characteristics as*E coli* colonies and no growth of microorganism occurs on the plate of test sample, or the appearance of the microbial colonies does not match the description in table 47 –1, *E. coli* is absent in the product.

Table 47 –1　Morphologic characteristics of *E. coli* colonies

Culture medium	Colony characteristics
MacConkey agar medium	Brilliant pink or pale red, deep pink at center of the colony, circular, flat, regular margin, smooth surface, moist

When the colonies on the sample plate share the similarities with *E. coli*, pick up 2 ~ 3 colonies to inoculate on tryptic soy agar slants and incubate for 18h for further tests.

(5) Microscopic examination

After incubation, examine cellular morphology with Gram stain. *E. coli* should be gram – negative brevis bacillus without endospore.

(6) Biochemical tests

Inoculate the bacteria from the slant culture to biochemical culture media (lactose fermentation and IMViC tests) and then incubate for 24 ~48h.

Positive control: *E. coli* can produce acid and gas when fermenting lactose. The IMViC tests (represent indole test, methyl red test, V – P test and citrate test) result should be " + + – – ".

Negative control: no growth appears.

Test sample: In Gram stain, if the sample is gram – negative bacterium without endo – spore, and produces acid with " + + – – " or " – + – – " in IMViC tests, *E. coli* is detected.

(7) Report the examination result

The test cough syrup complies with the microbial limits of *E. coli* or not.

Results and Discussion

(1) Calculate the average colony number of every dilution and report the total numbers of aerobes, molds or yeasts count according to the report rules. Estimate if the examination results comply with the microbial limits or not.

(2) Record the results of *E. coli* examination and report it.

(3) How to estimate whether a pharmaceutical preparation complies with the microbial limits? Give an example.

扫码"练一练"

第八部分　综合性实验

微生物在自然界分布广泛，在药品生产的各个环节都有可能受到微生物的污染，因此，微生物的污染及其预防是药物生产和保藏中的重要问题。所以，在药物生产中应予以高度重视，同时在药物的质量管理中必须严格进行药物的微生物学检验，以保证药物制剂达到卫生学标准。

本部分主要包括以下内容：①筛选微生物产生抗生素、淀粉酶、重组人干扰素的相关实验设计与研究；②污水中大肠埃希菌噬菌体的分离；③抗药细菌的分离鉴定。

实验四十八　土壤中抗生素产生菌的分离、鉴定和抗菌活性测定

扫码“学一学”

【实验目的】

（1）掌握从土壤中分离与纯化放线菌的基本原理及常用方法。

（2）了解放线菌产生抗生素的抗菌谱测定方法。

【实验原理】

放线菌是重要的抗生素产生菌，许多临床应用的抗生素均由土壤中分离的放线菌产生的。放线菌一般在中性偏碱性、有机质丰富、通气性好的土壤中含量较多。由于土壤中的微生物是各种不同种类微生物的混合体，必须把各种放线菌从这些混杂的微生物群体中分离出来，从而获得某一放线菌的纯培养。根据放线菌对营养、酸碱度等条件要求，常选用合成培养基或有机氮培养基，也可采用选择性培养基或加入某种抑制剂，使细菌、霉菌出现的数量大大减少，从而分离土壤中的放线菌；再通过稀释法，使放线菌在固体培养基上形成单独菌落，并可得到纯菌株。

抗生素是放线菌的次级代谢产物，放线菌经液体培养后，其分泌的抗生素多数存在于离心所得的上清液中，可采用微生物方法进行检测，从而筛选到所需的抗生素产生菌。

【实验材料】

1. **菌种**　金黄色葡萄球菌（*Staphylococcus aureus*）和大肠埃希菌（*Escherichia coli*）牛肉膏蛋白胨液体培养物。

2. **培养基与试剂**　高氏1号合成培养基，肉汤琼脂培养基，灭菌的生理盐水。

3. **土壤**　校园土，空气中干燥，磨碎。

4. **仪器**　恒温培养箱，超净工作台，游标卡尺等。

5. **其他**　镊子，药敏试纸片，无菌平皿，无菌玻璃铲，无菌涂布棒，无菌移液管等。

【实验方法】

从校园土壤中分离培养放线菌，采用移块法初筛抗生素产生菌，测定抗菌谱。

1. 土壤中放线菌的分离

（1）采集土样　土壤的种类和自然条件影响着放线菌的种类和分布数量。链霉菌主要存在于干燥、偏碱而营养丰富的土壤里；而小单孢菌多分布在潮湿土壤或湖底泥土中。因此在采土时，应注意地区、时间和植被情况。采土季节以春秋二季为宜，雨季不宜采土。一般认为，南方地区的土壤和北方地区土壤相比，南方地区的土壤链霉菌的种类较多，而某些特殊土壤或地区也可能存在一些特殊菌种。采集的土样最好随即分离，否则要放在阴凉通风处，防止变潮生霉。

在选定的采土地点，用小铲除去 5cm 厚表层土，用酒精棉球擦拭过的铁锹深挖 15～20cm 处，将采得的土放入一个无菌纸袋或培养皿内，并按要求记录有关土样的内容，包括土壤编号、采集日期、采集地点及土壤基本特征。

（2）土壤悬液梯度稀释

①将土样放入用酒精擦拭过的乳钵中，除去石块、草根，研磨压碎后，称取 5.0g 放入盛有 50ml 灭菌的生理盐水的三角瓶中。振荡 5 分钟，即 10^{-1} 的土壤悬液，静置 30 秒。

② 取 1ml 土壤悬液，加入到 9ml 灭菌生理盐水中 10 倍稀释。

③ 按 1∶10 梯度稀释至 10^{-4}、10^{-5} 和 10^{-6}，见图 48－1。

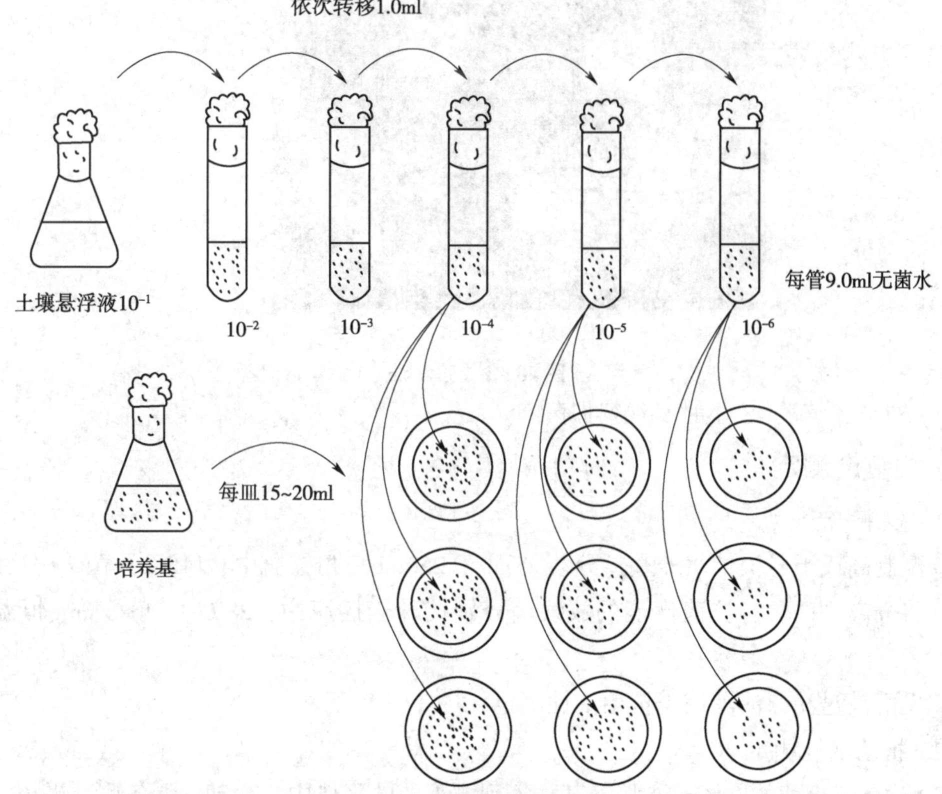

图 48－1　土壤放线菌的分离

（3）制备培养基平板

① 准备 9 个无菌玻璃平皿，分别标记 10^{-4}、10^{-5} 和 10^{-6}，每个稀释度平行三皿。

② 配制高氏 1 号琼脂培养基并于 115℃灭菌 20 分钟，待其冷却至 50℃左右后，将其倒入无菌平皿中，每个平皿加 1～20ml，待冷凝制成无菌平板。

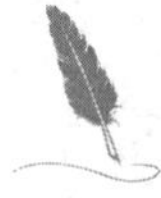

（4）分离培养：从对应稀释度（10^{-4}、10^{-5} 和 10^{-6}）的土壤悬液中分别吸取 0.5ml 稀

释液加到冷凝好的高氏 1 号平板中，用无菌涂布棒将加在平板培养基上的土壤稀释液在整个平板表面涂匀（每个稀释度换一支无菌涂布棒）。平板倒置于培养箱 28℃恒温培养 1 周。

（5）纯化培养：分别挑取平板上的放线菌单菌落，接种于高氏 1 号琼脂培养基斜面，28℃恒温培养 1 周，用于观察放线菌生长特征和产抗生素能力的测定。

2. **移块法粗筛抗生素产生菌**　移块法适合检测膏状体或斜面琼脂培养物的抑菌活性，还可用于土壤放线菌的初筛和抗菌活性测定。

（1）在灭菌的平皿中加入金黄色葡萄球菌肉汤培养液 4 ~ 5 滴，倒入溶化并冷却到 50℃左右的肉汤琼脂培养基约 20ml，混匀。

（2）在培养基表面贴上 1cm^{2}的放线菌琼脂块 4 块，其中一块为阳性对照菌，另三个为土壤中分离放线菌琼脂菌块，见图 48－2。

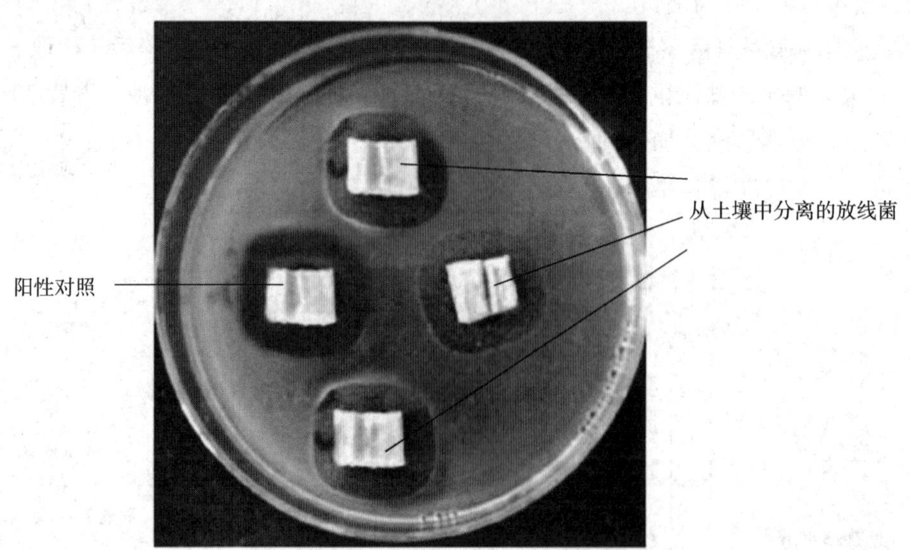

图 48－2　移块法

（3）37℃，培养 48 小时，观察抑菌圈。

3. 抗菌谱测定

（1）发酵培养

① 配制高氏 1 号液体培养基，分装 25ml 于 250ml 三角摇瓶中，115℃灭菌 20 分钟。

② 将分离到的具有抗菌性能的放线菌分别接种于摇瓶中，28℃、240 r/min 恒温培养 1 周。

③ 发酵液过滤，滤液用于抗菌活性测定。

（2）抗菌活性测定

① 将 10ml 灭菌的肉汤琼脂培养基加入到已灭菌的平皿中、冷却，制备底层平板。

② 取培养 8 小时的金黄色葡萄球菌或大肠埃希菌液体培养物 2ml 分别加到 200ml 无菌的肉汤琼脂培养基中（注意培养基应冷却到约 50℃），振荡混匀，吸取 6ml 加入到底层平板上，制备双层平板（每种菌株平行做 2 皿）。

③ 用无菌镊子将一系列吸附有放线菌发酵液的无菌滤纸片分别置于含金黄色葡萄球菌和大肠埃希菌的双层平板上，37℃培养 24 小时。

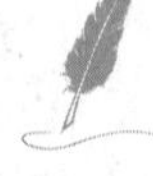

④ 观察并测量抑菌圈，判断放线菌是否产生抗生素，见图 48－3。

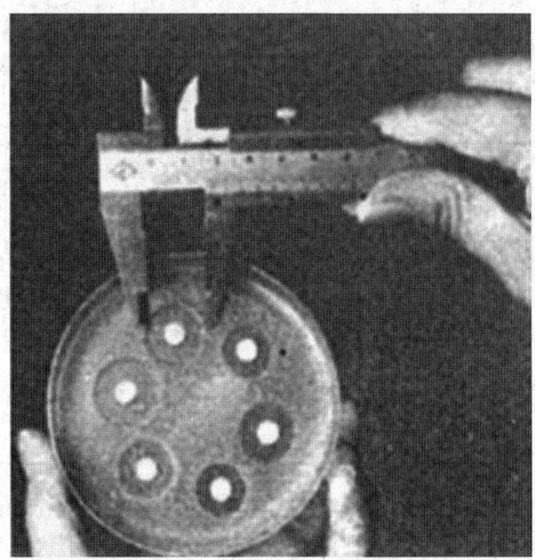

图 48 - 3 抗菌谱的测定

【结果与讨论】

(1) 记录各稀释度平板中分离到的放线菌菌落数并描述放线菌菌落的形态特征。

(2) 记录 4 ~6 株分离的放线菌所产生的抗生素的抗菌谱。

(3) 在分离土壤中放线菌时，如何避免细菌和真菌的生长？

PART EIGHT Integrated Experiments

Microbes are widespread in the nature so prevention of contamination from microbes are of great importance in pharmaceutical production process. Microbial examination in drug quality management must be strictly performed to ensure that pharmaceutial preparations meet hygiene standards.

This part includes three sections: ①experiments on screening microbes which can produce antibiotics, amylase and recombinant human interferon. ②Isolation of phage of *E. coli* from sewage. ③screening of drug - resistant microbes.

EXPERIMENT 48 Isolation and Identification of Antibiotic - Producing Actinomycetes from Soil, and Determination of its Antimicrobial activity

Purposes

(1) To grasp the principles and methods of how to isolate and purify actinomycetes from soil.

(2) To be familiar with the determination of anti - bacterial spectrum of antibiotics.

Principles

Actinomycetes are important antibiotic - producing bacteria. A lot of useful clinic antibiotics are derived from actinomycetes in soil. Actinomycetes are usually found in the soil with neutral or alkaline pH, adequate organics and good ventilation. Since the microorganisms in soil are always a mixture of different species, it is necessary for us to isolate different species of actinomycetes from the mixture to get pure culture of a certain actinomycete. Synthetic medium or organic nitrogen culture is commonly used. You can isolate actinomycetes from soil by using selective culture media or medium

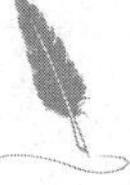

with addition of certain inhibitor to substantially reduce the growth of bacteria and molds. After that, you can get individual colony of actinomycetes on solid culture media by dilution, and then obtain pure culture.

Antibiotics are the secondary metabolites of actinomycetes. After fermentation in liquid media and centrifugation, antibiotics secreted by antibiotics – producing actinomycetes appear in the supernatant can be determined by microbial method. As a result, the antibiotic – producing strain is successfully screened.

Materials and Apparatus

1. Strains Nutrient broth culture of *Staphylococcus aureus* and *Escherichia coli.*

2. Media and Reagents Gauss' No. 1 defined medium, nutrient agar media, sterilized normal saline, *etc.*

3. Soil Obtained from campus by air dry and powdering.

4. Apparatus Incubator, clean bench, vernier caliper, *etc.*

5. Others Tweezer, paper slip, sterile dish, sterile glass spade, sterile glass spreader, sterile pipette, *etc.*

Procedures

Isolate actinomycetes from campus soil, screen primarily the antibiotic – producing actinomycetes by moving – agar block method and measure the anti – bacterial spectrum.

1. Isolation of Actinomycetes from Soil

(1) Soil sample collection

Actinomycetes species and their distribution vary with species and natural conditions of the soil. Streptomycetes mainly exist in dry, alkaline and nutrient – rich soil, while Micromonospora mainly distribute in damp soil or lake – bottom clay. Therefore, region, time and condition of vegetation should be considered when collecting soil samples. It is appropriate to collect the samples in spring and autumn, but not in rainy days. The species of actinomycetes in South China are more abundant than those in the North. Certain special soil or region may contain some special species of actinomycetes. It is better to isolate the strains from the sample soil right after sampling, or preserve the soil in cool places to prevent from mildewing.

In the selected region, remove the surface soil of 5cm depth and then dig into 15 ~ 20cm deep with alcohol cleaned spade. Put the collected soil in a sterile paper bag or plate, and record the sample No. , sample name, collection date, and place of sampling and the basic characteristic of the soil.

(2) Prepare a serial dilution of the soil samples

① Put the sample soil to a mortar which is cleaned by alcohol, remove stones, grass roots, grind the soil. Weigh 5.0g soil and put it into the flask containing 50ml sterile normal saline. Mix thoroughly for 5min to make a uniform soil – water suspension.

② Transfer 1ml soil suspension to 9ml sterile normal saline for 10 times dilution.

③ Repeat the 1:10 dilution to obtain 10^{-4}, 10^{-5} and 10^{-6} diluted solution (Fig. 48 – 1).

(3) Prepare culture media plates

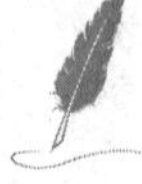

① Prepare 9 sterile glass plates, label three sets of sterile plate with the dilutions (10^{-4}, 10^{-5}

and 10^{-6}).

② Prepare Gauss' No. 1 agar media and sterilize at 115℃ for 20min, cool off to 50℃ ~55℃, add 15 ~20ml of it to each plate and wait to cool down.

(4) Isolation and incubation

Transfer 0.5ml diluted solution of 10^{-4}, 10^{-5} and 10^{-6} to three sterile plates respectively and spread it. Incubate all plates in an inverted position at 28℃ for one week.

(5) Purification

Aseptically pick actinomycetes colonies, streak on Gauss' No. 1 agar slant and incubate at 28 ℃ for one week for the observation of growth features of actinomycetes and the determination of antibiotics.

2. The moving – agar block method This method is applicable to test the inhibitory ability of ointment or slant culture, and it can be used to preliminarily screen actinomycetes isolated from soil and its antibiotic – producing antibiotic ability.

(1) Add 4 ~ 5 drops of broth culture of *S. aureus* to an sterile plate, and then pour 15 ~ 20ml of broth agar media which has been melt and then cooled to 50℃. Mix well.

(2) Attach the surface of the culture media with four $1cm^3$ sizes of agar blocks of actinomycetes, one is as positive control, the other three are isolated from soil (Fig. 48 –2).

(3) Incubate at 37℃ for 48h and observe the inhibitory zone.

3. Determination of Antibiotic Spectrum

(1) Fermentation cultivation

① Prepare starch media and pour 25ml to a 250ml shaking flask, sterilize at 115℃ for 20min.

② Inoculating each agar slant cultures of actinomycetes with antimicrobial activity to each shaking flask, incubate at 28℃ 240r/min for one week.

③ Filtrate the fermentation broth for the determination of antimicrobial activity.

(2) Determination of Antimicrobial activity

① Pour 10ml sterile nutrient agar media to a sterile plate and allow it to cool off in order to prepare the bottom plate.

② Transfer 2ml of 8h cultures of *S. aureus* or *E. coli* to 200ml sterile nutrient agar media (50℃ ~55℃) respectively, mix well and pour 6 ml to the bottom plate to make double – layered agar plate (two plates for each screened strain).

③ Add a series of paper slip absorbed with the culture broth of actinomycetes on the surface of double – layered agar plate of *S. aureus* and *E. coli*, incubate at 37 ℃ for 24h.

④ Observe the inhibitory zone and determine whether actinomycetes can produce antibiotics (Fig. 48 –3).

Results and Discussion

(1) Count the number of actinomycete colonies in every plates and describe their characteristics.

(2) Record the anti – bacterial spectrum of 4 ~6 antibiotics.

(3) How to avoid the growth of bacteria and fungi when isolating antibiotic – producing actinomycetes from the soil?

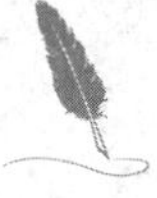

扫码“学一学”

实验四十九 重组人干扰素 α 工程菌的构建、培养和诱导表达

【实验目的】

(1) 了解基因工程在生物制药领域的应用。

(2) 掌握基因工程菌的构建、培养和诱导表达。

(3) 学会酶联免疫法检测 IFN－α。

【实验原理】

干扰素（IFN）是一种广谱抗病毒剂，主要是通过细胞表面受体作用使细胞产生抗病毒蛋白，从而抑制病毒的复制，其类型分为三类：α－型、β－型、γ－型；同时还可增强自然杀伤细胞、巨噬细胞和 T 淋巴细胞的活力，从而起到免疫调节作用，并增强抗病毒能力。

基因工程技术可以按照人们的期望，将外援基因整合入宿主基因组中，表达具有生物学活性的蛋白药物，极大解决了生物药物的药源性问题。本实验将外源的 IFN－α 基因全合成后，插入到以 λ 噬菌体的 pLpR 为强启动子的 pBV220 质粒中，构建的IFN－α 表达工程菌只须改变培养温度即可控制目的基因的表达。

表达产物 IFN－α 经亲和层析纯化后，可采用双抗体夹心 ELISA 法进行测定。用抗人 IFN－α 抗体包被于酶标板上，实验时样品或标准品中的人 IFN－α 会与包被抗体结合，游离的成分被洗去。依次加入生物素化的抗人 IFN－α 抗体和辣根过氧化物酶标记的亲和素。抗人 IFN－α 抗体与结合在包被抗体上的人 IFN－α 结合、生物素与亲和素特异性结合而形成免疫复合物，游离的成分被洗去。加入显色底物（TMB），TMB 在辣根过氧化物酶的催化下呈现蓝色，加终止液后变成黄色。用酶标仪在 450nm 波长处测 OD 值，IFN－α 浓度与 OD_{450} 值之间成正比，通过绘制标准曲线计算出样品中 IFN－α 的浓度。

【实验材料】

1. **菌株与质粒** *E. coli* BL21（DE3），温控型质粒 pBV220。

2. **培养基** LB 液体培养基：1% 胰蛋白胨，0.5% 酵母提取物，1% NaCl，pH 7.0，使用前加入氨苄青霉素使得终浓度为 100μg/ml。

3. **主要试剂** 低相对分子质量蛋白质 marker，胰蛋白胨，酵母提取物，溶菌酶，PMSF，Triton X－100，丙烯酰胺，甲叉丙烯酰胺，镍柱亲和层析试剂盒（Gene script），人 α 干扰素-α 酶联免疫分析试剂盒（Elab science）。

4. **主要仪器** PCR 仪，水浴锅，培养箱，摇床，层析，稳压电泳仪，电泳槽，凝胶成像系统，752 紫外分光光度计，高压灭菌锅，超净工作台，部分收集器，高速台式离心机等。

【实验方法】

1. **BL21/pBV220－cIFN 工程菌的构建** 设计的 DNA 双链均由化学方法合成，经过退火，限制性酶切处理后，插入载体 pBV220 载体。步骤如下：

将该质粒转化到大肠埃希菌 BL21（DE3）中，得到工程菌 BL21/pBV220/IFN。

2. **工程菌的诱导表达** 挑取保存在甘油管中保存的工程菌 BL21/pBV220/IFN 菌液，划线于含氨苄青霉素的 LB 平板上，37℃过夜培养后，挑取单菌落接种于 5ml LB 培养液中，

37℃，200r/min 活化过夜。

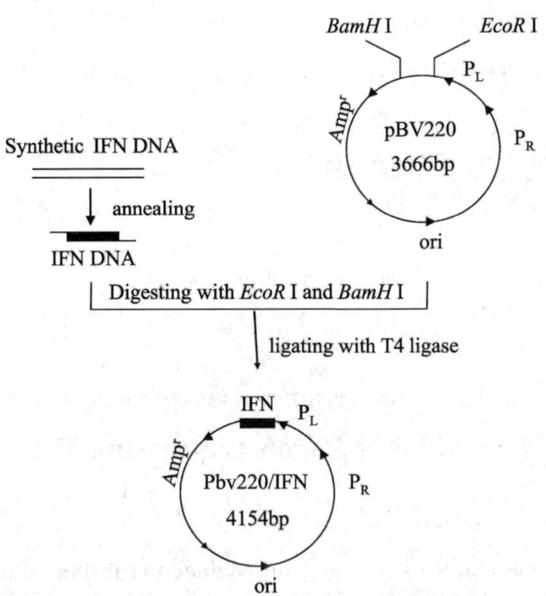

取已经活化的菌液 5ml，加入 100ml 含有氨苄青霉素的 LB 液体培养基中，30℃，220r/min 培养 5.5 小时，然后立刻升温到 42℃诱导培养 3 小时，SDS－PAGE 检测干扰素的表达量。

3. 重组干扰素-α 的分离纯化　取 50ml 诱导表达液，4℃、5000r/min 离心 5 分钟，收集细胞，加入 8ml LE Buffer 重新悬浮细胞。在冰上操作，超声破碎细胞，总时间为 30～45 分钟。4 ℃、12000 r/min 离心裂解液 15 分钟，收集上清液过 Ni－NTA 亲和层析介质。将含多聚 his 标签的澄清样品上样至柱中，流速控制为 0.5～1ml/min，收集流出液以待后续分析。以流速为 1ml/min 的洗涤缓冲液洗涤柱子以去除杂蛋白，用 5～10 倍柱体积的洗脱缓冲液以 0.5～1ml/min 的流速洗脱，收集洗脱液，或根据流出液 A_{280} 值判断，当数值陡然上升时开始接收洗脱液，直到 A_{280} 数值降至最低且稳定停止收集。收集液对 20mM Tris－HCl，pH 8.0 或 1 × PBS，pH 7.4 进行透析，冻干保存备用。

4. 重组干扰素 α 的检测　实验开始前，各试剂均应平衡至室温；或样品配制时需充分混匀并尽量避免起泡。

（1）加样　分别设空白孔、标准待测品 100μl。

（2）弃去液体，甩干，不用洗涤。每个孔中加入生物素化抗体工作液 100μl（在使用前 15min 内配制），酶标板加上覆膜，37 ℃温育 1 小时。

（3）弃去孔内液体，甩干，洗板 3 次，每次浸泡 1～2 分钟，大约 350μl/孔，甩干并在吸水纸上轻拍将孔内液体拍干。

（4）每孔加酶结合物工作液（临用前 15 分钟内配制）100μl，加上覆膜，37 ℃温育 30 分钟。

（5）弃去孔内液体，甩干，洗板 5 次，方法同步骤 3。

（6）每孔加底物溶液（TMB）90μl，酶标板加上覆膜，37℃避光孵育 15 分钟左右。当标准孔出现明显梯度时，即可终止。

（7）每孔加终止液 50μl，终止反应此时蓝色立转黄色。

（8）立即用酶标仪在 450nm 波长测量各孔的光密度（OD 值）。

（9）每个标准品的 OD 值减去空白孔的 OD 值后作图，如设置复孔，则应取其平均值计

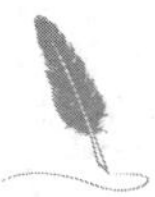

算。以标准品的浓度为横坐标，OD 值为纵坐标，绘出准曲线。亦可以 OD 值为横坐标，标准品的浓度为纵坐标，绘出准曲线。

推荐使用专业的曲线制作软件，如 curve expert 1.4，在软件界面既可根据样品 OD 值，由标准曲线查出相应的浓度，乘以稀释倍数；亦可将样品 OD 值代入标准曲线的拟合方程式，计算出样品浓，再乘以稀释倍数，即为样品的实际度。

【结果与讨论】

（1）比较工程菌表达的干扰素和天然来源的干扰素的不同。

（2）基因工程手段生产生物药物有哪些局限性？

EXPERIMENT 49 Construction, Expression and Cultivation of Recombinant *E. coli* Expressing INF – α

Purpose

(1) To understand the application of genetic engineering in the field of biomedicine.

(2) To grasp the construction of engineered bacteria, the expression and purification of target protein.

(3) Learn to detect interferon alpha by enzyme – linked immunoassay.

Principle

Interferons are a group of signaling proteins produced and released by host cells in response to the presence of pathogens, such as viruses, bacteria, parasites, or tumor cells. In a typical scenario, a virus – infected cell will release interferons causing nearby cells to heighten their anti – viral defenses. Three classes of interferons have been identified: alpha, beta and gamma. Each class has many effects, though some of their effects overlap. The mechanism of action of interferon is complex and is not well understood. Interferons modulate the response of the immune system to viruses, bacteria, cancer, and other foreign substances that invade the body.

Using genetic engineering technology, we can integrate foreign genes into the host cell to produce protein drugs and solves the problems of limited sources for biological drugs. In this experiment we synthesize the gene of human interferon alpha and insert it into the plasmid pBV220 with a strong promoter lambda phage pLpR. The induced expression of interferon alpha in engineered *E. coli* can be easily controlled by temperature change.

Purified by affinity chromatography, the expressed interferon alpha can be determined by using ELISA kit. The micro ELISA plate provided in this kit has been precoated with an antibody specific to Human IFN – α. Standards or samples are then added to the appropriate micro ELISA plate wells and bind to the specific antibody. Then a biotinylated detection antibody specific for Human IFN – α and Avidin – Horseradish Peroxidase (HRP) conjugate is added to each micro plate well and incubated. Free components are washed away. The substrate solution is added to each well. Only those wells that contain Human IFN – α, biotinylated detection antibody and Avidin – HRP conjugate will appear blue in color. The enzyme – substrate reaction is terminated by the addition of a sulphuric acid solution and the color turns yellow. The optical density (OD) is measured spectrophotometrically at a wavelength of 450nm. The OD value is proportional to the concentration of Human IFN –

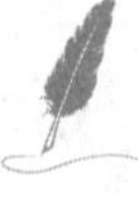

α.

Materials and apparatus

1. Strains and plasmids *E. coli* BL21 (DE3), plasmid pBV220.

2. Medium LB medium with 100μg/ml Ampicillin.

3. Reagents and kit Low molecular weight protein marker, peptone, yeast extract, lysozyme, PMSF, Triton X - 100, Acrylamide, N, N′- Methylenebisacrylamide, High Affinity Ni - NTA Resin (Gene script), Human IFN - α ELISA Kit (Elab science).

4. Apparatus PCR amplifier, water bath, incubator, shaker, chromatography column, electrophoresis apparatus, electrophoresis tank, gel imaging system, ultraviolet spectrophotometer, autoclave, clean bench, fraction collector, high - speed centrifuge.

Procedures

1. The construction of pBV220/IFN Designed Human IFN - α gene DNA was inserted into the plasmid pBV220 after synthesis, annealing, restriction enzyme digestion. The step is illustrated in the following diagram:

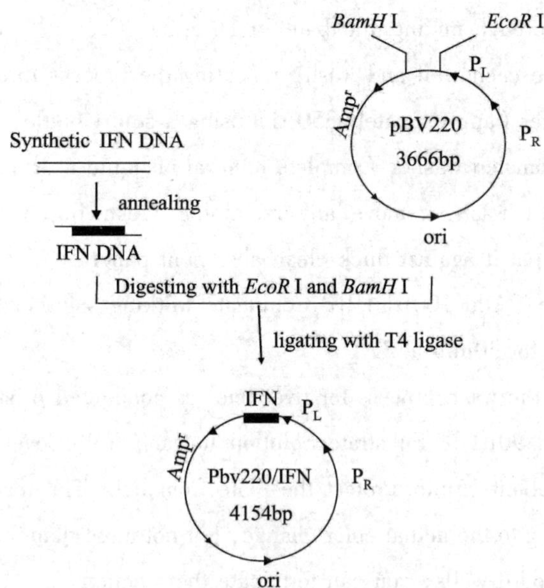

Construction of plasmid pBV220/IFN

2. Induced expression of the engineered strain Take a small amount of BL 21/pBV 220/IFN culture from glycerin tube and streak it on the LB plate supplemented with 100 u/ml ampicillin. Place the plate inverted in a 37℃ incubator for 24h. Pick a single colony in LB broth. The cultures were grown at 37℃ with shaking (200r/min) overnight.

LB medium was inoculated with 5 ml cultures in 250ml flasks. The culture was grown at 30℃ with shaking (200 r/min) for 5. 5h. Then the temperature was regulated to 42℃ to induce the gene expression. 3h later, the level of IFN - α was assayed by SDS - PAGE.

3. The separation and purification of recombinant IFN - α Harvest cells from a 50ml induced culture by centrifugation at 4℃ (5,000 r/min for 5 minutes). Resuspend the cells in 8 ml of LE buffer with appropriate amount of PMSF or other protease inhibitors. Sonicate the solution on ice using 180 one - second bursts at high intensity with a three - second cooling period. Centrifuge the ly-

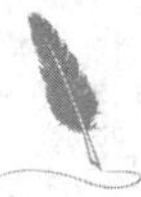

sate at 12,000 r/min for 15 min at 4 ℃ to pellet the cellular debris.

Apply the supernatant onto a Ni^{2+} column with a flow – rate of 0.5 ~ 1ml per minute. Collect and save the flow – through for analysis. Wash the column with 8 × bed volumes of wash buffer or until A_{280} is stable at the flow – rate of 1 ml per minute. Elute the polyhistidine – tagged protein with 5 to 10 × bed volumes of Elution Buffer at a flow – rate of 0.5 ~ 1ml per minute. Collect the elute and dialyze it against 20 mM Tris – HCl, pH 8.0 or 1 × PBS, pH 7.4. Freeze – dry and preserve for further use.

4. The Assay of recombinant IFN – α Assay procedure is as below:

(1) Add Sample: Add 100μl Standard, Blank, or Sample into the well. The blank well is added with Reference Standard & Sample Diluent. Solutions are added to the bottom of micro ELISA plate well, avoid touching the inside wall and formation of foams as far as possible. Mix it gently. Cover the plate with the sealer provided. Incubate for 90min at 37℃.

(2) Biotinylated Detection Ab: Remove the liquid of each well, don't wash. Immediately add 100μl Biotinylated Detection Ab working solution to each well. Cover with the plate sealer. Gently tap the plate to ensure thorough mixing. Incubate for 1h at 37 °C.

(3) Wash: Aspirate each well and wash, repeating the process three times. Wash by filling each well with Wash Buffer (approximately 350μl) using a squirt bottle, multi – channel pipette, manifold dispenser or automated washer. Complete removal of liquid at each step is essential to good performance. After the last wash, remove any remaining Wash Buffer by aspirating or decanting. Invert the plate and pat it against thick clean absorbent paper.

(4) HRP Conjugate: Add 100μl HRP Conjugate working solution to each well. Cover with the Plate sealer. Incubate for 30min at 37℃.

(5) Wash: Repeat the wash process for five times as conducted in step 3.

(6) Substrate: Add 90μl of Substrate Solution to each well. Cover with a new Plate sealer. Incubate at 37°C for about 15min. Protect the plate from light. The reaction time can be shortened or extended according to the actual color change, but not more than 30minutes. When apparent gradient appeared in standard wells, you can terminate the reaction.

(7) Stop: Add 50μl of Stop Solution to each well. Color turns to yellow immediately. The addition order of stop solution should be the same as the substrate solution.

(8) OD Measurement: Determine the optical density (OD value) of each well at once, using a microplate reader set at 450nm. You should open the microplate reader beforehand, preheat the instrument, and set the testing parameters.

After experiment, put all the unused reagents back into the refrigerator according to the specified storage temperature respectively.

Result and discussion

(1) Compare the differences between recombinant interferon and natural interferon.

(2) What are the limitations of genetic engineering technology for the production of biodrugs?

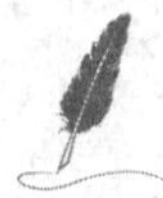

实验五十　产淀粉酶枯草芽孢杆菌的选育

【实验目的】

（1）掌握紫外线的诱变原理。

（2）了解紫外线对枯草芽孢杆菌的诱变效应。

【实验原理】

紫外线（ultraviolet ray，UV）作为物理诱变剂用于工业微生物菌种的诱变处理具有悠久的历史，尽管几十年来各种新的诱变剂不断出现和被应用于诱变育种，紫外线作为诱变因子还是有其特殊的意义。到目前为止，对于诱变处理后得到的高单位抗生素产生菌株中，有80%左右是通过紫外线诱变后经筛选而获得的，因此，对于微生物菌种选育工作者来说，紫外线作为首选诱变剂。

紫外线的波长在200～400nm，但对于诱变最有效的波长仅仅是在253～265nm。日常生活中，紫外灯是产生紫外线的主要方式，其波长为254nm。紫外线在空气中穿透能力强，在液体中穿透能力较弱，在固体介质中几乎不能穿透，所以诱变时，一定要将目标直接暴露在紫外线下，才能取得较好的诱变效果。

265～266nm的紫外线杀伤作用最强。其主要作用机制是：紫外线穿过微生物细胞时，DNA吸收了紫外线，引起DNA分子中相邻的胸腺嘧啶借助共价键形成胸腺嘧啶二聚体，影响了DNA复制功能。

【实验材料】

1. 菌种　枯草芽孢杆菌BF7658。

2. 培养基及试剂　牛肉膏蛋白胨固体培养基，淀粉培养基，碘液，0.85%无菌生理盐水。

3. 仪器　培养箱，30W紫外灯，磁力搅拌器，离心机等。

4. 其他　无菌培养皿，无菌试管，无菌移液管，无菌三角耙，无菌带玻璃珠的锥形瓶，量筒，烧杯，离心管等。

【实验方法】

利用紫外线诱变枯草芽孢杆菌BF7658，研究产生高淀粉酶活力的菌株的诱变效应。

1. 诱变

（1）菌悬液的制备

① 取一支经20小时培养活化的枯草芽孢杆菌斜面。

② 用5ml 0.85%生理盐水将菌苔轻轻洗下，此过程重复两次，并倒入盛有玻璃珠的锥形瓶中。

③ 强烈振荡10分钟，将此菌悬液用无菌移液管吸至10ml离心管中，3000r/min离心15分钟。

④ 弃去上清液，将菌体用生理盐水10ml洗涤2次（每次3000r/min离心10分钟），最后用10ml无菌生理盐水制成菌悬液。

（2）菌悬液计数　用无菌移液管将菌悬液移入另一个锥形瓶中，调整细胞浓度为10^8/ml。

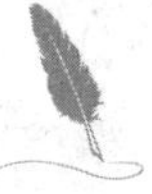

（3）淀粉琼脂平板制作　制备淀粉琼脂培养基灭菌备用，将其融化后，冷至50℃左右，倒平皿，凝固后待用。

（4）诱变处理

① 正式照射前开启紫外灯，预热20分钟。

② 取制备好的菌悬液4ml移入直径为6cm的无菌培养皿中，在30W紫外灯下30cm处进行预照射1分钟。

③ 开盖照射：诱变时间在1～5分钟（学生可自由选择3个时间梯度）。所有操作必需在红光灯下进行。

（5）稀释涂平板

① 在红光灯下，分别将未诱变的菌悬液和已诱变的菌悬液进行系列稀释。

② 分别取10^{-5}、10^{-6}和10^{-7}3个稀释度的稀释液各0.1ml，涂于淀粉培养基平板上；每个稀释度涂3个平板，用无菌三角耙涂匀。

③ 用黑布包好照射过的平板，37℃培养48小时。

注意：在每个平板背面要标明处理时间、稀释度、组别、姓名等。

2. 计算存活率及致死率

（1）存活率计算公式

$$存活率 = \frac{处理后1ml菌液中活菌数}{对照1ml菌液中活菌数} \times 10$$

（2）致死率计算公式

$$致死率 = \frac{对照1ml菌液中活菌数 - 处理后1ml菌液中活菌数}{对照1ml菌液中活菌数} \times 10$$

对照样品1ml中活菌数：将培养48小时后对照平板取出，进行细胞计数。根据平板上菌落数，计算出对照样品1ml菌落中的活菌数。

处理后1ml样品中活菌数：同上，计算照射相应时间后样品1ml菌液中的活菌数。

3. 观察诱变效应

（1）观察菌落透明圈　对平板中菌落进行计数后，选择菌落数在5个左右的平板分别向平板内滴加碘液数滴，观察菌落周围出现的透明圈。

（2）计算比值（HC值）　分别测量透明圈直径与菌落直径并计算比值（HC）。

（3）解读结果　与对照平板进行比较，根据结果说明紫外线对枯草芽孢杆菌产淀粉酶诱变的结果。

（4）接种纯培养　选取HC比值大的菌落，挑取单菌落并到接种到新鲜牛肉膏斜面培养基上培养，备进一步复筛用。

【结果与讨论】

（1）记录各平板中的菌落数，并分别算出存活率、致死率。

（2）测量并记录经UV处理后的枯草芽孢杆菌菌落（6个）周围的透明圈直径（mm值）与菌落直径，并计算比值（HC值），与对照菌株进行比较。

$$HC值 = \frac{透明圈直径（mm）}{菌落直径（mm）}$$

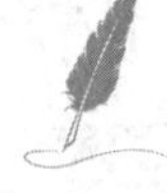

（3）紫外线诱变需注意的事项是什么？

（4）紫外线诱变的机制是什么？

（5）总结实验结果，哪一种照射时间的诱变效果最好？它的存活率、致死率和 HC 值各为多少？

EXPERIMENT 50 Screening of *Bacillus subtilis* with High Productivity of Amylase

Purposes

（1）To grasp the principle of ultraviolet radiation.

（2）To understand the mutagenic effects of *Bacillus subtilis* by ultraviolet radiation.

Principles

Ultraviolet radiation, as a physical mutagen, has been used in industrial microorganism breeding for many years. Although all kinds of new mutagens appear constantly and are used in mutation breeding in recent years, UV radiation has its special significance. So far, among the high - yield antibiotics producing strains obtained by mutagenic breeding, about 80% of them were obtained by UV radiation. So, UV radiation is still one of the best choices for microbial breeders.

Ultraviolet radiation (UV) ranges in wavelength from approximately 100nm to 400nm. It is most lethal from 253nm to 265nm. In everyday practice, the source of UV radiation is the germicidal lamp, which generates radiation at 254nm. Because UV radiation passes readily through air, slightly through liquids, and only poorly through solids, the objects to be induced must be directly exposed to it for better effects.

The most lethal UV radiation has a wavelength of 265 ~ 266nm. As UV radiation passes through a microbial cell, it is most effectively absorbed by DNA. The major mechanism of UV damage is the formation of thymine dimers in DNA. Two adjacent thymines in a DNA strand are covalently joined to inhibit DNA replication and function.

Materials and Apparatus

1. Strains *Bacillus subtilis* BF7658.

2. Media and Reagents Nutrient agar media, starch agar media, iodine solution, 0. 85% sterile normal saline.

3. Apparatus Incubator, 30 W germicidal lamp, magnetic stirrer, centrifuge.

4. Others sterile petri dish, sterile tube, sterile pipette, sterile glass spreader, sterile flask with glass bead, cylinder, beaker, centrifuge tube.

Procedures

The mutagenic effects on the activity of amylase will be investigated with *Bacillus subtilis* irradiated by UV irradiation.

1. Mutation

（1）Preparation of bacterial suspension

① Take an activated *Bacillus subtilis* BF7658 slant incubated for 20h.

② Gently scratch off the lawn on the surface of the slant and wash it with 5ml 0. 85 % normal saline twice, and then transfer the suspension to a sterile triangular flask with glass beads.

③ After vigorous shaking for 10min, transfer the suspension to a 10ml centrifuge tube and

centrifuge at 3000r/min for 15min.

④ Discard the supernatant. Wash and centrifuge twice with 10ml 0.85 % normal saline, and the finial liquor volume reaches 10ml.

(2) Cell counting of bacterial suspension

Using a sterile pipette, transfer a certain volume of the bacterial suspension to another sterile flask, dilute it properly to reach 10^8 cells per milliliter.

(3) Prepare sterile starch agar plates

Melt the sterilestarch agar media and cool down to 50℃ ~55℃ , add 15 ~20ml to each dish and allow it to cool down.

(4) Mutation treatment

① The UV lamp (30 W) should be turned on 20 min before the experiment.

② 4 ml of the suspension was added onto a sterilized Petri dish (the diameter was 6cm). Put the Petri dishes on a magnetic stirring apparatus which is 30 cm (vertical distance) away from the UV lamp, irradiate for 1 min at first.

③ Uncap the Petri plate and expose the plate to ultraviolet for 1 ~5min (student may randomly choose 3 of them) under shaking. All operations should be performed under red light.

(5) Diluting and spreading plate

① Under the red light, dilute the suspension of mutated and parental bacteria without irradiation into certain concentration gradient (10^{-4}, 10^{-5}、$10^{-6}$and 10^{-7}) .

② Transfer 0.5ml of diluted solution of 10^{-5}、$10^{-6}$and 10^{-7} to three sets of sterile dishes respectively, and spread with sterile glass spreader

③ Wrap the plates with black paper, incubate in dark at 37℃ 48h.

Notice: Label the bottom of the plate with your irradiation time, dilution rate, lab section, and your name。

2. Calculate the survival rate and the lethal rate

(1) The formula for survival rate

$$\text{the survival rate} = \frac{\text{the viable counts of bacteria in Check sample for one milliliter}}{\text{the viable counts of bacteria in control group for one milliliter}}$$

(2) The formula for the lethal rate

$$\text{the lethal rete} = \frac{\text{the viable counts of bacteria in Check sample for one milliliter} - \text{the viable counts of bacteria in control group for one milliliter}}{\text{the viable counts of bacteria in control group for one milliliter}}$$

The viable counts of bacteria in check sample: After incubation for 48h, take the plates, count the number of the colony on each plate, and calculate the viable counts of bacteria in milliliter of the control sample.

The viable counts of bacteria in test group: After incubation for 48h, take the plates, count the number of the colony on each plate, and calculate the viable counts of bacteria in one milliliter of different test groups.

3. Observe the mutagenic effects

(1) Observe the flat transparent circle

Choose appropriate plates on which colony number is no more than five. Add a few drops of iodine solution onto the plates and observe the flat transparent circle around the colony.

(2) Calculate the HC

Measure the diameter of the transparent circle and the colony. Calculate the ratio of flat transparent circle diameter to colony diameter (HC).

(3) Interpretation of the results

Compared with the control plates, explain the mutagenic effects of ultraviolet radiation on *Bacillus subtilis*.

(4) Inoculation for purification

Choose some colonies with a bigger HC value, pick the colonies and transfer them to fresh nutrient broth agar slants, incubate and preserve them for further screening.

Results and Discussion

(1) Count the colony number on each plate and calculate the survival rate and the lethal rate.

(2) Measure and record the transparent circle diameter and colony diameter of 6 colonies. Calculate the ratio of flat transparent circle diameter to colony diameter (HC), meanwhile compare with the control plates.

$$\text{HC value} = \frac{\text{the transparent circle diameter}}{\text{the colony diameter}}$$

(3) What are the general considerations in mutagenesis by UV radiation?

(4) What is the underlying mechanism of UV radiation?

(5) Generally speaking, which irradiation time has a better mutagenic effect? How about the survival rate, the lethal rate and the HC value?

实验五十一　β－内酰胺酶抗药菌株的分离和鉴定

扫码“学一学”

【实验目的】

(1) 熟悉抗药菌株的分离方法。

(2) 熟悉β－内酰胺酶的简单鉴定法。

(3) 熟悉药敏试验方法。

【实验原理】

β－内酰胺类抗生素是目前临床抗感染治疗最普遍应用的一类抗生素，随着这类药物的广泛使用（特别是滥用和误用）和致病菌的变迁，产生了病原菌对药物的耐药性，而且耐药发生率相当高。细菌产生β－内酰胺酶是细菌对β－内酰胺类抗生素耐药的主要机制之一。

【实验材料】

1. **菌种**　金黄色葡萄球菌临床标本。
2. **培养基**　营养琼脂培养基。
3. **试剂**　氯化钠，蒸馏水，青霉素。
4. **器材**　平皿，吸管，小试管，记号笔，接种环，酒精灯，培养箱，高压灭菌锅等。

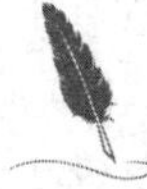

【实验方法】

1. **抗药菌株的分离** 梯度平板法分离抗药菌株，平板划线法分离单菌落，重复多次，分离纯化金黄色葡萄球菌抗青霉素菌株。

2. **MIC 测定** 试管系列稀释法测定青霉素对已分离菌株的 MIC。

3. **β－内酰胺酶的简单鉴定** 碘淀粉法对菌株产生青霉素酶能力进行简单鉴定。

4. **抗产 β－内酰胺酶的抗药菌株的抗菌物质筛选** 平板稀释法测定候选物质对分离的多株产 β－内酰胺酶的抗药菌株的 MIC。

【结果与讨论】

（1）青霉素对已分离菌株的 MIC 结果。

（2）β－内酰胺酶的鉴定结果。

（3）候选物质对分离的多株产 β－内酰胺酶的抗药菌株的 MIC 结果。

（4）怎样应对 β－内酰胺酶介导的抗药性问题？

EXPERIMENT 51 Isolation and Identification of beta－lactamase producing *Staphylococcus aureus*

Purposes

(1) To be familiar with the isolation of drug－resistant strains.

(2) To be familiar with the simple identification of beta－lactamase.

(3) To be familiar with drug sensitivity test.

Principles

Beta－lactam antibiotics are a class of antibiotics most commonly used in clinical treatment of infection. With the wide use of this class of antibiotics (especially the abuse and misuse), more and more drug－resistance strains have been discovered and the resistance rate is quite high. Production of beta－lactamase is one of the main mechanisms for resistance to beta－lactam antibiotic.

Materials and apparatus

1. Cultures *Staphylococcus aureus* from clinical specimen.

2. Media Nutrient agar.

3. Reagents Sodium chloride, distilled water, penicillin.

4. Apparatus Petri dish, tube, pipette, marker pen, inoculating loop, burner, incubator, autoclave, *etc*.

Procedures

1. Separation of drug－resistant strains Separate drug－resistant strain with gradient plate method and isolate pure culture with repeat streaking－technique to obtain penicillin resistant strains of *Staphylococcus aureus*.

2. Determination of MIC Determine the MIC value of penicillin for isolated drug－resistant strains with broth dilution method.

3. Simple identification of beta－lactamase Identify beta－lactamase of the isolated strains with iodine－starch plate method.

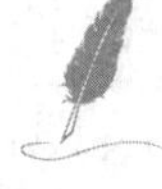

4. Screening of antibacterial substance Determine the MIC value of candidate antibacterial substance for multiple strains of beta – lactamase producing bacteria with plate dilution method.

Results and discussion

(1) Record the results of penicillin MIC for the isolated strain.

(2) Record the results of I_2 – starch test.

(3) Record the MIC value of the candidates for multiple strains of beta – lactamase producing bacteria.

(4) How to deal with the problem of drug – resistance mediated by beta – lactamase ?

扫码“练一练”

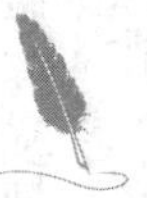

第九部分　设计性实验

实验五十二　药品微生物学质量标准的建立

扫码“学一学”

【实验目的】

熟悉利用药典对不同药物进行微生物学质量控制与检测的方法。

【实验原理】

药典作为我国保证药品质量的法典，在保持科学性、先进性、规范性和权威性的基础上，着力解决制约药品质量与安全的突出问题，提高药品标准质量控制水平。

药品的微生物学质量标准的建立一般来自以下几个方面：

药典的要求（我国历经2005版－2010版－2015－2020版的变化）；

新药送审的要求；

药品GMP的要求。

不同制剂的微生物学检验要求不完全相同。药品的无菌检查和微生物限度检查是指按照一定的检验程序和质量控制措施，确定要求无菌的待验样品中是否含有活的微生物，或者确定单位样品中存在的微生物的数量，以及是否含有某种致病菌。因此，药品微生物学质量标准的建立对于准确反映所检样品的微生物状况意义重大。学会使用药典进行药品的微生物学质量控制与检测，可以对保证药品质量提供参考依据。

本书实验四十六与实验四十七介绍了不同药品的相关检测方法，在本实验中，应学会按实际情况对不同药品进行相关检测。

【实验内容】

请查找最新版药典，按药品类别对下列药品进行相应的无菌检查或/及微生物限度检查。

（1）注射用头孢拉定。

（2）复方磺胺甲噁唑胶囊。

（3）安眠补脑糖浆。

（4）白凡士林。

PART NINE　Designed Experiments

EXPERIMENT 52　Microbial Quality Control of Pharmaceuticals

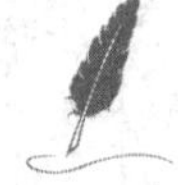

Purposes

To be familiar with the examination methods for microbial quality control of pharmaceuticals with the use of Pharmacopoeia.

Principles

The Chinese pharmacopoeia is the official collection of authoritative standards for medicinal products and pharmaceutical substances. It focuses on the solution of prominent problems about quality control and safety in use.

Usually, the establishment of standards on microbial quality control is from the following aspects:

1. Demands of Pharmacopoeia（2005 edition ~ 2010 edition ~ 2015 edition ~ 2020 edition）;
2. Demands of submission of new pharmaceuticals for approval;
3. Demands for GMP.

Microbial testing demands for different pharmaceuticals are not always the same. Sterility test and microbial limit test provide the instructions to ensure the existence of viable microbes, specific pathogens or the quantity of microbes in casual inspection. It plays an important role in the standard - setting process in quality control of pharmaceuticals.

In this book, experiments 46 and 47 have introduced the basic principles of sterility test and microbial limit test. In this experiment, students should practice to do essential inspections on different pharmaceuticals according to Chinese Pharmacopoeia.

Contents

Perform sterility test or/and microbial limit test on the following pharmaceuticals according to Chinese Pharmacopoeia.

（1） Cefradine for injection.

（2） Compound sulfamethoxazole capsule.

（3） The sleeping brain syrup.

（4） Albolene.

实验五十三　营养缺陷型菌株的筛选和鉴定

扫码“学一学”

【实验目的】

熟悉筛选和鉴定枯草芽孢杆菌的营养缺陷型。

【实验原理】

营养缺陷型菌株是指野生型菌株由于某些物理因素或化学因素处理，使编码代谢途径中某些酶的基因突变，丧失了合成某些代谢产物（如氨基酸、维生素）的能力，必须在基本培养基中补充该种营养成分，才能正常生长的一类突变株。营养缺陷型在氨基酸、核苷酸生产和微生物代谢途径的研究广泛使用，在遗传学分析和分子水平基因重组研究中作为供体和受体细胞的遗传标记。营养缺陷型筛选一般分四个环节，即诱变剂处理、营养缺陷型浓缩、检出和鉴定。

诱变：可以采用物理或化学诱变剂，如紫外线、硫酸二乙酯等。

浓缩：可采用青霉素法，也可采用加热法，利用芽孢和营养体对热敏感性的差异，诱变后的细菌形成芽孢后，把处在芽孢阶段的细菌移到基本培养液中，振荡培养一定时间，野生型芽孢萌发，而营养缺陷型芽孢不能萌发。此时将培养物加热到80℃，维持一定时间，

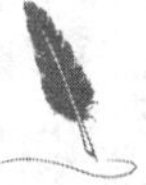

野生型细胞大部分被杀死，缺陷型则得以保留。

检出：包括影印法、夹层法、限量补充法、逐个检出法。

鉴定：采用生长谱法。

【实验内容】

请采用适当方法，筛选和鉴定枯草芽孢杆菌的营养缺陷型。

EXPERIMENT 53 Isolation and Identification of Auxotroph

Purposes

To be familiar with isolation and identification of *Bacillus subtilis* auxotroph.

Principles

A mutant with a nutritional requirement for growth is called an auxotroph. Auxotroph lost the ability of synthesis of some metabolites (such as amino acids, vitamin) due to gene mutation of the wild type strain and cannot grow on medium lacking these nutrient factors.

Auxotroph has been widely used in the production of amino acids and nucleotides and the study of microbial metabolic pathway. Auxotroph is useful genetic marker for donor and recipient cells in genetic analysis and gene recombination. Auxotrophic screening is generally divided into four steps: mutagenesis, enrichment, detection and isolation, auxanograms identification.

Physical or chemical mutagen can be used for mutagenesis, such as UV light, diethyl sulfate, *etc*. Penicillin method and heating method can be used for enrichment. The vegetative cells are more sensitive to heat than endospores and can be killed at 80 °C. Auxotroph can be detected and isolated by random isolation, replica plating, layer plating and limited supply method. Growth spectrum method can be used to identify auxanogram.

Contents

Please isolate and identify *Bacillus subtilis* auxotroph.

实验五十四 葡萄中酵母菌的分离、培养和鉴定

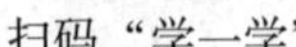
扫码“学一学”

【实验目的】

（1）从天然材料中分离具有特定功能的微生物。

（2）微生物的形态学观察方法和微生物鉴定的方法。

（3）了解 BIOLOG 微生物鉴定系统的原理和方法。

【实验原理】

大多数酵母菌为腐生，其生长最适 pH 为 4.5～6，常见于含糖分较高的环境，如果园土、菜地土及果皮、植物表面等。酵母菌喜欢酸性环境，使用酸性液体培养基以及青霉素等可抑制细菌的生长，而酵母菌得以富集和增殖。然后在固体培养基上用划线法进行分离，可获得酵母菌的纯培养。

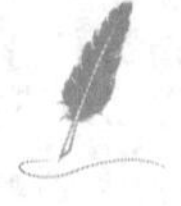

利用微生物对不同碳源进行呼吸代谢的差异，BIOLOG 微生物鉴定系统可以准确鉴定环境和病原微生物，其原理是在 96 孔板内培养的微生物进行呼吸代谢过程中产生的氧化还原

物质与显色物质发生反应而导致颜色变化，产生“代谢指纹”。菌悬液在预设置的板块指导下进行测试，经过培养、读取结果和数据库进行比对。96 孔板的反应结果通过 BIOLOG 配套软件的解释，可以得到比分子方法更准确的鉴定结果。

【实验内容】

（1）从新鲜葡萄中分离酵母菌。

（2）酵母菌的形态学观察。

（3）酵母菌的鉴定。

EXPERIMENT 54　Isolation, Culture and Identification of Yeast in Grapes

Purposes

1. To be familiar with isolation of microorganisms with specific functions from the natural material.

2. To be familiar with the methods of microbial morphology observation.

3. To understand the species and applications of the different microbes.

Principle

Most yeast is saprophytic. Its growth optimum pH is 4. 5 ~ 6 and can be found in the environment with high sugar, such as the orchard soil, vegetable garden soil, and the skin of fruits or vegetables. Yeast is especially fond of acid environment. In the acidic medium or the medium supplemented penicillin the bacteria can be inhibited, so the yeast can be enriched and proliferate. Streaking the sample of grape on the solid medium, we can get the pure culture of yeast.

Based on the differences of carbon source utilization or respiratory metabolism, BIOLOG's can accurately identify environmental and pathogenic microorganisms by producing characteristic chromogenic reactions or "metabolic fingerprint" from redox reactions in a 96 well microplate. Culture suspensions are tested with a panel of pre – selected assays, then incubated, read and compared to extensive databases. The scope of the 96 assay reactions, coupled with sophisticated interpretation software, delivers a high level of accuracy that is comparable to molecular methods.

Contents

(1) Separate yeast from fresh fruit of grape picked from vine yard.

(2) Morphological observation of yeast.

(3) Yeast identification.

实验五十五　菌种的复壮

扫码“学一学”

【实验目的】

（1）了解菌种衰退的原因。

（2）熟悉菌种复壮的方法。

【实验原理】

菌种在培养或保藏过程中出现某些原有优良生产性状的劣化、遗传标记的丢失等现象，

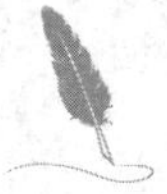

称为菌种的衰退。菌种衰退不是突然发生，而是从量变到质变逐步演变而成。菌种衰退的原因主要有以下几方面：基因突变、表型延迟、质粒丢失、连续传代、不适宜的培养和保藏条件。使衰退的菌种恢复原来优良性状称为菌种的复壮。狭义的复壮是指在菌种已发生衰退的情况下，通过纯种分离和生产性能测定等方法，从衰退的群体中找出未衰退的个体，以达到恢复该菌原有典型性状的措施；广义的复壮是指在菌种的生产性能未衰退前就有意识的经常进行纯种的分离和生产性能测定工作，以期菌种的生产性能逐步提高。

菌种复壮常用方法有：平板分离单菌落，一些寄生性的菌株在寄主体内生长，采用各种外界不良理化条件杀死淘汰已衰退的个体，对带抗生素标记质粒的菌株复壮采用在含抗生素的平板上划线分离法。菌种要采用有效的菌种保藏方法。

【实验内容】

请采用适当方法，对以下已衰退的菌种进行复壮。

（1）生产人干扰素-α 的重组大肠埃希菌。

（2）链霉素产生菌。

（3）青霉素产生菌。

（4）致病性肺炎链球菌。

（5）产淀粉酶的枯草杆菌。

（6）谷氨酸棒状杆菌。

（7）啤酒酵母。

（8）氧化醋酸杆菌。

EXPERIMENT 55 Strain Rejuvenation

Purposes

（1）To understand the reasons for microbial degeneration.

（2）To be familiar with the methods for strain rejuvenation.

Principle

Degeneration is the process that the microbial strains lose the good producing character and genetic marker during cultivation and preservation. The degeneration doesn't happen suddenly but in accumulation. The main reasons are: gene mutation, phenotypic lag, plasmid loss, continuous passage for too many times, unsuitable culture and preserve condition. To gain the good character back is called rejuvenation. Narrowly speaking, rejuvenation is to find the strain not degenerate and renew the typical character. Widely speaking, rejuvenation is to isolate the good strain and test its character often to keep and promote the producing ability.

The methods for strain rejuvenation include: single colony isolation through streaking - plate, virulence restoration with suitable host, elimination by killing the degenerated individuals with hard condition, *etc.* For the engineered strains carrying antibiotics labeled plasmid, streaking on the plate containing antibiotics will work.

Contents

Please rejuvenate the following degenerated strains with appropriate methods.

（1）*Escherichia coli* producing human recombinant α - interferon.

（2）Actinomycetes producing streptomycin.

（3）*Penicillium* producing penicillin.

（4）Pathogenic *Streptococcus pneumoniae.*

（5）*Bacillus subtilis* producing amylase.

（6）*Corynebacterium glutamicum.*

（7）*Saccharomyces cerevisiae.*

（8）*Acetobacter oxydans.*

实验五十六　基因工程菌种子库的构建

【实验目的】

了解建立和检定生产生物制品所用的基因工程菌种子库。

【实验原理】

种子库的构建是一项系统的实验，任何一种基因工程菌的生产都需要构建种子库。种子库分为原始种子库、主种子库和工作种子库。所有种子库建立的前提是严格的无菌意识和无菌操作。

原始种子库一般在实验室构建菌株时已经建立，需要对它们进行遗传稳定性分析，明确传代的次数。对遗传背景要有分析。还要分析蛋白表达量等如果是核酸疫苗则要检测拷贝数、无噬菌体和其他外源因子的污染。

对原始种子库扩大培养后液氮冻存，分别建立主种子库和工作种子库。主种子库种子管数和工作种子管数比例可以控制在1：20～30。甘油冻存，液氮、-80℃保存即可。

主种子库和工作种子库的菌种需要检测的项目：遗传背景、细菌形态学、导入基因的存在即没有突变和表达量等、无噬菌体和其他外源因子感染等。

【实验内容】

（1）构建生产重组人干扰素 α 的大肠埃希菌种子库（参考实验四十九），并进行检定。

（2）以大肠埃希菌为宿主细胞，构建生产重组 *L-Asp* 的基因工程菌种子库，并进行检定。

EXPERIMENT 56　Establishment of Seed Bank of Genetic Engineered Bacteria

Purposes

To understand how to establish three-tier seed bank of genetic engineering bacteria for production of biologicals and evaluate its stability.

Principles

It is always necessary to establish a seed bank before industrial production with genetically engineered bacteria. A three-tier seed bank is usually composed of a primary seed bank, a master seed bank and a working seed bank. The establishment of three-tier seed bank of genetically engineered bacteria is a systematic experiment. Attention must be paid to sterile operation during the whole process.

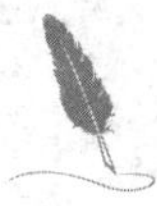

Generally, primary seed bank is prepared after the construction of the genetically engineered bacteria. The primary seed bank needs to be subjected to analysis of genetic stability and determination of passage times. The genetic background as well as expression stability of the strains should not show significant difference. DNA vaccine also needs to be tested for its copy number and whether it had been contaminated by bacteriophage and exogenous factors.

Then, seeds from primary seed bank are subcultured, propagated and subjected to overall control tests, while the qualified ones are lyophilized as master seed bank. The seeds from master seed bank are subcultured, propagated and subjected to overall tests, and the qualified ones are cryopreserved in glycerol and serve as working seed bank. They can be preserved in liquid nitrogen or -80℃.

The three - tier seed bank should be subjected to overall control tests, and the strains need to be evaluated for stability after lyophilization and cryopreservation in glycerol as well as the genetic background. The established three - tier seed bank should be qualified in overall control tests. The growth characteristic as well as genetic stability and expression stability of the strains should not show significant difference.

Contents

(1) Please establish a three - tier seed bank of human recombinant interferon - α producing *Escherichia coli* (referring to experiment 49) and evaluate its stability.

(2) Please establish a three - tier seed bank of L - Asp producing *Escherichia coli* and evaluate its stability.

实验五十七　环境中微生物的检测

扫码“学一学”

【实验目的】

(1) 了解环境中微生物的存在。

(2) 熟悉常用的微生物培养基的制备。

(3) 掌握微生物的分离纯化方法。

(4) 掌握不同类型微生物的菌落形态特征。

(5) 掌握无菌操作，培养微生物学工作者必须的“无菌”概念。

【实验原理】

微生物种类繁多且无处不在，但个体微小、肉眼不可见。从混杂的微生物群体中获得只含有某一种或某一株微生物的过程称为微生物的分离纯化，常用的是平板分离法。

将取自不同来源的样品适当稀释成单个细胞，接种于适宜的固体平板培养基上，在适宜的温度下培养一段时间后，单个微生物繁殖形成肉眼可见的菌落。一个单菌落代表原样品中的一个单细胞，不同种类的微生物所形成的菌落都有自己的特点，可通过固体平板培养来检测环境中的微生物的类型和数量。

【实验内容】

分别制备细菌、放线菌和真菌的固体培养基，并制备无菌平板。

分别从自来水、空气、手指（洗前、洗后、酒精消毒后）、头发、嘴唇、牙垢、酸奶、豆浆、奶茶、剩饭、纸巾、硬币、纸币、树叶、接种环（灭菌前后）等取样，检测周围环

境中微生物的数量和菌落形态，记录实验结果。

采集土样、适当稀释、活菌计数、记录稀释和计数结果。

EXPERIMENT 57　Detection of Environmental Microorganisms

Purposes

(1) To understand the existence of environmental microorganisms.

(2) To be familiar with the preparation of microbial media.

(3) To grasp the technique of microbial isolation and purification.

(4) To grasp the colonies of microorganisms.

(5) To grasp aseptic operation and establish the concept of "sterile" as microbiologists.

Principle

There are many different kinds of microorganisms almost everywhere, but the individual is tiny and invisible to the naked eye. The samples from different sources are diluted into single cell and inoculated onto solid plate of suitable media. The single colony will be obtained after cultivation under appropriate temperature. A single colony represents a single cell in the original sample and has its own characteristics. The quantity and categories of environmental microorganisms can be detected by plate cultivation. The common technique to isolate and purify a single species from the complex and mixed microbial population is streaking - plate.

Contents

Prepare media for bacteria, actinomycetes and fungi.

Take samples from tap water, finger (before and after washing, after alcohol disinfection), hair, lips, tartar, yogurt, milk - tea, soybean milk, leftovers, paper towels, coins, paper money, leaves, inoculating loop (before and after sterilization), and other environment, respectively. Detect the amount and observe the morphology of colonies formed by surrounding environmental microorganisms.

Collect sample soil and calculate the microbial quantity with viable count method.

实验五十八　利用 BIOLOG 自动分析系统分离鉴定人体正常菌群

扫码"学一学"

【实验目的】

(1) 掌握利用 BIOLOG 自动微生物分析系统进行微生物鉴定的原理。

(2) 了解利用 BIOLOG 自动分析系统分离鉴定人体正常菌群。

【实验原理】

正常菌群是指正常人体的体表及与外界相通的黏膜上，都存在着不同种类和数量的微生物。在正常情况下，这些微生物对人类无害，成为正常菌群。

正常菌群通常对人体有益无害，只有在特殊情况下，这些微生物才可能引发疾病。一般而言，人体正常菌群的种类与其定居的部位有关，正常菌群的种类、数量变化受人体生

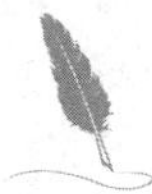

理因素和环境条件的影响。因此，人体特定部位正常菌群的分离与鉴定，具有重要的意义，可以为某些感染性疾病的诊断提供参考数据。

BIOLOG 自动微生物分析系统是美国 BIOLOG 公司于 1989 年研制开发的新型自动化快速微生物鉴定系统。作为目前应用最广泛的微生物鉴定系统之一，BIOLOG 自动微生物分析系统可鉴定包括细菌、放线菌、酵母菌和丝状真菌在内的 392 属，2000 种以上的微生物。

BIOLOG 微生物自动分析系统以微生物与 96 孔微平板上多种脱水碳源进行氧化实验和同化实验为基础进行鉴定。BIOLOG 系统可以测定待测微生物对 95 种碳源的利用能力。通过将待测微生物的特征性碳源利用类型（代谢图谱）与标准数据库作比对，可以在 24h 内得出鉴定结果。

96 孔微平板的横排标记为：1、2、3、4、5、6、7、8、9、10、11、12；纵排为：A、B、C、D、E、F、G、H。A1 孔内为水，作为阴性对照，其他 95 孔是 95 种不同的碳源。96 孔中均含有四唑类氧化还原染色剂和胶质。

BIOLOG 系统利用微生物对不同碳源代谢率的差异，针对每一类微生物筛选 95 种不同碳源，配合四唑类显色物质，固定于 96 孔板上（ A1 孔为阴性对照），接种菌悬液后培养一定时间（4h 或过夜培养），细菌利用碳源时，会将四唑类氧化还原染色剂从无色还原成紫色，从而在微生物鉴定板上形成该微生物特征性的反应模式或“指纹”，通过读数仪来读取颜色变化，并将该反应模式或“指纹”与数据库相比就可在瞬间得到鉴定结果。

BIOLOG 微生物鉴定系统由微生物自动分析仪、计算机分析软件、浊度计、和鉴定板组成，其中鉴定板分五大类，即 GN 板（鉴定革兰阴性好氧菌）、GP 板（鉴定革兰阳性好氧菌）、AN 板（鉴定厌氧菌）、YT 板（鉴定酵母菌）和 FF 板（鉴定丝状真菌）。鉴于咽喉和皮肤的正常菌群以革兰阳性和革兰阴性细菌为主，故选用 GN、GP 鉴定板。

【实验内容】

为了让学生了解人体咽喉、皮肤正常菌群种类和数量的差异，本实验采用最新的 BIOLOG 自动分析系统鉴定从皮肤、咽喉分离纯化的微生物。

EXPERIMENT 58 Isolation and Identification of Normal Flora in Human Body Using BIOLOG Automatic Analysis System

Purposes

(1) To grasp the principle of microbial identification by BIOLOG Automatic Analysis System.

(2) To understand how to isolate and identify normal flora in human body using BIOLOG Automatic Analysis System.

Principles

In a healthy human, the surface tissues, i. e., skin and mucous membranes in direct contact with the outside, are constantly exposed to environmental microorganisms and become readily colonized by certain microbial species. The mixture of microorganisms regularly found at any anatomical site is referred to normal microbiota or normal flora.

While most of the activities of the normal flora benefit their host, some are pathogenic (capable of producing disease) underparticular circumstances. Generally, most members of the normal

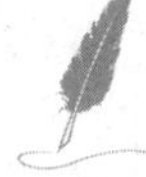

flora prefer to colonize specific tissues. The makeup of the normal flora may be influenced by physiological factors (including genetics, age, sex) and environmental factors (including stress, nutrition, diet of the individual, *etc*), Therefore, acquiring knowledge of normal flora in human is of great significance as it gives perspective on the possible sources and significance of microorganisms isolated from the infection site.

BIOLOG Microbial Identification System, which was developed by BIOLOG in 1989, is a new automated technology for rapid identification of microorganisms. BIOLOG Microbial Identification System, as one of the most widely used microbial identification system, can identify 2000 species of microorganisms within 32 genera, including bacteria, yeasts and filamentous fungi.

The system is based on a 96 well microplate containing a range of dehydrated carb on sources for oxidation and assimilation tests by microorganism. BIOLOG system tests the ability of bacteria to utilize 95 various carbon sources. Identification of the test bacterium by comparing its utilization pattern (metabolic fingerprint) to the BIOLOG database can generally be achieved within 24 h.

For a 96 - well microplate, the horizontal well is labeled with 1, 2, 3, 4, 5, 6, 7, 8, 9, 10, 11, 12; The vertical well is labeled with A, B, C, D, E, F, G, H. A1 is filled with water , as a negative control, the other wells are filled 95 kinds of different carbon sources. Tetrazolium violet is added into each of the 96 wells.

The BIOLOG microplate is a 96 - well dehydrated panel containing tetrazolium violet, a buffered nutrient medium, and a different carbon source for each well except the control, which does not contain a carbon source. The microwells are rehydrated with a cell suspension and read at either 4 h or overnight (16 to 24 h) for the ability of the bacteria to utilize the carbon source. Reduced tetrazolium violet is a purple formazan. When a carbon source is not used, the micro well remains colorless, as does the control well. The resulting pattern of purple wells yields a " metabolic fingerprint" of the bacterium tested. After incubation, the phenotypic fingerprint of purple wells is compared to BIOLOG's extensive species library. If a match is found, identification of the isolate at the species level is made.

The BIOLOG automated system consists of microplate reader, DOS - based IBM - compatible PC, a turbidimeter and BIOLOG microplates. BIOLOG microplates can be divided into five categories, namely, GN (for identification of aerobic gram - negative bacteria), GP (for identification of aerobic gram - positive bacteria), AN (for identification of anaerobic bacteria), YT (for identification of yeasts) and FF (for identification of filamentous fungi) . As skin or throat microbes are either gram - positive or gram - negative, GN and GP microplates should be chosen in this experiment.

Contents

This experiment aims at isolating and identifying normal flora in human body using the latest BIOLOG Automatic Analysis System. In this way, the students can understand the differences in species and number of normal flora on human skin and in the throat.

扫码“学一学”

实验五十九 药物对流感病毒的抑制作用

【实验目的】

熟悉对不同药物进行流感病毒体内外抑制作用检测的实验方法。

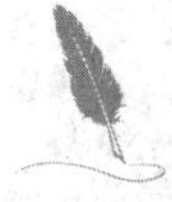

【实验原理】

病毒是传染性疾病的主要病原。抗病毒药物的研制，是新药开发的热点。

流感病毒可通过侵犯人的呼吸道上皮细胞，引起流行性感冒，严重威胁人类生命和健康。现有药物及疫苗无法彻底预防和治疗流感病毒的感染。通过研究药物对流感病毒的抑制作用，可以帮助我们找到更有针对性的有效抑制流感病毒感染的药物。

药物对流感病毒抑制作用的研究，可分为体内和体外两部分实验进行。在实验中，需要有明确药效的药物作为阳性对照。

体外实验中，病毒感染细胞出现的 CPE（细胞病变效应）、病毒空斑等病毒指标或者细胞活力等毒性指标可作为观察检测内容。根据这些指标，计算 IC50（半数有效浓度），来初步评价药物在体外抑制流感病毒复制的能力（可参考本书实验二十四）。

细胞水平的实验结果需要在动物水平进行验证。体内实验中，根据流感病毒感染小鼠后，所引起的小鼠死亡率和肺部病变程度，计算半数有效量（ED50）和 TI（治疗指数）等指标，可明确药物对流感病毒的抑制作用。

【实验内容】

请分别对下列药品进行相应的体内外病毒抑制作用检测。

（1）利巴韦林注射液。

（2）板蓝根颗粒。

EXPERIMENT 59 *In Vitro* Inhibition of Influenza Virus by Antivirals

Purposes

To be familiar with the methods of determining inhibition on influenza virus by antivirals.

Principles

Viruses are the main pathogens of infectious diseases. Development of antiviral drugs is a hot spot in new drug development.

Through the infection of human airway epithelial cells, influenza virus can cause influenza and pose a threat to human life and health. Existing drugs and vaccines cannot completely prevent and treat influenza virus infection. Researches on influenza inhibition can help us find antivirals with different targets and inhibitory efficacy.

Studies on drugs' inhibitory effect on influenza virus can be divided into two parts, *in vivo* and *in vitro*. During the experiment, positive drugs are needed as control.

By *in vitro* studies, CPE (cytopathic effect), viral plaques and other viral index or toxicity index (such as cell viability) can be observed. Based on these indicators, IC_{50} (the median inhibitory concentration) is calculated to evaluate the *in vitro* inhibitory ability of drugs on the replication of influenza virus. (see experiment 24).

Experimental results at cellular level require validation in animals. By *in vivo* studies, mortality and lung lesions in mice caused by influenza virus infection are used for calculation of median effective dose (ED 50), TI (therapeutic index) and other indicators to determine drugs' inhibitory effect on influenza virus.

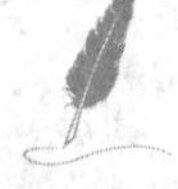

Contents

Perform inhibition test on influenza virus with the following antivirals.

(1) Ribavirin injection.

(2) Banlangen granules.

实验六十 实验药物对机体的免疫调节作用

【实验目的】

熟悉药物对机体免疫调节作用的检测方法。

【实验原理】

实验药物对机体的免疫调节作用研究一般采用体外和体内相结合的方式。体外试验研究可明确药物对免疫应答某一特定环节的具体影响，而体内研究则可探讨药物对机体免疫应答水平，对正常免疫应答、异常免疫应答等的综合影响。研究药物对机体免疫系统和免疫功能的作用，不仅能够深入揭示药物的作用机制，更为疾病的药物治疗奠定基础。

实验药物对机体的免疫调节作用研究主要包含四部分：建立动物模型；药物对固有性免疫功能的影响（可参考本书实验三十六和实验三十七）；药物对获得性体液免疫功能的影响（可参考本书实验三十八~实验四十）和药物对获得性细胞免疫功能的影响（可参考本书实验四十一~实验四十三）。

实验动物的选取，除正常动物外，往往选取一种以上的免疫抑制（多采用环磷酰胺、氢化可的松等抑制剂）或功能低下（通过辐射等方法可获得）的动物模型，以评价药物的作用。

【实验内容】

评价香菇多糖和 IFN－γ 的免疫调节功能。

EXPERIMENT 60 Regulatory Effects of Pharmaceuticals on Immunity

Purposes

To be familiar with methods of measuring pharmaceutical effect on immune regulation.

Principles

The efficacy of immunomodulatory drugs have been generally studied by a combination of *in vitro* and *in vivo* approaches. *In vitro* studies can be used to determine which aspect of the immune response is affected by the drug. *In vivo* studies can explore the total effects of the drug on the level of immune response, normal immune response and abnormal immune responses. Studies on drugs effect on immune system and immune function not only reveal the mechanism of drugs but also provide a basis for disease treatment.

The initial study of immunomodulatory drugs mainly contains four parts: the establishment of animal models, innate immune functions (see experiment 36 and 37), acquired humoral immunity functions (see experiment 38 ~40), acquired cellular immunity functions (see experiment 41 ~43) .

To evaluate the role of drugs, the selection of experimental animals, in addition to the normal animals, tends to cover more than one type of animal models, such as models of immune suppres-

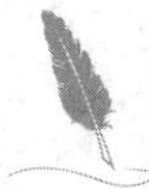

sion (by use of immunosuppressors such as cyclophosphamide and hydrocortisone) and immuno-compromised models (by radiation or other methods).

Contents

Evaluate the immuno-regulating functions of lentinan and IFN-γ.

扫码“学一学”

实验六十一　抗原抗体反应在伤寒疫苗制备中的应用

【实验目的】

根据药典或药品标准，熟悉进行生物制品质量评估和监测过程中的抗原抗体检测方法。

【实验原理】

疫苗在传染性疾病的预防中起重要作用。疫苗制备过程中，利用抗原抗体反应，可对疫苗的特异性、免疫力和抗原性等进行检测，以达到评估和监测疫苗质量的目的。

伤寒疫苗制备过程中，检测伤寒沙门菌的特异性可通过玻片凝集反应进行；伤寒疫苗的免疫力可通过加温处理后的菌液免疫小鼠所引起的小鼠存活率变化判断；疫苗的抗原性检测结果则体现为疫苗免疫家兔后所获得的血清效价（方法参见实验三十九）。

【实验内容】

请查找最新版药典，采用抗原抗体反应，进行伤寒沙门菌疫苗制备过程中的质量评估和监测。

EXPERIMENT 61　Application of Antigen-Antibody Reaction in Preparation of Typhoid Vaccine

Purposes

To be familiar with antigen-antibody reaction methods stipulated in Pharmacopoeia or standards for quality assessment and monitoring of biological products.

Principles

Vaccines play an important role in the prevention of infectious diseases. During the preparation of the vaccine, antigen-antibody reaction is used to detect the specificity, immunity and immunogenicity of a vaccine, and thus to assess and monitor the quality of a vaccine.

In the preparation process of typhoid vaccine, slide agglutination reaction can be used to detect the specificity of *Salmonella typhi*. The immunity of typhoid vaccine can be judged by the survival rate of mice immunized by heat-treated bacteria. The immunogenicity of typhoid vaccine is reflected by the serum titer of immunized rabbits (see experiment 39).

Contents

Find the latest edition of Chinese Pharmacopoeia, use the antigen-antibody reaction to assess and monitor the quality of typhoid salmonella vaccine during its preparation.

附　录

Ⅰ. 微生物实验室规则

微生物学实验材料，有的是病原微生物，在实验中稍有不慎，便有发生人身感染的可能。要求同学认真遵守下列各点：

1. 进入实验室须穿好实验服，离室时脱下；
2. 个人物品应放到指定地点，实验台上只能放实验指导、记录本和文具；
3. 保持肃静，不得随便走动；
4. 如果留有长发，请将长发挽起，扎在后面；整个实验过程中，必须穿鞋；
5. 禁止饮食，不能用手抚摩头面，以防感染；
6. 实验中若发生割破（灼伤）皮肤、实验材料破损及污染事故，应立即报告教师，并做适当处理；
7. 用过的有菌器材和培养物应放于指定位置；
8. 注意节约实验药品，爱护实验器材；
9. 易燃物品（如酒精、二甲苯等）不准接近火源，如遇火险，先关掉电源，再用湿布或灭火器灭火；
10. 实验结束后，做好室内清洁卫生，实验台收拾整洁，再洗手消毒后方可离去；
11. 离开实验室前，检查水、电、煤、气等开关是否关好。

Ⅱ. 常用无菌玻璃仪器的准备和废品处理

1. 无菌仪器的准备　准备试验中常用的无菌吸管、平皿、试管、锥形瓶等时，应先将所需仪器洗涤干净，干燥后用棉花、纱布、纸等包起来，至烘箱中经160℃、2小时灭菌后方可使用，不怕水汽的仪器可用高压灭菌法灭菌。各种仪器的包扎方法如下。

（1）吸管　口吸的一端塞入少许棉花，用纸条从吸管尖端开始紧紧的将吸管全部裹缠起来，使不与外界接触。如一次大批使用吸管时，可用特制的金属桶，将大批吸管的尖端向下轻轻插入桶中，盖紧后灭菌。如一次未用完，必须重新灭菌后再用。

（2）平皿　用纸将整个平皿包起，或几个一包，亦可装入有盖的金属桶内灭菌。

（3）试管　用棉花做成棉塞，将管口塞紧后灭菌。棉塞必须松紧适宜，管内的棉塞较露出管外的棉塞长，管外的棉塞应较粗、较紧，能够将管口沿盖住。

（4）锥形瓶　用外包纱布的棉塞紧塞瓶口，再包以纱布或纸，用细麻绳扎住。

2. 废品处理　试验中被微生物污染的仪器及各种培养物，必须经过适当的处理后方可洗涤，以免微生物散布或造成感染。

（1）吸取菌液的吸管　用后轻轻插入有5%酚溶液或1%新洁尔灭溶液的玻璃桶内，浸泡1天，取出后用流水冲洗，冲洗时应不断有流水从管中通过。

（2）盛过微生物的平皿、试管、锥形瓶等一般先经高压灭菌后再用去污剂洗涤。

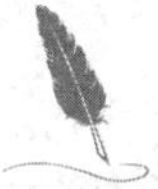

（3）标本片　不需保留的标本片，浸入5%的酚或1‰的新洁尔灭中1天或煮沸半小时后再洗刷，玻璃器皿洗涤后有时尚需再用清洁液浸泡。

Ⅲ. 教学用菌种

1. 细菌和放线菌

Bacillus pumilus［（CMCC（B）63202）］.	短小芽孢杆菌［CMCC（B）63202］
Bacillus subtilis	枯草杆菌
Bacillus tetani	破伤风杆菌
Clostridium sporogenes［CMCC（B）64941］	生孢梭菌［CMCC（B）64941］
Clostridium tetani	破伤风梭菌
Clostridium sp	梭菌
Enterobacter aerogenes	产气杆菌
Escherichia coli	大肠埃希菌
E. coli K12W1485	大肠埃希菌 K12W1485
E. coli C600	大肠埃希菌 C600
E. coli K12	大肠埃希菌 K12
Proteus vulgaris	普通变形杆菌
Pseudomonas aeruginosa	铜绿假单胞菌
Salmonella typhi	伤寒沙门菌
Salmonella species	沙门氏菌
Salmonella typhimurium TA97	鼠伤寒沙门菌 TA97
Salmonella typhimurium TA98	鼠伤寒沙门菌 TA98
Salmonella typhimurium TA100	鼠伤寒沙门菌 TA100
Salmonella typhimurium TA102	鼠伤寒沙门菌 TA102
Staphylococcus aureus	金黄色葡萄球菌
Streptococcus pneumoniae	肺炎链球菌
Vibrio cholerae	霍乱弧菌
Streptomyces sp.	链霉菌

2. Fungi

Aspergillus niger	黑曲霉
Candida albicans［CMCC（F）98001］	白色念球菌［CMCC（F）98001］
Mucor	毛霉
Penicillium	青霉
Rhizopus	根霉

Ⅳ. 培养基

1. 普通肉汤琼脂培养基

牛肉膏	5g
蛋白胨	10g
NaCl	5g

琼脂	15～20g
水	1000ml
pH	7.41

$1kg/cm^2$高压蒸汽灭菌20分钟

2. 放线菌、真菌常用培养基

（1）高氏1号培养基

可溶性淀粉	20 g
KNO_3	1.0g
NaCl	0.5g
K_2HPO_4	0.5g
$MgSO_4$	0.5g
$FeSO_4$	0.01g
琼脂	15～20g
水	1000ml
pH	7.2～7.4

$1kg/cm^2$高压蒸汽灭菌20分钟

（2）改良沙氏培养基

蛋白胨	10g
葡萄糖	40g
琼脂	15～20g
水	1000ml
pH	自然

$0.56kg/cm^2$高压蒸汽灭菌15～20分钟

（3）麦芽汁琼脂培养基　大麦或小麦用水洗净，浸泡6～12小时，置15℃阴暗处发芽，上面盖一层纱布，每天用水淋3次，麦根生长至麦粒的两倍时，即可停止发芽，烘干备用。将麦芽粉碎，加4倍水，于65℃水浴中糖化3～4小时，4～6层纱布过滤。如果滤液浑浊，可用鸡蛋白澄清，即将一个鸡蛋白加水20ml，调匀至产生泡沫为止，然后倒在糖化液中搅拌煮沸后再过滤。将滤液稀释至5～6波美度，pH约为6.4，加入2%琼脂即可。

（4）葡萄糖－醋酸盐培养基

葡萄糖	1g
酵母膏	2.5g
醋酸钠	8.2g
琼脂	15～20g
水	1000ml
pH	4.8

$0.70kg/cm^2$（10磅/英寸^2，115.2℃）灭菌20分钟

3. 病毒组织培养用营养液等的配制

（1）营养液

牛血清	2.0ml
0.5%乳蛋白水解物	97ml

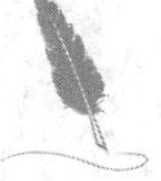

抗生素	1.0ml

(2) 维持液

0.5%乳蛋白水解物	98ml
醋酸钠 (240mg/ml)	1.0ml
抗生素	1.0ml

每管加入1ml维持液，可维持6~7天。抗生素系青霉素与链霉素的混合液，每毫升含青霉素10000U，链霉素10000U。

(3) Hanks液　制备本溶液需用双蒸水，第二次蒸馏必须在玻璃蒸馏器内进行，所用化学药品应为分析纯试剂（A.R.），配制步骤如下：

①原液甲

NaCl	160g
KCl	8g
$MgSO_4 \cdot 7H_2O$	2g
$MgCl_2 \cdot 6H_2O$	2g
$CaCl_2$	2.8g
双蒸水定容至	1000ml

加2ml三氯甲烷作为防腐剂保存于4℃备用

②原液乙

$Na_2HPO_4 \cdot 12H_2O$	3.04g
KH_2PO_4	1.2g
葡萄糖	20g
0.4%酚红液	100ml
双蒸水定容至	1000ml

加2ml三氯甲烷作为防腐剂保存于4℃备用

③使用时，按下列比例配成Hanks液：原液甲1份，原液乙1份，双蒸水18份，混合后于0.56 kg/cm^{2}高压蒸汽灭菌10分钟，溶液保存于4℃，可使用1个月。用前于20ml上述液体中加入1.4% $NaHCO_3$液0.5ml（1.4% $NaHCO_3$液是等渗液，制备后也以0.56kg/cm^{2}高压蒸汽灭菌10分钟，保存于-20℃），或把$NaHCO_3$配成3.5%的浓溶液，每100ml Hanks液加灭菌的3.5% $NaHCO_3$1.0ml。

4. 各种生化反应用培养基

(1) 糖发酵培养基

①制备“蛋白胨-水”培养基（蛋白胨1%，氯化钠0.5%，pH7.6）备用。

②配制各种单糖（葡萄糖、乳糖、麦芽糖、甘露醇、蔗糖共5种）的20%水溶液，0.56~0.7kg/cm^{2}高压蒸汽灭菌20分钟。

③取上述蛋白胨-水培养基100ml，加1.6%溴甲酚紫0.1ml，混匀，分装于小试管中，内倒置一杜氏小管，0.56~0.7kg/cm^{2}高压蒸汽灭菌，以无菌操作加入相应的灭菌单糖溶液于每管中，使最终浓度为0.5%~1.0%。

(2)“磷酸盐-葡萄糖-蛋白胨-水”培养基（甲基红-VP试验培养基）

蛋白胨	0.5g
磷酸氢二钾	0.5g

葡萄糖 0.5g

蒸馏水 100ml

pH 7.2~7.6

0.56~0.7kg/cm^{2}高压蒸汽灭菌20分钟

（3）枸橼酸盐琼脂培养基

枸橼酸钠（无水） 0.2g

氯化钠 0.5g

硫酸镁 0.02g

磷酸氢二钾 0.1g

磷酸二氢铵 0.1g

琼脂 2g

蒸馏水 100ml

以上成分加热融化，调pH至6.8~7.0，加入1%溴麝香草酚蓝1ml，混匀，分装试管，经0.7kg/cm^{2}高压蒸汽灭菌20~30分钟后制成斜面即可。

（4）蛋白胨－水培养基（吲哚试验用）

蛋白胨 1g

氯化钠 0.5g

蒸馏水 100ml

pH7.2~7.4

1kg/cm^{2}高压蒸汽灭菌20分钟

（5）醋酸铅培养基

1.5%~2.0%普通肉汤琼脂培养基 100ml

硫代硫酸钠 0.25g

10%醋酸铅溶液 1ml

将琼脂培养基加热融化，冷却至约60℃，加入硫代硫酸钠，混合，高压灭菌。冷却至约50℃，无菌操作加入醋酸铅溶液，混匀，分装试管，每管3~5ml，直立待凝即可。醋酸铅溶液预先经0.56 kg/cm^{2}高压蒸汽灭菌15分钟。

（6）明胶培养基 肉汤培养基100ml加入明胶12~18g，加热融化，分装试管，每管2~3ml，0.56 kg/cm^{2}高压蒸汽灭菌30分钟，最终pH为7.2~7.4，直立待凝。

（7）淀粉琼脂培养基

琼脂 12.0g

可溶性淀粉 10.0g

牛肉膏 13.0g

pH 7.5

1kg/cm^{2}高压蒸汽灭菌20分钟

（8）尿素琼脂培养基

尿素 20.0g

琼脂 15g

氯化钠 5.0g

磷酸二氢钾 2.0g

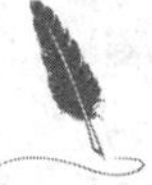

蛋白胨	1.0g
葡萄糖	1.0g
酚红	0.012g

5. 抗生素微生物检查用培养基

（1）培养基Ⅰ

胨	5g
牛肉浸出粉	3g
磷酸氢二钾	3g
琼脂	15～20g
水	1000ml

除琼脂外，混合上述其余成分，调节 pH 使比最终的 pH 略高 0.2～0.4，加入琼脂，加热溶化后过滤，调节 pH 使灭菌后为 7.8～8.0 或 6.5～6.6，115℃灭菌 30min。

（2）培养基Ⅱ

胨	6g
牛肉浸出粉	1.5g
酵母浸出粉	6g
葡萄糖	1g
琼脂	15～20g
水	1000ml

除琼脂和葡萄糖外，混合上述其余成分，调节 pH 使比最终的 pH 略高 0.2～0.4，加入琼脂，加热溶化后过滤，加葡萄糖溶解后摇匀，调节 pH 使灭菌后为 7.8～8.0 或 6.5～6.6，115℃灭菌 30 分钟。

6. 无菌检查用培养基

（1）需气菌、厌气菌培养基（硫乙醇酸盐流体培养基）

酪胨	15.0g
葡萄糖	5g
L－胱氨酸	0.5g
硫乙醇酸钠（或硫乙醇酸 0.3ml）	0.5g
酵母浸出粉	5.0g
氯化钠	2.5g
0.1%刃天青（新配制）	1.0ml
琼脂粉	0.5～0.75g
水	1000ml

除葡萄糖和刃天青溶液外，取上述其余成分加入水中，微温溶解，调节 pH 至弱碱性，煮沸后过滤，加葡萄糖和刃天青溶液，摇匀，调节 pH 使灭菌后为 7.1 ± 0.2，分装，灭菌。

（2）真菌培养基

胨	5.0g
酵母浸出粉	2.0g
葡萄糖	20g
磷酸氢二钾	1g

硫酸镁	0.5g
水	1000ml

除葡萄糖外，取上述其余成分加入水中，微温溶解，调节 pH 约为6.8，煮沸，加葡萄糖溶解后摇匀，调节 pH 使灭菌后为6.4 ± 0.2，分装，灭菌。

7. 微生物限度检查用培养基

（1）玫瑰红钠琼脂培养基

胨	5.0g
葡萄糖	10.0g
磷酸二氢钾	1g
硫酸镁	0.5g
玫瑰红钠	0.0133g
琼脂	15 ~ 20g
水	1000ml

除葡萄糖、玫瑰红钠外，取上述其余成分混合，加热溶化后，过滤，加葡萄糖、玫瑰红钠后分装，灭菌。

（2）酵母浸出粉胨葡萄糖琼脂培养基

胨	10.0g
酵母浸出粉	5g
葡萄糖	20.0g
琼脂	15 ~ 20g
水	1000ml

除葡萄糖外，取上述其余成分混合，加热溶化后，过滤，加葡萄糖后分装，灭菌。

（3）胆盐乳糖培养基

胨	20.0g
乳糖	5g
氯化钠	5g
磷酸氢二钾	4.0g
磷酸二氢钾	1.3g
去氧胆酸钠	0.5g
水	1000ml

除乳糖、去氧胆酸钠外，取上述其余成分混合，加热溶化后，过滤，加乳糖、去氧胆酸钠后分装，灭菌。

（4）曙红亚甲基蓝琼脂培养基

营养琼脂培养基	100ml
20% 乳糖溶液	5ml
曙红钠指示剂	2ml
亚甲基蓝指示剂	1.3 ~ 1.6ml

取营养琼脂培养基，加热溶化后，冷却至60℃，按无菌操作加入灭菌的其他3种溶液，摇匀，倾注平板。

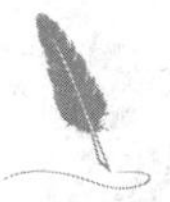

V. 染色液的配制

1. 常用染料的溶解度

染料	溶于100ml溶剂的染料量（g）	
	水	95%乙醇
结晶紫	1.68	13.87
伊红	44.2	2.18
碱性复红	1.03	3.20
孔雀绿	7.60	7.52
亚甲蓝	3.55	1.48
沙黄（番红）	5.45	3.41
甲苯胺蓝	3.82	0.57

一般配法系将染料加入到玻璃研磨内，加入95%乙醇后放置孵箱内数日（每日振摇数次），然后用滤纸过滤备用。

2. 革兰染液

（1）结晶紫染液　结晶紫14g，溶于95%乙醇100ml中使成饱和液备用，取该饱和液200ml与1%草酸胺水溶液80ml混合即成。

（2）路哥碘液　碘化钾2g溶于100ml蒸馏水中，再加碘1g，至全溶后徐徐加蒸馏水至300ml即成。

（3）稀释复红溶液　用蒸馏水将石炭酸复红染液（如下）稀释10倍，即为稀释复红染液。

3. 鞭毛染色液

（1）鞭毛染色液甲　将明矾饱和液20ml、20%鞣酸10ml、95%乙醇15ml、蒸馏水10ml和复红酒精饱和液3ml混合即可。

（2）鞭毛染色液乙　1.0 g硼砂、1.0 g亚甲蓝溶于200ml蒸馏水中。

4. 抗酸染色液

（1）石炭酸复红染液　碱性复红4g溶于100ml 95%的乙醇中制成饱和液备用，取该饱和液10ml与5%石炭酸溶液90ml混匀即成。

（2）3%盐酸酒精　取浓盐酸3ml缓缓滴入97ml 95%的乙醇中。

（3）吕氏亚甲蓝染液　取亚甲蓝2g溶于100ml 95%乙醇中使成饱和溶液备用，取此饱和液30ml与0.01%的KOH水溶液100ml混匀即成。

5. 方他那染液的配制

（1）方他那甲液　冰醋酸1ml和40%甲酸2ml溶于100ml蒸馏水。

（2）方他那乙液　鞣酸5g加热溶于100ml蒸馏水中。

（3）方他那丙液　硝酸银4g，溶于200ml蒸馏水中，取50ml硝酸银溶液，滴加浓氨水，使先有沉淀发生复而溶解，然后再加入硝酸银溶液少许，至振荡后仍显轻度浑浊为止。澄清的溶液不能使用。

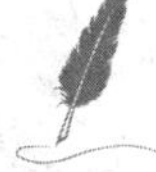

Ⅵ. 试剂及缓冲液配制

1. 常用指示剂的配制 称取指示剂0.1g，置于研钵中磨成粉末，按下表所示滴加0.01mol/L NaOH，加蒸馏水至规定量（250ml）即可。

指示剂	色调变更 酸→碱	稀释0.1g指示剂所需0.01mol/L NaOH量（ml）	总体积（ml）	浓度（%）	10ml培养基所需量（ml）
溴甲酚蓝	黄→紫	1.85	250	0.04	0.5
溴酚蓝	黄→蓝	1.49	250	0.04	0.5
溴麝香草酚蓝	黄→蓝	1.60	250	0.04	0.5
甲基红	红→黄	–	500	0.02	0.5
酚红	黄→红	2.82	500	0.02	0.5
麝香草酚蓝	黄→蓝	2.15	250	0.04	0.5

2. 各种生化反应用试剂的配制

（1）甲基红试剂 取甲基红0.1g，溶于300ml 95%乙醇中，蒸馏水定容至500ml。

（2）寇氏试剂 5.0g对二甲基氨基苯甲醛加至75 ml戊醇中，置50℃～60℃水浴中，搅拌使之完全溶解，冷却，将25ml浓盐酸一滴滴徐徐加入，边加边摇，配制后装棕色瓶并放暗处保存。

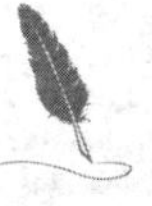

APPENDIX

Ⅰ. Microbiology Laboratory Rules

The experimental materials of microbiology contain pathogenic microorganism. If any accident occurs in the laboratory, it may have the possibility of personal infection. Students are required to observe the following rules:

1. Laboratory coats are essential for protection of clothing during the experiment. Laboratory coats must be worn in the laboratory. When you leave the laboratory, don't forget to take off your laboratory coat.

2. Personal belongings should be placed at the designated area. Only the experiment manual, notebooks and stationery can be brought into the laboratory.

3. Keep quiet and do not move casually.

4. If you have long fair, tie it back. Wear shoes at all times.

5. Eating and drinking in the laboratories is not permitted. In order to avoid the infection, do not touch your face with your hands.

6. All accidents must be reported to the teacher and handled properly. This includes incised wound, burn, chemical spill or any other accident.

7. Contaminated equipment and culture should be placed in designated area.

8. Pay attention to saving experimental materials and taking care of experimental equipment;

9. Keep flammable materials (e. g. ethanol, xylene) far away from fire. If any accident occurs causing fire, turn off the power immediately and then use wet cloth and fire extinguisher to put out the fire.

10. Ensure the experiment table is clean and tidy after experiment. Keep the laboratory clean and wash your hands.

11. Before leaving the laboratory, ensure the water, electricity, coal gas and other switches are turned off.

Ⅱ. Sterilization of Glass Apparatus and Treatment of Waste

1. Preparation and Sterilization of Glass Apparatus

Sucker, petri dish, tubes and flask should be washed before they are desiccated. The desiccated vessels should be packed with cotton, gauze or paper, placed in oven and heated 2 hours under 160℃. The apparatus which can tolerate vapor can be autoclaved. The methods of package of apparatus are these:

(1) Sucker Stuff a little cotton in the end of sucker, wrap the sucker with paper strip, heat 2h under 160℃.

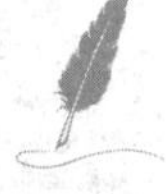

(2) Petri dish Package the petri with paper and heat 2h under 160℃.

(3) Tube Stuff the jaws of tube with silica gel tuck and heat 2h under 160℃.

(4) Flask Stuff the jaws of tube with silica gel tuck and heat 2h under 160℃.

2. Treatment of Waste the culture and apparatus, which contaminated microbial should be treated before they can be cleaned.

(1) Sucker Treat with 5% hydroxybenzene a day, wash it with water.

(2) Petri, tube and flask Autoclave.

(3) Specimen Treat with 5% hydroxybenzene a day.

Ⅲ. Microorganisms

1. Bacteria and Actinomycetes

Bacillus pumilus [CMCC (B) 63202]

Bacillus subtilis

Bacillus tetani

Clostridium sporogenes [CMCC (B) 64941]

Clostridium tetani

Clostridium sp.

Enterobacter aerogenes

Escherichia coli

E. coli K12 W1485

E. coli C600

E. coli K12

Proteus vulgaris

Pseudomonas aeruginosa

Salmonella typhi

Salmonella species

Salmonella typhimurium TA97

Salmonella typhimurium TA98

Salmonella typhimurium TA100

Salmonella typhimurium TA102

Staphylococcus aureus

Streptococcus pneumoniae

Vibrio cholerae

*Streptomyces*sp.

2. Fungi

Aspergillus niger

Candida albicans [CMCC (F) 98001]

Mucor

Penicillium

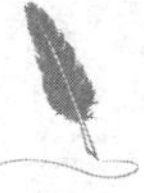

Rhizopus

Ⅳ. Culture Media

1. Nutrient Broth Agar

Beef extract	5g
Peptone	10g
NaCl	5g
Agar	15 ~ 20g
Water	1000ml
pH	7.4

Autoclave for 20min at $1kg/cm^2$

2. Media for Actitomycetes and Fungi

(1) Gauze's synthetic medium No. 1

Soluble starch	20g
KNO_3	1.0g
NaCl	0.5g
K_2HPO_4	0.5g
$MgSO_4$	0.5g
$FeSO_4$	0.01g
Agar	15 ~ 20g
H_2O	1000ml
pH	7.2 ~ 7.4

Autoclave for 20min at $1kg/cm^2$

(2) Improved Sabouraud's medium

Peptone	10g
Glucose	40g
Agar	15 ~ 20g
water	1000ml
pH	natural

Autoclave for 15 ~ 20min at $0.56kg/cm^2$

(3) Wort agar

Agar	15g
Malt extract	15g
Maltose	12.75g
Dextrin	2.75g
Glycerol	2.35g
K_2HPO_4	1g
NH_4Cl	1g
Pancreatic digest of gelatin	0.78g

pH	4.8

Autoclave for 15 ~ 20min at 0.56kg/cm^2.

Preparation of Medium: Add components to distilled/deionized water and bring volume to 1.0 L. Mix thoroughly. Gently heat and bring to boiling. Boil for 1 min with mixing. Distribute into tubes or flasks. Autoclave for 15 min at 15 psi pressure or 121℃. Do not overheat as this will result in hydrolysis of the agar. An additional 5.0g of agar can be used to make a firmer agar. Pour into sterile Petri dishes or leave in tubes Reaction: The low pH of the agar selectively inhibits bacterial growth and permits the growth of yeast.

(4) glucose – acetate agar

Glucose	1g
Yeast extract.	2.5g
Natriumacetate	8.2g
Agar	15 ~ 20g
Water	1000ml
pH	4.8

Autoclave for 20min at 0.7kg/cm^2

3. Virus Culture Broth

(1) nutrient broth

Beef serum	2.0ml
0.5% milk protein	97ml
Antibiotin solution	1.0ml

(2) maintain solution

0.5% digest of casein	98ml
Natrium acetate (240mg/ml)	1.0ml
Antibiotin solution	1.0ml

1ml maintain solution per tube. Antibiotic solution contains penicilium 10000U and streptomycin 10000U.

(3) Hank's solution

(a) Solution A

NaCl	160g
KCl	8g
$MgSO_4 \cdot 7H_2O$	2g
$MgCl_2 \cdot 6H_2O$	2g
$CaCl_2$	2.8g
ddH_2O	1000ml

Add chloroform 2ml to the solution. preserved at 4℃

(b) Solution B

$Na_2HPO_4 \cdot 12H_2O$	3.04g
KH_2PO_4	1.2g
Glucose	20g

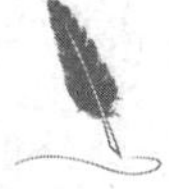

0.4% bromcresol blue	100ml
ddH_2O	1000ml

Add chloroform 2ml to the solution. preserved at 4℃

(c) Preparation Add solution A 10ml and solution B 10ml to ddH_2O 18ml, mixed and autoclave for 20min at 0.56kg/cm^2. The solution can be preserved in 4℃. Before use, add 0.5ml 1.4 % $NaHCO_3$.

4. Media for Biochemistry Test

(1) Carbohydrate fermentation medium.

(a) Peptone - water medium (g/100ml): (peptone 1g, NaCl (sodium chloride) 0.5g, pH7.6).

(b) Sugars solutions: 2g glucose (or lactose, maltose, mannitol, sucrose) in 10ml water. autoclave for 20min at 0.56kg/cm^2.

(c) In the tubes of sterile peptone – water medium (about 5ml) with inverted Durham tubes, Add 10μl 1.6% Bromocresol Purple to the medium. autoclave for 20min at 0.56kg/cm^2. Add 200μl 20% sugar to every medium.

(d) MRVP broth

Peptone	0.5g
KH_2PO_4	0.5g
Glucose	0.5g
Distilled water	100ml
pH	7.2 ~ 7.6

Autoclave for 20min at 0.56 ~ 0.7kg/cm^2

(2) Simmons' citrate agar

Citrate	0.2g
NaCl	0.5g
$MgSO_4$	0.02g
K_2HPO_4	0.1g
$NH_4H_2PO_4$	0.1g
Agar	2g
Distilled water	100ml

Melt the components, adjust the pH to 6.8 ~ 7.0. Add bromthymol blue 1 ml to the solution, distribute to tubes. autoclave for 20min at 0.7kg/cm^2.

(3) Peptone – water medium (for indole test)

Peptone	1g
NaCl	0.5g
Distilled water	100ml
pH	7.2 ~ 7.4

Autoclave for 20min at 1.0kg/cm^2.

(4) Lead acetate agar

1.5% ~ 2.0% broth agar	100ml

$Na_2S_2O_3$	0. 25g
10 % lead acetate solution	1ml

Melt the broth agar, cooling to 60℃. Add $Na_2S_2O_3$ to solution, mix solution, autoclave for 20min at 1. 0kg/cm^2. Cooling to 50℃, add 10 % lead acetate solution to broth agar, distribute to tubes (3ml per tube), erect the tubes, let the broth agar freeze to the solid state.

(5) glutin medium Add glutin 12 ~ 18g to 100ml broth, melt the broth, distribute to tubes (3ml per tube), autoclave for 20min at 1. 0kg/cm^2, erect the tubes, let the broth agar freeze to the solid state.

(6) starch agar (g/L)

Agar	12. 0g
Soluble starch	10. 0g
Beef extract	3. 0g
pH	7. 5

Autoclave for 10min at 1. 0kg/cm^2.

(7) Urea agar (g/L)

Urea	20. 0g
Agar	15. 0g
NaCl	5. 0g
KH_2PO_4	2. 0g
Peptone	1. 0g
Glucose	1. 0g
Phenol red	0. 012g
pH	6. 8

Autoclave for 15min at 1. 0kg/cm^2.

5. Media for Biological Assay of Antibiotics

(1) Medium A

Peptone	6 g
Beef extract	3 g
Dipotassium hydrogen phosphate	3 g
Agar	15 ~ 20g
Water to produce	1000ml

Dissolve the solids in the water except agar, Add 1M sodium hydroxide so that the value of solution pH is 0. 2 ~ 0. 4 higher than the value of sterilized medium. Add the agar, boil and filtrate the solution, adjust the pH so that the solution will have a pH of 7. 8 ~ 8. 0 or 6. 5 ~ 6. 6 after sterilization. Sterilize the medium at 115℃ for 30min.

(2) Medium B

Peptone	6g
Beef extract	1. 5g
Yeast extract	6g
Glucose monohydrate	1g

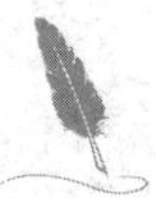

Agar	15 ~ 20g
Water to produce	1000ml

Dissolve the solids in the water except glucose and agar, Add 1M sodium hydroxide so that the value of solution pH is 0.2 ~ 0.4 higher than the value of sterilized medium. Add the agar, boil and filtrate the solution, add the glucose, shake up and adjust the pH so that the solution will have a pH of 7.8 ~ 8.0 or 6.5 ~ 6.6 after sterilization. Sterilize the medium at 115℃ for 30 min.

6. Media for Sterility Test

(1) Aerobes and anaerobes medium (Fluid thioglycollate medium)

Pancreatic digest of casein	15.0g
Glucose monohydrate	5g
L - Cystine	0.5g
Sodium thioglycollate 0.5 gor Thioglycollic acid	0.3ml
Yeast extract (water - soluble)	5.0g
Sodium chloride	2.5g
Resazurin sodium solution (Freshly prepared, 1 in 1000)	1.0ml
Agar, granulated (moisture content not in excess of 15%)	0.75g
Water	1000ml

pH 7.1 ± 0.2 after sterilization

Dissolve the solids in the water except glucose and resazurin sodium solution, warm slightly to effect solution. Add 1M sodium hydroxide so that the solution will be weakly basic. Boil and filtrate the solution, add the glucose and resazurin sodium solution, shake up and adjust the pH so that the solution will have a pH of 7.1 ±0.2 after sterilization. Distribute and sterilize the medium.

(2) Fungi medium

Peptone	5.0g
Yeast extract	2.0g
Glucose	20g
Dipotassium hydrogen phosphate	1g
$MgSO_4$	0.5g
Water	1000ml

pH6.4 ± 0.2 after sterilization

Dissolve the solids in the water except glucose, warm slightly to effect solution. Add 1M sodium hydroxide so that the solution will have a pH of 6.8. Boil the solution and add the glucose, adjust the pH so that the solution will have a pH of 6.4 ±0.2 after sterilization.

7. Media for Microbial Contamination Test

(1) Rose Bengal agar

Peptones (meat and casein)	5.0g
Glucose	10.0g
Dipotassium hydrogen orthophosphate	1g
Magnesium chloride	0.5g
Rose Bengal Sodium	0.0133g

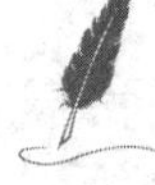

Agar 15 ~ 20g

Water 1000ml

Dissolve the solids in the water except glucose and rose bengal sodium, warm slightly to effect solution. Filtrate the solution, add glucose and rose bengal sodium, sterilize the medium.

(2) Yeast extract peptone dextrose medium (YPD)

Peptones (meat and casein) 10.0g

Yeast extract 5g

Glucose 20.0g

Agar 15 ~ 20g

Water 1000ml

Dissolve the solids in the water except glucose, warm slightly to effect solution. Filtrate the solution, add glucose and sterilize the medium.

(3) Bile salt lactose medium (BL)

Peptones (meat and casein) 20.0g

Lactose 5g

Sodium chloride 5g

Dipotassium hydrogen phosphate 4.0g

Potassium dihydrogen phosphate 1.3g

Bile salt Sodium (or deoxycholate 0.5g) 2g

Water 1000ml

Dissolve the solids in the water except lactose and sodium deoxycholate, warm slightly to effect solution. Add 1M sodium hydroxide so that the solution will have a pH of 7.4 ±0.2 after sterilization. Boil and filtrate the solution, add lactose and sodium deoxycholate, sterilize the medium.

(4) EMB

Nutrient Broth 100ml

20% Lactose solution 5ml

Eosin 2ml

Methylene blue solution 1.3 ~ 1.6ml

Melt the nutrient broth agar and cool to 60℃, add the other solutions by aseptic technology, shake up and sterilize. Pour the petri disks.

V. Staining Solutions

1. Solubility of Dye

Dyes	Solubility (g/100ml solvent)	
	Water	95% Ethyl alcohol
Crystal violet	1.68	13.87
Eosin	44.2	2.18
Fuchsin basic	1.03	3.20

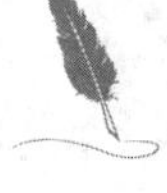

续表

Dyes	Solubility (g/100ml solvent)	
	Water	95% Ethyl alcohol
Malachite green	7.60	7.52
Methylene blue	3.55	1.48
Safranin	5.45	3.41
Toluiden blue	3.82	0.57

Preparation: grounded in the mortar, the dye was dissolved with 95% ethanol under 37℃ (shake every day). Before use, the solution must be filtrated with filter paper.

2. Gram's Stain Solutions

(1) Crystal violet solution A: 2g crystal violet in 20ml 95% ethanol. solution B: 0.8g ammonium oxalate in 80ml distilled water. Mix solution A and solution B and let stand for 24hours. filter through paper.

(2) Iodine solution 1g iodine and 2g potassium iodide in 300ml water.

(3) Safranin 2.5g safranin in 100ml of 95% ethyl alcohol. Add 1000ml of distilled water.

3. Flagella Stain Solutions

(1) Solution A Saturated $KAl(SO_4)_2$ solution 20ml, 20% tannic acid solution 10 ml, 95% ethanol 15 ml, distilled water 10 ml and saturated safranin solution 3 ml. Mix thoroughly.

(2) Solution B Boron 1.0 g and methylene blue 1.0g in distilled water 200ml.

4. Acid-Fast Stain Solution

(1) Carbol fuchsin stain Basic fuchsin 0.4g in 95% ethanol 10ml. Then mix with 5% phenol 90ml.

(2) 3% acid alcohol Concentrated HCl 3ml in 97ml 95% ethanol.

(3) Methylene blue solution 2g methylene blue in 100ml 95% ethanol. Add the solution 30ml to 0.01% KOH 100ml.

5. Fontana Solution

(1) Fontana solution A Acetate 1ml and 40% formic acid 2ml in 100ml distilled water.

(2) Fontana solution B Tannic acid 5g in 100ml distilled water.

(3) Fontana solution C $AgNO_3$ 4g in 200ml distilled water. add concentrated ammonia to the 50ml $AgNO_3$ solution, the precipitation will be produced, then add a little $AgNO_3$ solution, shake the solution to leave little precipitation in it.

Ⅵ. Solutions and Buffers

1. Indicators

0.1g grinded indicator dissolved in 0.01mol/L NaOH, add distilled water to 250 ml.

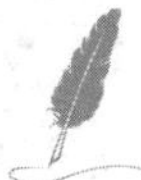

Indicator	Color change Acid →basic	Volume of NaOH to dissolve indicator (ml)	Total volume	Concentration (%)	Volume in 10ml medium (ml)
bromocresol blue	yellow→violet	1. 85	250	0. 04	0. 5
bromocresol blue	yellow→blue	1. 49	250	0. 04	0. 5
bromocresol blue	yellow→blue	1. 60	250	0. 04	0. 5
methyl red	red→yellow	-	500	0. 02	0. 5
phenol red	yellow→red	2. 82	500	0. 02	0. 5
thymolsulfonphthalein	yellow→blue	2. 15	250	0. 04	0. 5

2. Sulutions for Biochemistry Test

(1) Methyl red indicator methyl red 0. 1g is dissolved in 300ml 95% ethanol. Add distilled water to 500ml.

(2) Kovac's reagent 5. 0g dimethyl - alpha - naphthylamine is dissolved in 75ml amyl alcohol. Heat at 55℃ in water bath until crystal is dissolved. Cool and add 25ml concentrated hcl. Preserve it in umber bottle.

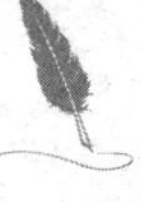

专用名词表

α - naphthol solution	α - 萘酚
acetate agar	醋酸琼脂
acetate buffer	醋酸缓冲液
acid and gas production	产酸产气
acid - fast bacteria	抗酸细菌
acid - fast stain	抗酸染色法
acridine orange stain	吖叮黄染色
actinomycete	放线菌
aerial filament	气生菌丝
aerobes	需氧微生物
aerosol	气雾剂
agar	琼脂
agarose gel	琼脂糖凝胶
agglutination	凝聚反应
air dry	空气干燥
Ames test	艾姆斯实验
amplification	扩增
amylase	淀粉酶
anaerobes	厌氧微生物
anaerobic bacteria	厌氧细菌
anaerobic culture techniques	厌氧培养技术
antibiotic	抗生素
antimicrobial activity	抗菌活性
antimicrobial spectrum	抗菌谱
antibiotic medium	抗生素培养基
antibiotic resistance	抗生素抗性
antibiotic - resistant mutants	抗生素抗性突变
antiseptic	防腐
annulus	环状物
asepsis	无菌
aseptic	无菌的
aseptic technique	无菌技术
Aspergillus	曲霉菌
autoclave	高压灭菌

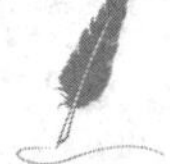

auxanogram	生长谱
auxanography	生长谱法
azithromycin	阿奇霉素
Bacillus	杆菌
Bacillus pumilus	短小芽孢杆菌
Bacillus tetani	破伤风杆菌
back mutation	回复突变
bacteria	细菌
bacterial classification	细菌分类
morphology	形态
bacterial endospore stain	细菌芽孢染色
bacterial identification	细菌鉴定
bacterial reproduction	细菌繁殖
bacterial slant	细菌斜面
bacterial stab	细菌穿刺
bacterial transformation	细菌转化
bacteriophage	噬菌体
bacteriophage enrichment	噬菌体富集
barbital buffer	巴比妥缓冲液
beta lactam	β-内酰胺环
barritt's reagent	Barritt 试剂
basal synthetic medium	基础合成培养基
basophils	嗜碱性细胞
bauer-kirby disk method	B-K 法
beef extract	牛肉膏
binary fission	二分裂
biomass	生物量
BL (Bile Lactose)	胆盐乳糖
blood agar	血琼脂
blood type	血型
brewer jar	广口瓶
bright-field microscope	亮视野显微镜
bromcresol purple broth	溴甲酚紫肉汤
brown's motion	布朗运动
broth medium	肉汤培养基
calcium chloride	氯化钙
Candida albicans, CMCC (F) 98001	白色念珠菌
capsule	荚膜，胶囊
capsule stain	荚膜染色
carbohydrate fermentation	糖发酵试验

carbol fuchsin	石炭酸品红
carbon source	碳源
carcinogen	致癌物质
casein hydrolysate	水解酪蛋白
catabolite repression	代谢物抑制
catalase	触酶，过氧化氢酶
carcinogen	致癌因子，致癌剂
carcinogenic	致癌的
carcinogenicity	致癌性
cedar wood oil	香柏油
cell wall	细胞壁
cellulose decomposition	纤维素降解
centrifugation	离心
centrifuge	离心，离心机
cesium chloride	氯化铯
chloramphenicol（cm）	氯霉素
chromogen	发色基团
chromosome	染色体
chlamydia	支原体
citrate agar	枸橼酸盐琼脂
citrate utilization	枸橼酸盐利用
chook embryos	鸡胚
Clostridium	梭菌
Clostridium sporogenes	生孢梭菌
colony	菌落
colony forming unit（CFU）	菌落形成单位
coliform bacteria	肠道菌
competent bacterium	感受态细菌
competent cells	感受态细胞
complex medium	合成培养基
concavity slide	凹玻片
conjugation	接合
contamination	污染
continuous streak	连续划线
correlation	相关性
counterstain	复染
counting chamber	血球计数板
counting chamber	计数室
cover slip	盖玻片
crystal violet stain	结晶紫

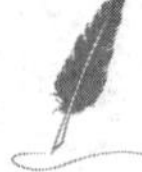

crossover	交换
culture	培养物
cultivation of bacteria	细菌培养
culture	培养
culture morphology	培养状态
culture preservation	培养物保存
cysteine desulfurase	半胱氨酸脱硫酶
cytochrome oxidase	细胞色素氧化酶
dark – field microscope	暗视野显微镜
daunomycin	正定霉素
deaminase	脱氨酶
decarboxylase	脱羧酶
decolorizing	脱色
decolorizing agent	脱色剂
decline or death phase	衰退期
stationary phase	稳定期
defined medium	限制性培养基
degrade	降解
detergent	去污剂
diethyl sulfate（DES）	硫酸二乙酯
disk diffusion	平板扩散
donor	供体
dropper	滴管
drug – resistant	抗药性
denitrification	脱氮
desiccation	干燥
deoxycholate agar	双氧胆酸盐琼脂
desoxycholate – citrate agar（DCA）	双氧胆酸盐 – 枸橼酸盐琼脂
dextran	葡聚糖
differential media	鉴别培养基
direct counts	直接计数
dimethylsulfoxide	二甲基亚砜
disinfectant	消毒剂
disinfectant effectiveness	消毒剂效果
disinfectants	消毒剂
donor DNA	供体 DNA
dry heat sterilization	干热灭菌
ear drops	滴耳剂
electrophoresis	电泳
EMB agar	EMB 琼脂

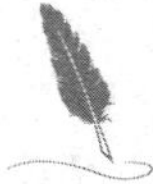

endospore stain	芽孢染色
emulsions	乳剂
enteric gram - negative rods	革兰阴性肠道菌
Enterobacter aerogenes	产气肠杆菌
Enterobacter species	产气杆菌属
environmental microbiology	环境微生物
exonuclease	内切酶
enzyme assays	酶分析
enzyme induction	酶诱导
enzyme - linked immunosorbent assay	酶联免疫分析
eosin methylene blue agar	依红亚甲蓝琼脂
eosinophils	曙红
error - prone	倾向差错的
Escherichia coli	大肠埃希菌
ethidium bromide staining	EB 染色
experimental design	实验设计
eye drops	一般滴眼剂
eye ointments	一般眼膏剂
eukaryote	真核细胞
F - pili	性菌毛
F - plasmid	F 质粒
facultative anaerobes	专性厌氧菌
Fermentation	发酵
films	膜剂
fixation	固定
flagella	鞭毛
flagella stain	鞭毛染色
fluorescein - conjugated antibody	荧光结合抗体
fluorescent antibody staining (FAB)	荧光抗体染色
freeze - drying	冷冻干燥
fuchsin	复红
fungus	真菌
fungal classification	真菌分类
galactose	半乳糖
gel	凝胶剂
gelatin hydrolysis	明胶水解
gelatinase	明胶酶
generalized transduction	普通转导
genome	基因组
germicides	杀菌剂

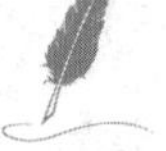

glass slides	载玻片
glycolysis	糖酵解
gonococcus	淋病双球菌
Gram stain	革兰染色
gram – negative	革兰阴性
gram – positive	革兰阳性
granules	颗粒剂
growth curve	生长曲线
hand washing	手洗
hanging drop method	悬滴法
heat killing	加热杀死
heavy metals	重金属
histidine	组氨酸
Hfr strain	高频重组菌株
homogenate	匀浆
hydrogen sulfide production	硫化氢产生实验
immune response	免疫应答
immunofluorescence	免疫荧光
immunoglobulins	免疫球蛋白
immunology	免疫学
incubation time	接种时间
incubator	培养箱
indicator microorganisms	指示微生物
indirect counts	间接计数
indirect immunofluorescence	降解免疫荧光反应
indole production	吲哚产生实验
inoculate	接种
inhibition zone	抑菌圈
inoculating loop	接种环
inoculating needle	接种针
inoculum	接种量
insecticide	杀虫剂
integration	整合
irradiation	照射
isoelectric point	等电点
isolation of bacteriophage	噬菌体分离
kirby – bauer antibiotic susceptibility test	K – B 法
Klebsiella	克雷伯菌
Klebsiella pneumoniae	肺炎克雷伯菌
Kovac's reagent	寇氏试剂

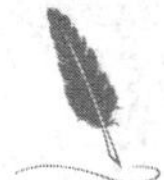

lactose	乳糖
lactose - fermenting bacteria	乳酸发酵细菌
lag phase	延迟期
lead acetate agar	醋酸铅琼脂
lens paper	擦镜纸
leukocytes	白细胞
levofloxacin	左旋氧氟沙星
liniments	搽剂
liquid paraffin	液体石蜡
liquid nitrogen	液氮
liquid medium	液体培养基
light microscope	光学显微镜
logarithmic (log) phase	对数生长期
lotions	洗剂
lyophilizing	冻干
lysozyme	溶菌酶
ligase	连接酶
lysogenic	溶源的
lysate	裂解物
lytic bacteriophage	烈性噬菌体
lytic phage replication cycle	烈性噬菌体复制循环
Macconkey agar	麦康凯培养基
malt extract	麦芽汁
mating	杂交
mean	平均
medium	培养基
medium preparation	培养基制备
membrane filter method	膜过滤技术
Meningococcus	脑膜炎球菌
metabolism	代谢
methyl red test	甲基红实验
methyl red - voges - proskauer broth	MRVP 肉汤
microaerophiles	微厌氧菌
microbial biomass	生物量
microbial classification	微生物分类
microscopic counts	显微计数
microbial genetics	微生物遗传
microbial growth	微生物生长
microbial identification	微生物鉴定
microbial metabolism	微生物代谢

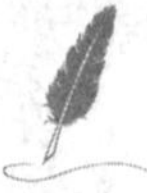

microbial nomenclature	微生物命名
microbial taxonomy	微生物分类
microbiological methods	微生物法
micrometer	测微尺
microscope	显微镜
minimal agar	基本培养基琼脂
MBC	最低杀菌浓度
minimal bactericidal concentration	最低杀菌浓度
minimal broth	基本培养基肉汤
MIC	最低抑菌浓度
minimal inhibitory concentration	最低抑菌浓度
mite	螨
minimal medium（MM）	最低限度培养基
mold	霉菌
mordant	媒染
morphology	形态学
most probable number method	MPN 法
Mucor	毛霉
M – H	M – H 培养基
Mueller – Hinton agar	M – H 琼脂
mutagen	突变剂
mutant	突变体
mycelia	菌丝
Mycobacterium	分枝杆菌
Mycoplasma	支原体
nasal drops	滴鼻剂
neutrophils	中性粒细胞
nitratase	硝酸还原酶
2 – nitrofluorene	2 – 氨基芴
nitrification	硝化作用
nitrogen fixation	固氮
normal growth curve	常规生长曲线
NTG	亚硝基胍
nucleotide	核苷酸
mycostatin	制霉菌素
numerical aperture	数值口径
nutrient agar	营养琼脂
nutrient agar slant	营养琼脂斜面
nutrient broth	营养肉汤
oil immersion lens	油镜

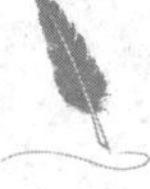

ointments	软膏剂
oral liquids	口服液
paper slips	纸片
Pasteurization	巴氏消毒
pathogenic bacteria	致病菌
penicillin	青霉素
penicillin G	青霉素 G
penicillinase	青霉素酶
penicilloic acid	青霉噻唑酸
Penicillium	青霉菌
petri dish	培养皿
pharmacopoeia	药典
physiological saline	生理盐水
pills	丸剂（滴丸、糖丸等）
plasmid DNA	质粒 DNA
plasmid	质粒
Pneumococcus pneumoniae	肺炎球菌
polypeptone	聚胨
polysaccharides	多糖
polypeptides	多肽
potato dextrose agar	PDA 培养基
pour plate method	倾注平板法
powders	散剂
powders for external use	外用散剂
precipitin lines	沉淀线
primary stain	初染
procaryote	原核细胞
proteose peptone	蛋白胨
Proteus species	变形杆菌
protoplasts	原生质体
prophage	前噬菌体
pure culture	纯培养
Pseudomonas aeruginosa	铜绿假单胞菌
Pseudomonas species	假单胞菌
pure culture	纯培养
pure culture techniques	纯培养技术
puncture	穿刺
quadrant streak	分区划线
recombinant DNA technology	重组 DNA 技术
replica plating	影印平板法

Rhizopus	根霉
Rickettsiaes	立克次体
Rose Bengal agar	玫瑰红钠琼脂
ruler	尺
Sabouraud agar	沙氏琼脂
Saccharomyces cerevisiae	啤酒酵母
safranin	沙黄
Salmonella typhimurium	伤寒沙门菌
Salmonella	沙门菌
Salmonella typhi	伤寒杆菌
Sarcina lutea	藤黄八叠球菌
screen	筛选
smear	涂片
solid medium	固体培养基
stain	染色
staining tray	染缸
stationary phase	稳定期
selective media	选择培养基
serological identification	血清学鉴定
semisolid medium	半固体培养基
Shigela species	志贺菌
Simmons' citrate agar	西蒙枸橼酸盐琼脂
simple staining	单染法
soya peptone	大豆蛋白胨
spectrophotometric	光比色法
specialized transduction	局限性转导
specimen	标本片
spheroplasts	球形体
spirochetes	螺旋体
spontaneous mutations	自发突变
spore	芽孢
sporebearing filament	孢子丝
spore stain	芽孢染色
spread plate method	平板划线法
staining	染色
standard error	标准差
Staphylococcus	葡萄球菌
Staphylococcus aureus	金黄色葡萄球菌
Staphylococcus. epidermidis	表皮葡萄球菌
starch	淀粉

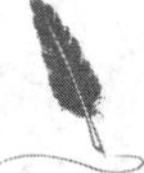

starch agar	淀粉琼脂
starch agar slant	淀粉琼脂斜面
starch hydrolysis	淀粉水解
statistics	统计学
sterilization	灭菌
streak plate	划平板
streptomycin	链霉素
subculturing	接种
substrate filament	基内菌丝
sucker	吸管
sudan black stain	苏丹黑染色
suppository	栓剂
susceptibility of antibiotics	抗生素敏感性
suspensions	混悬剂
syrups	糖浆剂
tablets	片剂
tellurite agar	亚碲酸盐
test for sterility	无菌检查
tetracycline	四环素
T－even phage	T－偶数序列噬菌体
tincture	酊剂
toluidine blue solution	甲苯胺蓝溶液
toothpick	牙签
transducing bacteriophage	转导噬菌体
transduction	转导
transformation	转化
transformant	转化子
Treponema pauidum	梅毒螺旋体
triple sugar iron agar（tsi）	三糖铁盐琼脂
tris－hydrochloride buffer	Tirs－HCl 缓冲液
tryptone	酪蛋白
tryptone agar	酪蛋白琼脂
tryptone broth	酪蛋白肉汤
tryptophan deaminase	色氨酸脱氨酶
tryptose	胰蛋白
tweezers	镊子
ultraviolet（UV）radiation	紫外辐射
ultra－cold frozen	超低温冷冻
urea agar	尿素琼脂
urease	脲酶

urease test agar	脲酶测试琼脂
variation	变异
virus	病毒
vaseline	凡士林
voges – proskauer test	V – P 试验
water – adsorption paper	吸水纸
wort agar	麦芽汁琼脂
wright' s stain	赖氏染色
xylene	二甲苯
yeast	酵母
yeast extract	酵母膏
YPD	酵母浸出粉胨葡萄糖琼脂

参考文献

[1] 周长林. 微生物学实验与指导. 2 版. 北京：中国医药科技出版社，2009.

[2] 周长林. 微生物学实验与指导. 3 版. 北京：中国医药科技出版社，2015.

[3] 周德庆，徐德强. 微生物学实验教程. 4 版. 北京：高等教育出版社，2019.

[4] 柳忠辉，吴雄文. 医学免疫学实验技术. 2 版. 北京：人民卫生出版社，2014.

[5] 蒋群，李志勇. 生物工程综合实验. 北京：科学出版社，2010.

[6] 吴根福. 发酵工程实验指南. 2 版. 北京：高等教育出版社，2013.

[7] 袁丽红. 微生物学实验. 北京：化学工业出版社，2010.

[8] 徐威. 微生物学实验. 2 版. 北京：中国医药科技出版社，2014.

[9] Ted R. Johnson, Christine L. Case. Laboratory Experiments in Microbiology (10th Edition). Benjamin Cummings, 2015.

[10] Ted R. Johnson, Christine L. Case. Laboratory Experiments in Microbiology (11th Edition). Benjamin Cummings, 2015.

[11] Park Talaro, Foundation in Mirobidlogy (8th Edition). Hither Education Press. 2013.